PUBLIC HEALTH, ETHICS, AND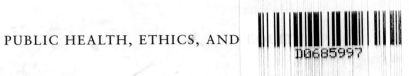

Public Health, Ethics, and Equity

Edited by
SUDHIR ANAND
FABIENNE PETER
AMARTYA SEN

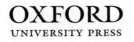

UNIVERSITY PRESS

OXFORD

UNIVERSITY PRESS

Great Clarendon Street, Oxford OX2 6DP

Oxford University Press is a department of the University of Oxford.
It furthers the University's objective of excellence in research, scholarship,
and education by publishing worldwide in Oxford New York
Auckland Cape Town Dar es Salaam Hong Kong Karachi
Kuala Lumpur Madrid Melbourne Mexico City Nairobi
New Delhi Shanghai Taipei Toronto

With offices in

Argentina Austria Brazil Chile Czech Republic France Greece
Guatemala Hungary Italy Japan Poland Portugal Singapore
South Korea Switzerland Thailand Turkey Ukraine Vietnam

Oxford is a registered trade mark of Oxford University Press
in the UK and in certain other countries

Published in the United States
by Oxford University Press Inc., New York

© Oxford University Press, 2004

The moral rights of the authors have been asserted
Database right Oxford University Press (maker)

First published 2004
First published in paperback 2006

British Library Cataloguing in Publication Data

Data available

Library of Congress Cataloging in Publication Data

Data available

Typeset by Newgen Imaging Systems (P) Ltd., Chennai, India
Printed in Great Britain
on acid-free paper by
Antony Rowe Ltd, Chippenham, Wiltshire

ISBN 978–0–19–927636–3
ISBN 978–0–19–927637–0 (Pbk.)

3 5 7 9 10 8 6 4

Preface

This book originated in a set of workshops and seminars that we organised at Harvard University in 1998 and 1999. Our objective in launching this series of meetings was to initiate a wide investigation of the ethical issues underlying inequalities in health. We were moved by the recognition that the extensive empirical and policy literature on health inequalities had not been matched by an adequate appreciation of the normative underpinnings of health equity. We assembled, therefore, authors and commentators interested in these issues, from a variety of disciplines, and invited them to contribute to this important subject area. We were most encouraged by the wide interest generated by the workshops and the lively discussions at the meetings. We are also deeply grateful to the authors for their willingness to revise and restructure their papers, taking note of the discussions, comments and written exchanges. Moreover, the continuing involvement of many of the participants in the enquiry we initiated has been extremely gratifying. The respective contributions made in different chapters in this volume are briefly discussed in a separate Introduction.

The workshops and seminars were organised as part of the Global Health Equity Initiative, and funded by a grant from the Rockefeller Foundation to Harvard University. The later stages of the work in preparing, editing and producing the volume for publication were supported by a grant from the Rockefeller Foundation to St Catherine's College, Oxford. We are very grateful to the Foundation for its generous backing of this project.

SA, FP, AS
August 2004

Acknowledgements

Thanks are due to the following journals and publishers for giving us permission to reprint:

"The Concern for Equity in Health" by Sudhir Anand, which originally appeared in the *Journal of Epidemiology and Community Health* 56(7) 2002: 485–7; copyright BMJ publishing group

"Why Health Equity?" by Amartya Sen, which originally appeared in *Health Economics* 11(8) 2002: 659–66; copyright John Wiley & Sons

"Health Equity and Social Justice" by Fabienne Peter, which originally appeared in the *Journal of Applied Philosophy* 18(2) 2001: 159–70; copyright Blackwell Publishers

"Disability-Adjusted Life Years: A Critical Review" by Sudhir Anand and Kara Hanson, which originally appeared in the *Journal of Health Economics* 16(6) 1997: 685–702; copyright Elsevier

"Ethical Issues in the Use of Cost Effectiveness Analysis for the Prioritization of Health Care Resources" by Dan Brock, which originally appeared in *Handbook of Bioethics: Taking Stock of the Field from a Philosophical Perspective*, edited by George Khushf. Dordrecht: Kluwer, 2004; copyright Kluwer Academic Publishers.

Contents

List of Figures

List of Tables

List of Abbreviations

CEA   Cost effectiveness analysis
DALY   Disability-adjusted life year
HRQL   Health-related quality of life
HUI   Health utilities index
ICIDH International Classification of Impairments, Disabilities
       and Handicaps
PPP   Purchasing Power Parity
PYLL   Potential years of life lost
QALY   Quality-adjusted life year
QWB   Quality of well-being

List of Contributors

Vincanne Adams, University of California, San Francisco
Sudhir Anand, University of Oxford
Dan W. Brock, Harvard Medical School
John Broome, University of Oxford
Norman Daniels, Harvard School of Public Health
Kara Hanson, London School of Hygiene and Tropical Medicine
Frances M. Kamm, Harvard University
Ichiro Kawachi, Harvard School of Public Health
Bruce Kennedy, Cambridge, MA
Arthur Kleinman, Harvard University
Sir Michael Marmot, University College, London
Fabienne Peter, University of Warwick
Thomas W. Pogge, Columbia University and Australian National University
Amartya Sen, Harvard University
Philippe Van Parijs, Université Catholique de Louvain and Harvard University
Daniel Wikler, Harvard School of Public Health

Introduction

SUDHIR ANAND AND FABIENNE PETER

Impressive gains in average life expectancy have been achieved worldwide in the second half of the twentieth century. These gains have been attributed to a variety of socio-economic factors and public policies, and—to a lesser extent—to improved medical care. The changes in life expectancy, however, have not been distributed equally either among or within countries. Among countries, there have been advances in many, but some countries—especially in sub-Saharan Africa and the former Soviet Union—have seen reversals in life expectancy (United Nations Development Programme 2003: 262–5). Within countries, some social groups have benefited significantly but the health status of others has stagnated or worsened. Very large disparities in life expectancy are found within countries across different social groups and regions.[1] Thus, although average life expectancy worldwide has increased significantly, inequalities in health remain a matter of deep concern.

Research on the health status of populations and population subgroups has a long history in public health. The relationship between poverty and ill-health, in particular, has been recognised centuries ago. In contemporary public health research, poverty is still treated as a major factor behind health inequalities within and between countries[2], but it is becoming increasingly evident that significant inequalities exist even in the absence of (absolute) material deprivation and in countries that have universal access to health care (see Chapter 3 by Marmot, this volume).

Current research on social inequalities in health—differences in health outcomes between social groups defined by variables such as class, race, gender, and geographical location—has been much influenced by the publication of two reports in the United Kingdom around 1980. One was the Black Report, which documented extensive health inequalities among socio-economic groups in Britain (Black and Morris 1992 [1980]). The second was a study by Michael Marmot and his collaborators (the Whitehall study), which

---

[1] For example, see the US ethnic- and county-level estimates of life expectancy in Murray et al. (1998).

[2] For example, in cross-country regressions of life expectancy, Anand and Ravallion (1993) find that (absolute) income poverty is a very significant explanatory variable.

found that among British civil servants there is a significant inverse relationship between employment grade and mortality rate—the higher the grade, the
lower the mortality rate (Marmot et al. 1978). A huge literature has since
spawned on this question in many countries, which systematically documents
inequalities in health across social groups.[3]

Concern with health inequalities has figured on the policy agenda—
international and national—for some decades. Implicit recognition of the
importance of health inequalities led to the World Health Organization
(WHO) 'Health for All' initiative—proclaimed in Alma Ata in 1978 (World
Health Organization 1978). During the 1980s and 1990s, however, the policy
discourse continued to emphasise aggregate population health. Given the
mounting evidence of stagnation—and sometimes deterioration—in the health
status of many population groups, a renewed interest in health inequalities has
begun to emerge.

The current concern with health equity emphasises that health is influenced
by a wide range of social circumstances and public policies, and not just by
access to health care and traditional health-sector policies. Within the
discipline of public health, there is growing appeal to the social sciences and a
move towards more interdisciplinary analysis of the social processes underlying inequalities in health. This development is often labelled the *new public
health*, but as Ann Robertson (1998: 1419) stresses, '[m]any would argue that
this is not so much a new public health as a return to the historical commitments of public health to social justice'.[4]

This commitment of public health to social justice and to health equity
raises a series of ethical issues which, until recently, have received insufficient
attention. Why, if at all, should a concern with health equity be singled out
from the pursuit of social justice in general? Can existing theories of justice
provide an adequate account of health equity, or is there a need to rethink
what is unjust about inequalities in health? What is the extent of social—as
opposed to individual—responsibility for health? What ethical problems arise
in evaluating population health and health inequalities, and what are appropriate criteria to do so? How should universal aspirations be balanced with
contextual considerations in the evaluation of health and health equity?

These are some of the important questions that need to be addressed in
understanding the foundations of health equity. The extensive empirical and
policy research on health and health inequalities has yet to be matched by an
appreciation of the normative underpinnings of health equity. Philosophers
and applied ethicists have tended to remain silent on the topic of health

---

[3] Chapters 3 and 4 in this volume by Marmot and Daniels et al., respectively, provide good
summaries of this research.
[4] On this, see also Mann (1995) and Krieger and Birn (1998).

inequalities. John Rawls's theory of 'justice as fairness', for example, avoids any discussion of health.[5] Insofar as the topic of health equity is addressed at all, the focus has been restricted to access to *health care* (Daniels 1985). In this respect Charles Fried's (1975) argument that a right to health can only imply a right to health care was very influential (Marchand et al. 1998). Similarly, *bioethics* has tended to focus on medicine and individual life-and-death questions, but has neglected the variety of social forces that influence health. Access to medical care is certainly an important factor in the preservation and restoration of health and is one element in assessing health equity, but by no means the only one.

According to Daniel Wikler (1997) bioethics is now ready to move to a new phase and address the issues raised by the empirical literature on social inequalities in health. Indeed, over the past few years, several publications have appeared which deal with what may be called public-health ethics (Marchand et al. 1998; Beauchamp and Steinbock 1999; Daniels et al. 2000; Danis et al. 2002).

The present volume was conceived as an attempt to initiate this important subject area. It has been our aim to launch a wide investigation of the ethical issues underlying inequalities in health. In order to examine health equity from a variety of perspectives, contributions have been solicited from philosophers, anthropologists, economists, and public-health specialists. The contributions centre on five major themes: (1) what is health equity?; (2) health equity and its relation to social justice; (3) health inequalities and responsibilities for health; (4) ethical issues in health evaluation and prioritisation; and (5) anthropological perspectives on health equity.

HEALTH EQUITY

The two chapters in this part provide an introduction to health equity. Many of the issues raised in these chapters are subsequently addressed elsewhere in the volume. In Chapter 1 Sudhir Anand starts by asking the following questions: why are we concerned with health equity and what is its relation to equity in general? Should we be more concerned about inequalities in health than about inequalities in other dimensions such as income? Should we be more concerned with some types of health inequalities than with others? Should we be less tolerant of inequalities across certain population groups than across others? He argues that health should be treated as a special good

---

[5] '[S]ince the fundamental problem of justice concerns the relations among those who are full and active participants in society...it is reasonable to assume that everyone has physical needs and psychological capacities within some normal range' (Rawls 1993: 272n).

because it is a prerequisite to a person functioning as an agent. Inequalities in health thus constitute inequalities in people's capability to function—a denial of equality of opportunity.

Chapter 2 by Amartya Sen provides a multidimensional framework for investigating health equity. According to him, 'health equity is a broad and inclusive discipline', which consists of many aspects. It is concerned not only with equity in the dimensions of health care and health outcomes, but with broader considerations of social justice which have a bearing on health. The capability approach developed by Sen lends itself well to illuminate these different aspects of health equity. He further emphasises the distinction between outcome-related evaluation and process-related evaluation. In contrast to those who conceive of health equity as primarily an outcome-based concept, Sen emphasises the importance of procedural considerations such as nondiscrimination in the pursuit of equality of health outcomes and in the delivery of health care.

HEALTH, SOCIETY, AND JUSTICE

Chapter 3 by Michael Marmot provides an excellent introduction to the issues raised by research on social inequalities in health. It draws on his famous 'Whitehall' studies of British civil servants (Marmot et al. 1978, 1991) and similar studies, which show that health is positively correlated with socio-economic status. In his chapter, Marmot discusses why social gradients in health outcomes should be a matter of policy concern. He then critically examines a variety of explanations that have been offered for the occurrence of social inequalities in health. Marmot argues that the most promising approaches are those that attempt to uncover the social causes and pathways underlying differences in health outcomes between social groups.

In commenting on the observed correlation between social position and health, he questions explanations which give prominence to reverse causation (or 'endogeneity'). In particular, he rejects the 'health selection' argument, according to which social inequalities in health arise not because of social influences on health, but because individuals or families with a disposition to poor health are economically less successful and end up in the lower socio-economic groups.

The main thrust of Marmot's chapter is to emphasise the role of social factors in the production of ill-health and to underscore the need for policies that address these factors. He shows that even for those disparities in health that may be linked to individual lifestyle choices such as smoking, a social gradient in health outcomes remains after controlling for these choices. Hence such individual choices do not, according to Marmot, undermine the case for interventions to correct inequalities in health. In a later chapter, Daniel Wikler also discusses the extent to which society's obligation to correct inequalities in health is diminished by individual lifestyle choices, and concludes that responsibility for health cannot reside solely with the individual.

In Chapter 4 Norman Daniels, Bruce Kennedy, and Ichiro Kawachi take the same starting point as Marmot, viz., the observation of a social gradient in health outcomes. They seek to answer the question 'When are social inequalities in health unjust?', and argue that the Rawlsian conception of justice is applicable in this context. Their argument draws on an extension of Rawls's theory of justice developed by Daniels (1985) in the context of just health care. He invoked the Rawlsian principle of 'fair equality of opportunity' and broadened the definition of opportunity to include health. While Daniels (1985) saw health as being determined by health care, Chapter 4 by Daniels et al. recognises that there are many factors other than health care which affect a person's health. In consequence, they extend Rawls's principle of fair equality of opportunity to the entire range of factors that influence health.

Although this argument would seem to be a sufficient foundation for health equity, Daniels et al. introduce another reading of the relationship between Rawlsian justice and health equity. This approach brings to bear the entire edifice of 'justice as fairness' as developed by Rawls (1971). The first principle of justice requires equality of basic rights and liberties. The second principle consists of the subprinciples of 'fair equality of opportunity' and the 'difference principle'. These principles are applied by Rawls to the distribution of 'primary goods', which Daniels et al. claim happen to be coterminous with the social determinants of health. Thus, they argue that the application of Rawls's principles of justice will automatically solve the problem of social inequalities in health.[6] As expressed in the title of their chapter, they conclude that a just society 'is good for our health'.

Like the previous two chapters, Chapter 5 by Fabienne Peter also takes as its starting point the empirical findings of social inequalities in health, and examines how these relate to normative judgements about health equity. Her approach, an indirect one, embeds judgements about health equity within the pursuit of social justice generally. Most existing approaches to health equity are what she calls 'direct': they treat health as a special good and identify principles that should rule its distribution. An example is the application in Chapter 4 by Daniels et al. of Rawls's principle of fair equality of opportunity. According to Peter's 'indirect' approach, social inequalities in health are unjust when they are the result of injustices in the basic structure of society in Rawls's sense. This relationship explains why we are particularly concerned with certain inequalities in health—for example, those between the rich and the poor—and not with others. Conversely, knowledge of particular inequalities in health can be used to reveal how the basic structure of society is working, and thus inform judgements about social justice.

---

[6] See the commentary by Anand and Peter (2000) on the possible tension involved in simultaneously invoking both views of how Rawlsian justice might apply in dealing with health equity.

RESPONSIBILITY FOR HEALTH AND HEALTH CARE

Rawls's theory of justice has been criticised for neglecting the distinction between situations in which individuals carry no responsibility and situations where they do. As it is sometimes argued that social inequalities in health arise from health-compromising individual behaviours, it is important to scrutinise the moral relevance of personal responsibility. In Chapter 6, Daniel Wikler concedes that individual responsibility matters, but rejects the conclusion that this absolves society from an obligation to correct social inequalities in health. Wikler points out that health gradients exist independently of behavioural patterns. And even if health outcomes do vary with behaviour, he argues that it is difficult to establish whether the actions have been taken through free will—a necessary condition for attributing moral responsibility. Wikler concludes that personal responsibility for health should not be assigned more than a peripheral role in health equity.

Chapter 7 by Thomas Pogge discusses the theoretical question of how justice gives rise to social responsibility for health. He distinguishes between conceptions of justice that focus on 'distributional' factors and those that focus on 'relational' factors. Pogge argues that most existing conceptions of justice are of the distributional type, where judgements of justice and equity are concerned with bringing about a 'good distribution' of some entity that is judged to be morally relevant—for example, health. A relational conception of justice assesses not merely the outcomes but also the extent to which our actions are responsible for the outcomes. The more we are responsible for an outcome—the stronger the causal relation between our actions and the harms suffered—the stronger our obligation to help or intervene.

In the case of health, a relational perspective is concerned with more than a good distribution of health outcomes. Judgements of health equity must be concerned with an evaluation of the responsibility of agents in the production of health.[7] The stronger our involvement in bringing about adverse health outcomes, the greater our obligation to redress them. According to Pogge, such an evaluation—and our obligations—should not be confined to national boundaries.

Chapter 8 by Philippe Van Parijs is concerned with obligations for health care across regional boundaries. He discusses the case of Belgium, where the two main linguistic groups (the Flemish and the Walloon) are at odds over the allocation of the country's health-care resources. The per capita consumption of publicly-funded health care is significantly higher in Wallonia than in Flanders, which is economically better off, and the Flemish have objected to subsidising the Walloon's health-care expenses. For Van Parijs, this conflict raises the more general issue of what the requirements of justice should be between the two groups, or 'peoples'. His proposed solution draws on

---

[7] In contrast to Wikler's view, Pogge's line of reasoning would seem to imply a greater role for individual responsibility in judgements of health equity.

Rawls's *Law of Peoples* (1999), but is more demanding. Van Parijs rejects a dualist approach, with two largely independent systems and minimal transfers. Instead, he argues that we should avoid making 'a sharp dichotomy between solidarity within one people and solidarity across peoples' (p. 179, this volume).

ETHICAL AND MEASUREMENT PROBLEMS IN HEALTH EVALUATION

The fourth part of the volume is concerned with ethical and measurement problems in health evaluation. How should we aggregate health across people, time, and different types of health condition? What ethical problems arise with existing measures of population health and of the burden of disease? What are the consequences of using cost-effectiveness analysis for evaluating health interventions? What problems arise in incorporating longevity in the valuation of health at a point in time? These are some of the questions addressed in this part of the volume.

Most of the chapters focus on the 'disability-adjusted life year' (DALY), a measure adopted by the World Health Organization and the World Bank, and related metrics such as the quality-adjusted life year (QALY). Chapter 9 by Sudhir Anand and Kara Hanson and Chapter 10 by Dan Brock discuss a number of ethical problems with the use of DALYs and QALYs. They draw attention to questionable assumptions underlying these metrics—for example, concerning age-weighting and discounting future life in DALYs—and to the limitations of cost-effectiveness analysis in priority setting.

Anand and Hanson distinguish the use of DALYs for measuring the quantity of ill-health (the 'burden of disease') from their use for resource allocation or priority setting. They argue that the information sets required for the two exercises are quite different, and that the use of DALYs is flawed on both counts. Age-weighting and discounting of future life cannot be justified for either exercise. Weighting a year lived at age 70 at less than half of a year lived at age 25 (as the DALY formula implies) is ethically unacceptable. Similarly, discounting at a rate of 3 per cent per annum implies that one life saved today is worth more than five certain lives saved in 55 years, which the authors suggest is inequitable. Furthermore, the use of DALYs introduces a systematic bias against individuals with permanent disabilities: for a person with a preexisting disability, any illness independent of his disability will count for less than the same illness for an able-bodied person.

Given that DALYs are a measure of the burden of disease, Anand and Hanson examine the specific nature of the 'burden'. The 'burden' does not capture individuals' differential ability to cope with illness, and does not include indirect burdens on others. More seriously, the authors argue that the burden measured by DALYs is the burden of disease *and* underdevelopment, and not that of disease alone. This follows because DALYs quantify the potential life years lost to mordidity or premature mortality in each country with respect to a standardised maximum life expectancy—that of Japan—for all countries.

Chapter 10 by Brock expands on the ethical problems that arise with cost-effectiveness analysis (CEA) in health resource allocation. CEA represents a utilitarian moral standard for resource distribution, and hence is subject to the standard problems of this approach for distributive justice or equity. Brock organises his comments on existing approaches to prioritising health-care resources in terms of the construction of the metric (QALYs and DALYs) and its use in CEA, and problems of distributive justice raised by CEA. On top of Anand and Hanson's criticisms of the construction of the DALY, he raises the problem of determining disability weights. For example, whose preferences should be used to evaluate the degree to which disability is weighted—those of the healthy or those of the disabled (who typically have very different perspectives)?

Brock raises a number of questions on distributional issues in CEA. Should priority be given to the worst-off in health-care resource prioritisation and if so for what reasons? How should we decide between small benefits to large numbers of people and large benefits to a few? How should the conflict be resolved between using resources to produce the best overall health outcomes and giving all individuals in need of treatment a fair chance to receive it?

The last two issues are taken up in Chapter 11 by Frances Kamm, which is concerned with the allocation of scarce resources related to health. She discusses microallocation problems—for example, giving a health-care resource to one person rather than another—and macroallocation problems—for example, allocating money to production of one health-care service or product rather than another. She describes the possible theoretical foundations for giving priority to some factors and not to others when allocating resources. A number of principles (the Principle of Irrelevant Good, the Principle of Irrelevant Identity, the Causative Principle, the Treatment Aim Principle) and arguments (the Aggregative Argument, the Balancing Argument, the Major Part Argument, the Moral Importance Argument, the Only Available Option Argument) are stated with the ultimate aim of arriving at a decision procedure for whom to help. Kamm also uses the principles she identifies in her chapter to reveal specific ethical problems with QALYs and DALYs, and to make suggestions for dealing with these problems in priority setting.

In Chapter 12 John Broome investigates the theoretical problems that arise in incorporating longevity in the valuation of people's health. He argues that longevity poses a special difficulty for measurement because it cannot be pinned down to a point in time. Broome discusses two types of aggregation or separability: the well-being of a single person as an aggregate of her well-being at each of the separate times in her life; and the well-being of a population as an interpersonal aggregate of each individual's well-being. With the aid of a variety of Parfittian diagrams, he shows that a 'snapshot valuation' of the distribution of well-being across people at a given point in time cannot account for longevity differences. If we concentrate only on well-being at each point in time, we cannot detect any difference between the following possibilities, *ceteris paribus*: a single person living for a certain period, and two different people who each live for half that period where the second person is born immediately after the first one dies. The reason this problem arises is that the snapshot contains no information on the length-of-life of an individual, that is, the period for which a person's well-being continues. Broome concludes that there is no such thing as 'the health of a country at a particular time'.

EQUITY AND CONFLICTING PERSPECTIVES ON HEALTH EVALUATION

Any evaluation of health and inequalities in health, and any policy towards health equity, must rely on value judgements and be based on particular cognitive perspectives. The origins, therefore, of these value judgements and cognitive perspectives need to be investigated. The contributions of the first four parts of the volume have tended to assume a common approach to the nature of health, which has formed the basis for its evaluation. Given this approach, the assessment of health equity is directed at the weighting of different health conditions and the identification of criteria for the just distribution of health. In contrast, the chapters in the last part of the volume address the question of how to proceed if there are conflicting accounts or narratives of health and illness. One of the main challenges encountered here is the tension between the desire to address health problems and the need to accommodate a diversity of perspectives and socio-cultural circumstances.

The three chapters in this final part all seek to strike a balance, in different ways, between universal and culturally-specific perspectives on health and health equity. Chapter 13 by Amartya Sen addresses the role of medical anthropology in health assessment, and provides the link between the first four parts of the volume and the last two chapters by Arthur Kleinman and Vincanne Adams, both medical anthropologists.

Sen contrasts two types of approaches to health assessment: the 'internal' perspective—emphasised by anthropologists—of individual experience of illness; and the 'external' perspective of public-health experts, economists, and the like, that is based on aggregate mortality and morbidity data collected through statistical surveys and censuses. Since each has its strengths as well as its shortcomings, successful policies need to take both perspectives into account. Sen discusses the experience of pain and suffering as an example of a health-related phenomenon that cannot adequately be captured by the external perspective. Relying too much on the internal perspective may, however, be misleading as well. Since perception is socially contingent, certain states of disease or disability may be perceived as normal and unavoidable, even though they are preventable. Sen illustrates a further problem with relying on the internal perspective. For example, the state of Kerala reports the highest rates of self-perceived morbidity (internal perspective) of any state in India, while at the same time having the highest levels of life expectancy (external perspective).

Chapter 14 by Kleinman addresses a similar tension, but puts the emphasis on ethics rather than on epistemology. Kleinman contrasts the differences between the 'translocal' ethical discourse and local moral experiences and practices. He outlines what he calls an anthropological approach to health equity—a framework for health equity analysis that incorporates both perspectives. The chapter starts with an exploration of why both perspectives matter. On the one hand, the ethical discourse remains empty and will not fulfil its ambitions if it does not echo local moral experiences. On the other hand, local moral practices may be unethical, in which case a translocal perspective could serve as a useful corrective. The need for a translocal perspective is often endorsed by health policy-makers, but Kleinman argues that successful health policy should pay greater attention to local perspectives. With the aid of a theoretical and a practical example, he discusses how an anthropological approach would change the health equity discourse. The theoretical example relates to health rights, which are formulated on the basis of a notion of a uniform human nature. Anthropological research, however, questions this uniformity. According to Kleinman, this makes the standard discourse on health rights unviable. The practical example he discusses is that of suicide in China. Several cases bring to bear the diversity of circumstances and reasons which lead people to commit suicide. Against this backdrop Kleinman argues that without a serious engagement with local moral experience, health policy recommendations are bound to fail.

Adams' case study of Tibet in Chapter 15 illustrates and expands on Kleinman's framework. It examines how Tibetan life and health are affected by the secularist, modernist policies of the Chinese government. China had a leading role in the Health-for-All movement, whose goal was to secure universal access to primary health care. To achieve this goal, the Chinese government did not rely on biomedicine alone, but also made use of the practice of traditional medicine. Adams suggests that the efforts of the Chinese government should not be seen in isolation but, in the context of the broader politics of China, as a means towards the realisation of a socialist state.

She argues that a tension arises between the health policies of the Chinese government, which did allow a role for traditional medicine, and the larger agenda of modernisation and secularisation, which required the confinement of religious practices in public and social life. This tension is examined in the context of Tibet, where the repression of religious and cultural practices has curbed ethnomedicine.

Against this background, Adams discusses the link between culture and health in policies towards health equity. Through narratives of Tibetan ethnomedicine, her fieldwork documents how Chinese policies in Tibet may actually have produced stress and ill-health. Hence, she argues that the understanding of health equity should not be confined to 'scientized' medical theory, but needs to accommodate an 'equity of epistemologies'—that is of different approaches to health, to the body, and the body's relationship to the mind and the environment.

References

Anand, Sudhir and Fabienne Peter (2000). 'Equal Opportunity', in Joshua Cohen and Joel Rogers (eds.), *Is Inequality Bad for Our Health?* Boston: Beacon Press, pp. 48–52.

Anand, Sudhir and Martin Ravallion (1993). 'Human Development in Poor Countries: On the Role of Private Incomes and Public Services', *Journal of Economic Perspectives*, 7(1): 133–50.

Beauchamp, D. and B. Steinbock (1999). *New Ethics for the Public's Health*. New York: Oxford University Press.

Black, Douglas and J. N. Morris (eds.) (1992) [1980]. *Inequalities in Health: the Black Report and the Health Divide*, 2nd edn. London: Penguin.

Daniels, Norman (1985). *Just Health Care*. Cambridge: Cambridge University Press.

——, Bruce Kennedy, and Ichiro Kawachi (2000). 'Justice is Good for Our Health', in Joshua Cohen and Joel Rogers (eds.), *Is Inequality Bad for Our Health?* Boston: Beacon Press.

Danis, Marion, Carolyn Clancy, and Larry R. Churchill (eds.) (2002). *Ethical Dimensions of Health Policy*. New York: Oxford University Press.

Fried, Charles (1975). 'Rights and Health Care: Beyond Equity and Efficiency', *New England Journal of Medicine*, 253: 241–5.

Krieger, Nancy and Anne-Emanuelle Birn (1998). 'A Vision of Social Justice as the Foundation of Public Health: Commemorating 150 Years of the Spririt of 1848', *American Journal of Public Health*, 88(11): 1603–6.

Mann, Jonathan M. (1995). 'Human Rights and the New Public Health', *Health and Human Rights*, 1(3): 229–33.

Marchand, Sarah, Daniel Wikler, and Bruce Landesman (1998). 'Class, Health, and Justice', *The Milbank Quarterly*, 76(3): 449–68.

Marmot, Michael G., G. Rose, M. Shipley, and P. J. Hamilton (1978). 'Employment Grade and Coronary Heart Disease in British Civil Servants', *Journal of Epidemiology and Community Health*, 32(4): 244–9.

——, George Davey Smith, Stephen Stansfeld, Chandra Patel, Fiona North, Jenny Head, Ian White, Eric Brunner, and Amanda Feeney (1991). 'Health Inequalities among British Civil Servants: The Whitehall II Study', *The Lancet*, 337: 1387–93.

Murray, Christopher J. L., C. M. Michaud, M. T. McKenna, and J. S. Marks (1998). *U.S. Patterns of Mortality by County and Race: 1965–1994*. Cambridge, MA: Harvard Center for Population and Development Studies.

Rawls, John (1971). *A Theory of Justice*. Cambridge, MA: Belknap Press of Harvard University Press.

—— (1993). *Political Liberalism*. New York: Columbia University Press.

—— (1999). *The Law of Peoples*. Cambridge, MA: Harvard University Press.

Robertson, Ann (1998). 'Critical Reflections on the Politics of Need: Implications for Public Health', *Social Science and Medicine*, 47(10): 1419–30.

United Nations Development Programme (2003). *Human Development Report.* New York: Oxford University Press.

Wikler, Daniel (1997). 'Bioethics, Human Rights, and the Renewal of Health for All: An Overview', in Z. Bankowski, J. H. Bryant, and J. Gallagher (eds.), *Ethics, Equity and the Renewal of WHO's Health for All Strategy.* Geneva: CIOMS, pp. 21–30.

World Health Organization (1978). 'Health for All', *Basic Documents.* Geneva: World Health Organization.

PART I

HEALTH EQUITY

1

The Concern for Equity in Health

SUDHIR ANAND

In this chapter I would like to reflect on some foundational questions relating to health equity. Why are we concerned with equity in health, and what is its relationship to equity in general? Should we be more concerned about inequalities in health than about inequalities in other dimensions such as income? Should we be more concerned with some types of health inequalities than with others? Should we be less tolerant of inequalities across certain population groups than across others? Attempting to answer these questions might help sharpen our understanding of the priority we attach to combating inequalities in health.

Let me start with the welfare-economic approach to assessing the distribution of a good—for simplicity, let us call this good 'income'. A positive value attaches to higher total or average income, and a negative value to inequality of incomes around the average. The tradeoff between these two attributes of the distribution—labelled 'efficiency' and 'equity' by economists—is inferred from the society's social welfare function, which explicitly incorporates its distributional values.

I think it makes much sense to treat the distribution of health outcomes in a similar fashion. More aggregate or average health is positively valued as a good thing, and inequality of health around the average is negatively valued as a bad thing. Again there is a normative tradeoff where we might, if necessary, be willing to sacrifice some aggregate health for more equality of health. Of course, in any actual situation we may not be faced with a tradeoff: there may be policies that permit the achievement of both a higher average *and* more equality.

As a matter of valuation, however, we do need to acknowledge the existence of a tradeoff. As health egalitarians, we should not be evaluating health distributions solely in terms of inequality and without regard to the average. Consider a distribution of two groups of equal size, each of which has a life expectancy at birth of 50 years—so there is perfect equality in health achievement of the two groups. Now suppose that one group's life expectancy

Research support from the Rockefeller Foundation is gratefully acknowledged. Thanks are also due to Timothy Evans, Sanjay Reddy, Amartya Sen, and Barbara Starfield for their comments.

increases to 55 years while the other group's life expectancy increases to 65 years. In the new situation, average life expectancy has gone up from 50 to 60 years, but there is inequality now in health achievement between the two groups. Much as we might be concerned with health inequality, it would be difficult for us to judge the old situation of a 50-year life expectancy for each group as better than the new situation of a 55-year life expectancy for one group and a 65-year life expectancy for the other. Of course, what egalitarians would prefer is a distribution with an average life expectancy of 60 years where both groups have the *same* life expectancy of 60 years, instead of one having 55 and the other 65 years. Compared to the latter, we would even be willing to accept an equal distribution with both groups having a life expectancy *lower* than 60 years (but more than 55 years). (The amount of sacrifice of 'efficiency' for 'equity' that we are willing to accept—in proportionate terms—is the definition of the Atkinson index of inequality; see Atkinson 1970.)

The tradeoff between average achievement and relative equality around the average will be dictated by our aversion to inequality, or concern for equality. The terms of this tradeoff—indeed our aversion to inequality—may well be different in the health space compared with the income space. In the economic inequality literature the tradeoff has been formalised by use of a parameter ε of the social welfare function, which measures society's aversion to inequality (Atkinson 1970). The value of ε varies from zero, where there is *no* concern for inequality and a distribution is assessed entirely by its (arithmetic) average value, to infinity where there is an extreme concern for inequality and the distribution is assessed solely by its minimum value (the so-called Rawlsian case)—see Anand and Sen (1996). As ε increases, the weight in the social welfare function on someone who is less well-off increases relative to the weight on someone who is better-off.

I want to argue that we should be more averse to, or less tolerant of, inequalities in health than inequalities in income. The reasons involve the status of health as a special good, which has both intrinsic and instrumental value. Income, on the other hand, has only instrumental value. Health is regarded as being critical because it directly affects a person's well-being and is a prerequisite to her functioning as an agent. Inequalities in health are thus closely tied to inequalities in the most basic freedoms and opportunities that people can enjoy. In contrast, there are sometimes reasons to tolerate income inequalities.

There are economic reasons why we may be willing to accept certain income inequalities. Economists often assert—with some justification—that income incentives are needed to elicit effort, skill, enterprise, and so on. These incentives— or differences in reward—have the effect of increasing the size of total income (or the 'cake') from which, in principle, the society as a whole can gain (through taxation and possibly trickle-down). Thus the increase in the size of the cake has to be balanced against the income inequalities that must be tolerated to provide the appropriate incentives for 'efficiency'. Furthermore, effort, skill, enterprise, and so on are regarded as legitimate and fair reasons for some people to earn—perhaps even to *deserve*—more than others.

But this incentive argument would not seem to apply in the case of health. Inequalities in health do not directly provide people with similar incentives to improve their health from which society as a whole benefits. There thus seem to be no incentive reasons for accepting inequalities in health, other than those that might be derivative on tolerating income inequalities. As the empirical literature demonstrates, inequalities in income do produce inequalities in health—with richer people generally having better health. I will presently argue against tolerating inequalities in health for this derived reason.

Our willingness to accept some inequality in general incomes must, I believe, be tempered by what the Nobel laureate James Tobin (1970) called 'specific egalitarianism' some thirty years ago. This is the view that certain specific goods—such as health and the basic necessities of life—should be distributed less unequally than people's ability to pay for them. (Indeed, I regard this to be a central reason why many of us are concerned with socio-economic gradients in health.) We are more offended by inequalities in health, nutrition, and health care than by inequalities in clothes, furniture, motor cars, or boats. We should somehow remove health and the necessities of life from the prizes that serve as incentives for economic activity, and instead let people strive and compete for non-essential luxuries and amenities. In other words, we would like to arrange things so that crucial goods such as health are distributed less unequally than is general income—or, more precisely, less unequally than the market would distribute them given an unequal income distribution. This idea is the basis of specific—in contrast to general—egalitarianism.

1.1. WHY IS HEALTH A SPECIAL GOOD?

The rationale for specific egalitarianism in the health space rests on the premise that health is a special good. There is a related notion in public economics—that of a merit good—whose distribution, it is argued, should not be determined according to people's income.

That health is a special good has been recognised through the ages. We find this view in ancient Greek poetry, and in the Hippocratic texts. Democritus in his book *On Diet*, written in the fifth century BC, states:

[w]ithout health nothing is of any use, not money nor anything else.

Some 2,000 years later, René Descartes asserted that health is the highest good. In *Discours de la Méthode*, published in 1637, Descartes (1637 [1953: 168]) writes:

the preservation of health is...without doubt the first good and the foundation of all the other goods of this life.

The reason that health is so important is that (1) it is directly constitutive of a person's well-being; and (2) it enables a person to function as an agent—that is, to pursue the various goals and projects in life that she has reason to value. This view deploys the notion of health as 'well functioning', but it is not grounded in notions of welfare that are based on utility or some other consequential good, such as enabling the person to increase his or her 'human capital' and hence 'income'. It is, rather, an agency-centred view of a person, for whom ill-health reduces the full scope of human agency. In the terminology of Amartya Sen, health contributes to a person's basic capability to function (Sen 1985)—to choose the life she has reason to value.

If we see health in this way, then inequalities in health constitute inequalities in people's capability to function or, more generally, in their 'positive freedom' (in the language of Isaiah Berlin 1969). This is a denial of *equality of opportunity*, as impairments to health constrain what people can do or be. The principle of 'fair equality of opportunity' is one of three principles of John Rawls's 'justice as fairness' (Rawls 1971). Rawls assessed opportunity in terms of people's holdings of 'primary goods'—or resources such as income, wealth, and so on. In his book *Just Health Care*, Norman Daniels (1985) extended the principle to deal with fair access to health care (see also Daniels et al. 2000, and the commentary by Anand and Peter 2000). However, opportunity is best seen directly in terms of the extent of freedom that a person actually has—that is, by one's capability to achieve alternative 'beings' and 'doings' (Sen 1987)—most of which depend critically on one's health. Moreover, the capability to lead a long and healthy life must itself be regarded as a basic capability, since our ability to do things typically depends on our being alive. Thus if we apply Rawls's 'fair equality of opportunity' principle in the space of (basic) capabilities, the reduction of inequalities in health will follow as a direct requirement of justice.

1.2. DIMENSIONS OF HEALTH

I have ducked any attempt to define health and do not propose to offer a definition here. Earlier, I used a particular measure of health, namely life expectancy in years, to illustrate the equity–efficiency tradeoff in health. There are, of course, many different aspects or dimensions of health and ill-health, captured by various different measures. The reasons we adduce for disvaluing inequalities in health more than inequalities in income will also direct us to pay more attention to inequalities in some dimensions (measures) of health than to inequalities in others. Thus, equality of opportunity reasoning may lead us to be more averse to a twofold (that is, a 2-to-1) disparity in the infant mortality rate (IMR) or the child mortality rate (CMR) between groups than to a twofold difference in adult or old age mortality rates. The reasoning may also lead us to be especially concerned about disabilities in health (physical or mental) that prevent a person being mobile or gaining employment.

1.3. THE UNIT OF ANALYSIS

Before concluding, I would like briefly to address the question of the unit of analysis of inequality—in other words, the question of 'inequality among whom?'. This is distinct from the question we have been considering so far, which is 'inequality of what?'—income, health, or specific dimensions of ill-health.

Much of the existing empirical research on health inequalities—undertaken by epidemiologists—has been concerned with differences in health across socio-economic groups, typically defined by occupation, education, or income. Thus, social class 'gradients' have been estimated for Britain and several other European countries. Some researchers have tried to understand these gradients by controlling for factors such as smoking behaviour. Yet, the gradients persist, and much research is underway attempting to understand the social causes and pathways that produce them.

There is much merit in analysing differences in life expectancy, mortality, and morbidity among socio-economic groups. The classification by groups helps to explain how they might be generated. As tools for understanding the determinants of population health, the categories should obviously be extended to include not just socio-economic status but also race, gender, and geographical location. In many developing country contexts, these latter variables have been found to be powerful in identifying inter-group inequalities—for example, race in South Africa, gender in Bangladesh, region in China. Moreover, cross-classifications of socio-economic and other variables often provide further epidemiological clues.

Apart from explanation, there are at least two other reasons for investigating inter-group inequalities in health. First, it allows us to identify groups that are at high risk or suffer particularly poor health. Public policy and public health policy may thus be able to target them directly to effect health improvements. This is the case with the United Kingdom government's current initiative on inequalities in health.

Second, and no less importantly, it allows us to uncover those inequalities in health that we regard as particularly unjust. In the language that I have been using, we will be more averse to—or less tolerant of—certain inter-group inequalities in health, such as racial or gender inequalities, than to inequalities where the groups are randomly defined (say by the first letter of a person's surname). Likewise, we will be more averse to socio-economic inequalities in health than to *inter-individual* inequalities in health that are undifferentiated, or unconditional on information about individuals.

Group inequalities give rise to the suspicion that they derive from social rather than natural (e.g. genetic) factors—and may thus be avoidable through public intervention. Moreover, health inequalities stratified by relevant variables often reveal a compounding of disadvantage—to wit, the observation of a positive correlation between (low) socio-economic status and (poor) health.

Such inequalities will typically be less tolerable than health inequalities observed across randomly defined groups or across undifferentiated individuals. In identifying inequity or injustice, we must take into account—or stratify by—those categories across which we are most averse to health inequalities.

1.4. CONCLUSION

Any approach to conceptualising and analysing inequality must confront two fundamental questions: (1) inequality of what?; and (2) inequality among whom?

On the *what* question, I have tried to argue that our aversion to inequality in health is likely to be greater than our aversion to inequality in income. And within different dimensions of health or ill-health, I have tried to suggest that our aversion to inequality in some dimensions—such as infant and child mortality—is likely to be higher than it is in others (namely, those that do not constitute as serious a denial of lifetime opportunity).

On the *whom* question, I have tried to suggest that our aversion to inequality across certain population groups is likely to be greater than it is across others—for instance, undifferentiated individuals (who are not identified by systematic differences in opportunity).

In all of this I have tried to adapt and extend the framework and language of welfare economics to understand our concern for equity in health.

References

Anand, S. and F. Peter (2000). 'Equal Opportunity', in J. Cohen and J. Rogers (eds.), *Is Inequality Bad for Our Health?*. Boston, MA: Beacon Press.

——and A. K. Sen (1996). 'Gender Inequality in Human Development: Theories and Measurement', in *Background Papers: Human Development Report 1995*. New York: United Nations Development Programme, pp. 1–19. Reprinted in S. Fukuda-Parr and A. K. Shiva Kumar (eds.), *Readings in Human Development*. New Delhi: Oxford University Press, 2003: 186–203.

Atkinson, A. B. (1970). 'On the Measurement of Inequality', *Journal of Economic Theory*, 2(3): 244–63.

Berlin, I. (1969). *Four Essays on Liberty*. Oxford: Oxford University Press.

Daniels, N. (1985). *Just Health Care*. New York: Cambridge University Press.

——, B. Kennedy, and I. Kawachi (2000). 'Justice is Good for Our Health', in J. Cohen and J. Rogers (eds.), *Is Inequality Bad for Our Health?*. Boston, MA: Beacon Press.

Descartes, R. (1637). *Discours de la Méthode, Sixième Partie*, in Bridoux, A. (ed.), *Descartes: Œuvres et lettres*. Paris: Gallimard (Bibliothèque de la Pléiade), 1953.

Rawls, J. (1971). *A Theory of Justice*. Cambridge, MA: Harvard University Press.

Sen, A. K. (1985). *Commodities and Capabilities*. Amsterdam: North-Holland.

——(1987). *The Standard of Living*. The Tanner Lectures. Cambridge: Cambridge University Press.

Tobin, J. (1970). 'On Limiting the Domain of Inequality', *The Journal of Law and Economics*, 13(2): 263–77.

2

Why Health Equity?

AMARTYA SEN

'The world...is not an inn, but a hospital', said Sir Thomas Browne more
than three and half centuries ago, in 1643. That is a discouraging, if not
entirely surprising, interpretation of the world from the distinguished author
of *Religio Medici and Pseudodoxia Epidemica*. But Browne may not be
entirely wrong: even today (not just in Browne's seventeenth-century
England), illness of one kind or another is an important presence in the lives
of a great many people. Indeed, Browne may have been somewhat optimistic
in his invoking of a hospital: many of the people who are most ill in the world
today get no treatment for their ailments, nor the use of effective means of
prevention.

In any discussion of social equity and justice, illness and health must figure
as a major concern. I take that as my point of departure—the ubiquity of
health as a social consideration—and begin by noting that health equity
cannot but be a central feature of the justice of social arrangements in general.
The reach of health equity is immense. But there is a converse feature of this
connection to which we must also pay attention. Health equity cannot be
concerned only with health, seen in isolation. Rather it must come to grips
with the larger issue of fairness and justice in social arrangements, including
economic allocations, paying appropriate attention to the role of health in
human life and freedom. Health equity is most certainly not just about the distribution of *health*, not to mention the even narrower focus on the distribution
of *health care*. Indeed, health equity as a consideration has an enormously
wide reach and relevance.

I shall consider three sets of issues. First, I shall begin by discussing the
nature and relevance of health equity. Second, I shall go on to identify and
scrutinise the distinct grounds on which it has been claimed that health equity
is the wrong policy issue on which to concentrate. I hope to be able to argue
that these grounds of scepticism do not survive close scrutiny. Finally, in the

Text of Keynote Address to Third Conference of the International Health Economics Association
on 'The Economics of Health: Within and Beyond Health Care,' York, 23 July 2001. For helpful
discussions, I am most grateful to Sudhir Anand, Lincoln Chen, Anthony Culyer, and Angus
Deaton. I would also like to acknowledge support from the Rockefeller Foundation funded
project on Health Equity at Harvard University.

third section, I shall consider some difficult issues that have to be faced for an adequate understanding of the demands of health equity. It is particularly important in this context to see health equity as a very broad discipline which has to accommodate quite diverse and disparate considerations.

2.1. HEALTH EQUITY AND SOCIAL JUSTICE

I have tried to argue in an earlier work, *Inequality Reexamined*, that a theory of justice in the contemporary world could not have any serious plausibility if it did not value equality in some space—a space that would be seen as important in that theory (Sen 1992). An income egalitarian, a champion of democracy, a libertarian, and a property-right conservative may have different priorities, but each wants equality of something that is seen as valuable—indeed central—in the respective political philosophy. The income egalitarian will prize an equal distribution of incomes; the committed democrat must insist on equal political rights of all; the resolute libertarian has to demand equal liberty; and the property-right conservative must insist on the same right of all to use whatever property each has. They all treasure—and not just by accident—equality in terms of some variable which is given a central position in their respective theories of justice. Indeed, even an aggregative focus, as Benthamite utilitarianism has, involves a connection with equality in so far as everyone would have to be treated in the same way in arriving at simple aggregates (such as the utility total).

In fact, equality, as an abstract idea, does not have much cutting power, and the real work begins with the specification of what it is that is to be equalised. The central step, then, is the specification of the space in which equality is to be sought, and the equitable accounting rules that may be followed in arriving at aggregative concerns as well as distributive ones. The content of the respective theories turns on the answers to such questions as 'equality of what?' and 'equity in what form?'(Sen 1980, 1992).

This is where health becomes a critical concern, making health equity central to the understanding of social justice. It is, however, important to appreciate that health enters the arena of social justice in several distinct ways, and they do not all yield exactly the same reading of particular social arrangements. As a result, health equity is inescapably multidimensional as a concern. If we insist on looking for a congruence of the different aspects of health equity before we make unequivocal judgements, then often enough health equity will yield an incomplete partitioning or a partial ordering. This does not do away with the discipline of rational assessment, or even of maximisation (which can cope with incompleteness through reticent articulation), but it militates against the expectation, which some entertain, that in every comparison of social states there must be a full ranking that places all the alternative states in a simple ordering.[1] Indeed, even when two alternative states are ultimately

---

[1] I have discussed the need for incomplete orderings and reticent articulations in Sen (1970, 1997).

ranked in a clear and decisive way, that ranking may be based on the relative weighing—and even perhaps a compromise—between divergent considerations, which retain their separate and disparate relevance even after their comparative weights have been assessed.

So what, then, are the diverse considerations? First, health is among the most important conditions of human life and a critically significant constituent of human capabilities which we have reason to value. Any conception of social justice that accepts the need for a fair distribution as well as efficient formation of human capabilities cannot ignore the role of health in human life and the opportunities that persons respectively have to achieve good health—free from escapable illness, avoidable afflictions and premature mortality. Equity in the achievement and distribution of health gets, thus, incorporated and embedded in a larger understanding of justice.

What is particularly serious as an injustice is the lack of opportunity that some may have to achieve good health because of inadequate social arrangements, as opposed to, say, a personal decision not to worry about health in particular. In this sense, an illness that is unprevented and untreated for social reasons (because of, say, poverty or the overwhelming force of a community-based epidemic), rather than out of personal choice (such as smoking or other risky behaviour by adults), has a particularly negative relevance to social justice. This calls for the further distinction between health achievement and the *capability* to achieve good health (which may or may not be exercised). This is, in some cases, an important distinction, but in most situations, health achievement tends to be a good guide to the underlying capabilities, since we tend to give priority to good health when we have the real opportunity to choose (indeed even smoking and other addictive behaviour can also be seen in terms of a generated 'unfreedom' to conquer the habit, raising issues of psychological influences on capability—a subject I shall not address in this talk).

It is important to distinguish between the achievement and capability, on the one side, and the facilities socially offered for that achievement (such as health care), on the other. To argue for health equity cannot be just a demand about how health care, in particular, should be distributed (contrary to what is sometimes presumed). The factors that can contribute to health achievements and failures go well beyond health care, and include many influences of very different kinds, varying from genetical propensities, individual incomes, food habits, and lifestyles, on the one hand, to the epidemiological environment and work condition, on the other.[2] Recently, Sir Michael Marmot and others have also brought out the far-reaching effects of social inequality on health and survival.[3] We have to go well beyond the delivery and distribution of health care to get an adequate understanding of health achievement and

[2] The importance of the distinction between health and health care for the determination of public policy has been well discussed, among other issues, by Ruger (1998).

[3] See Marmot et al. (1984); Marmot et al. (1991); Marmot et al. (1995). See also Wilkinson (1996).

capability. Health equity cannot be understood in terms of the distribution of *health care*.

Second, in so far as processes and procedural fairness have an inescapable relevance to social justice, we have to go beyond health achievement and the capability to achieve health. As someone who has spent quite a bit of effort in trying to establish the relevance of the capability perspective (including health capabilities) in the theory of justice, I must also stress that the informational basis of justice cannot consist only of capability information, since processes too are important, in addition to outcomes (seen in isolation) and the capability to achieve valued outcomes (Sen 1985, 2000). For this reason, inequalities even in health *care* (and not just in health achievement) can also have relevance to social justice and to health equity, since the process aspect of justice and equity demand some attention, without necessarily occupying the centre of the stage.

Let me illustrate the concern with an example. There is evidence that largely for biological reasons, women tend to have better survival chances and lower incidence of some illnesses throughout their lives (indeed even female foetuses have a lower probability of spontaneous miscarriage). This is indeed the main reason why women predominate in societies with little or no gender bias in health care (such as West Europe and North America), despite the fact that more boys are born than girls, everywhere in the world (and an even higher proportion of male foetuses are conceived). Judged purely in terms of the achievement of health and longevity, this is a gender-related inequality, which is absent only in those societies in which anti-female bias in health care (and sometimes in nutrition as well) makes the female life expectancy no higher than male. But it would be morally unacceptable to suggest that women *should* receive worse health care than men so that the inequality in the achievement of health and longevity disappears (Sen 1992: chapter 6). The claim to process fairness requires that no group—in this case women—be discriminated against in this way, but in order to argue for that conclusion we have to move, in one way or another, away from an exclusive reliance on health achievement.

Third, health equity cannot only be concerned with inequality of either health or health care, and must take into account how resource allocation and social arrangements link health with other features of states of affairs. Again, let me illustrate the concern with a concrete example. Suppose persons A and B have exactly similar health predispositions, including a shared proneness to a particularly painful illness. But A is very rich and gets his ailment cured or completely suppressed by some expensive medical treatment, whereas poor B cannot afford such treatment and suffers badly from the disease. There is clearly a health inequality here. Also, if we do not accept the moral standing of the rich to have privileged treatment, it is plausible to argue that there is also some violation of health equity as well. In particular, the resources used to cure rich A could have been used instead to give some relief to both, or in the case of an indivisibility, to give both persons an equal chance to have a cure through some probabilistic mechanism. This is not hard to argue.

Now, consider a policy change brought about by some health egalitarians, which gives priority to reducing health inequality. This prevents rich A from buying a cure that poor B cannot buy. Poor B's life is unaffected, but now rich A too lives with that painful ailment, spending his money instead on, say, having consoling trips on an expensive yacht on esoteric seas. The policy change does, in fact, reduce the inequality of health, but can it be said that it has advanced health equity? To see clearly the question that is being asked, note that it is not being asked whether this is a better situation overall (it would be hard to argue that it is so), nor am I asking whether it is, everything considered, a just arrangement (which, again, it is not—it would seem to be a Pareto worsening change, given A's desire to use his money to buy heath, rather than a yacht). I am asking, specifically, is there more *health equity* here than in the former case?

I would argue that health equity has not been enhanced by making rich A go around exotic seas on his costly yacht, even though inequality in the space of health as such is reduced. The resources that are now used by rich A to go around the high seas on his yacht could have been used instead to cure poor B or rich A, or to give them each some relief from their respective painful ailments. The reduction of health inequality has not advanced health equity, since the latter requires us to consider further the possibility of making different arrangements for resource allocation, or social institutions or policies. To concentrate on health inequality only in assessing health equity is exactly similar to approaching the problem of world hunger (which is not unknown) by eating less food, overlooking the fact that any general resource can be used to feed the hungry better.

The violation of health equity cannot be judged merely by looking at inequality in health. Indeed, it can be argued that some of the most important policy issues in the promotion of health care are deeply dependent on the overall allocation of resources to health, rather than only on distributive arrangements within health care (e.g. the 'rationing' of health care and other determinants of health), on which a good deal of the literature on health equity seems, at this time, to concentrate. Resources are fungible, and social arrangements can facilitate the health of the deprived, not just at the cost of other people's health care or health achievement, but also through a different social arrangement or an altered allocation of resources. The extent of inequality in health cannot give us adequate information to assess health equity.

This does not, of course, imply that health inequality is not a matter of interest. It does have interest of its own, and it certainly is a very important part of our understanding of health equity, which is a broader notion. If, for example, there are gross inequalities in health achievement, which arise not from irremediable health preconditions, but from a lack of economic policy or social reform or political engagement, then the fact of health inequality would be materially relevant. Health inequalities cannot be identified with health inequity, but the former is certainly relevant to the latter. There is no contradiction here once we see health equity as a multidimensional concept.

2.2. CONTRARY ARGUMENTS

The claim that health equity is important can be resisted on various different grounds, involving empirical as well as conceptual arguments. In various forms these contrary arguments have been presented in professional as well as popular discussions. It is useful to examine the claims of these different arguments and to assess the relevance of health equity in the light of these critical concerns. I do this through posing some sceptical questions as a dialogic device.

2.2.1. *Are distributive demands, in general, really relevant?*

It could be argued that distributive requirements in general, including equity (not just health equity), lack ethical significance as a general principle. Utilitarians, for example, are not particularly bothered by inequality in utilities, and concentrate instead on maximising the distribution-independent sum-total of utilities. A fundamental rejection of inequality as a concern would *inter alia* reduce the relevance of health equity.

There are several different counterarguments that have to be considered in response. First, as John Rawls has argued in disputing the claims of utilitarianism, distribution-indifference does not take the distinction between persons adequately seriously (Rawls 1971). If a person remains miserable or painfully ill, her deprivation is not obliterated or remedied or overpowered simply by making *someone else* happier or healthier. Each person deserves consideration as a person, and this militates against a distribution-indifferent view. The Rawlsian counterargument is as relevant to health inequalities as it is to the inequality of well-being or utility.

Second, specifically in the field of health, there are some upper bounds to the extent to which a person can be made more and more healthy. As a result even the engineering aspect of the strategy of compensating the ill health of some by better and better health of another has some strict limits.

Third, even if we were somehow convinced by the distribution-indifferent view, there would still be some form of equity consideration in treating all persons in the same way in arriving at aggregate achievements (as utilitarianism does). Distribution-independent maximization of sum-total is not so much a denial of equity, but a special—and rather limited—way of accommodating equity within the demands of social justice.

2.2.2. *Are distributional demands really relevant for health achievement in particular?*

It could be argued that equity may be important in some fields, but when it comes to ill health, any reduction of illness of anyone must be seen to be important and should have the same priority no matter what a person's overall level of health, or of general opulence, is. Minimisation of a distribution-independent Disability-Adjusted Life Years (DALY), which is now used quite widely, is a good example of this approach.[4]

In responding to this query, it is useful to begin by explicitly acknowledging that any improvement in anyone's health, given other things, is an adequate ground for recognising that there is some social betterment. But this need to be responsive to everyone's health does not require that exactly the same importance be attached to improving everyone's health—no matter how ill they presently are. Indeed, as Sudhir Anand and Kara Hanson have argued, distribution-indifference is a serious limitation of the approach of DALY (Anand and Hanson 1997, 1998).The use of distribution-indifference in the case of DALY works, in fact, with some perversity, since a disabled person, or one who is chronically ill, and thus disadvantaged in general, also receives less medical attention for other ailments, in the exercise of DALY minimisation, and this has the effect of adding to the relative disadvantage of a person who is already disadvantaged. Rawls's criticism of the distribution-indifference of utilitarianism (in not taking the difference between persons sufficiently seriously) would apply here with redoubled force.

It is interesting to note in that context that the founders (such as Alan Williams and Tony Culyer) of the QALY approach, which has some generic similarity with the DALY approach, have been keen on adjusting the QALY figures by distributional considerations.[5] Indeed, Alan Williams notes, in the context of expounding his views on what he calls the 'fair innings' argument (on which, more presently), he had 'for a long time' taken 'the view that the best way to integrate efficiency and equity considerations in the provision of health care would be to attach equity weights to QALYs [Quality-Adjusted Life Years]'.[6] There is no particular reason to be blind to health equity while being sensitive to equity in general.

2.2.3. *Given the broad ideas of equity and social justice in general, why do we need the more restricted notion of health equity?*

It can be argued that equity-related considerations connected with health are conceptually subsumed by some broader notion of equity (related to, say, utilities or rights). Health considerations may figure *inter alia* in the overall analysis of social equity, but health equity, in this view, does not have a status of its own.

---

[4] See Murray (1994); Murray and Lopez (1996); World Health Organization (2000).

[5] The exponents of the QALY and DALY strategies have discussed their differences rather prominently in recent debates between York and Geneva. I shall not, however, go into those differences in this essay.

[6] Williams (1998). See also Culyer and Wagstaff (1993); and Culyer (1995).

This criticism would have considerable cogency if the idea of health equity were intended to be detached from that of equity and justice in general. But as has been already argued in this essay, the discipline of health equity is not confined to concentrating only on inequalities in health. Health equity may well be embedded in a broader framework of overall equity, but there are some special considerations related to health that need to come forcefully into the assessment of overall justice. In doing this exercise, the idea of health equity motivates certain questions and some specific perspectives, which enrich the more abstract notion of equity in general.

The fact that health is central to our well-being needs emphasis, as does the equally basic recognition that the freedoms and capabilities that we are able to exercise are dependent on our health achievements. For one thing, we are not able to do much if we are disabled or ceaselessly bothered by illness, and we can do very little indeed if we are not alive. As Andrew Marvel had noted in his 1681 poem 'To His Coy Mistress': 'The grave's a fine and private place,/ But none, I think, do there embrace.' The penalty of illness may not be confined to the loss of well-being only, but also include one's lack of freedom to do what one sees as one's agency responsibilities and commitments.[7] Health and survival are central to the understanding not only of the quality of one's life, but also for one's ability to do what one has reason to want to do. The relevance of health equity for social justice in general is hard to overstress.

2.2.4. *Is it not the case that health equity is subsumed by considerations of equity in the distribution of resources (such as incomes or what Rawls calls 'primary goods')?*

In this line of reasoning it is argued that health equity may have, in principle, some importance, but it so happens that this consideration is empirically subsumed by the attention we have to pay to equity in the distribution of resources or 'primary goods', since these economic and social resources ultimately determine the state of people's health.

In response, we can begin by noting that the state of health that a person enjoys is influenced by a number of different considerations which take us well beyond the role of social and economic factors. An adequate policy approach to health has to take note not only of the influences that come from general social and economic factors, but also from a variety of other parameters, such as personal disabilities, individual proneness to illness, epidemiological hazards of particular regions, the influence of climatic variations, and so on. A proper theory of health equity has to give these factors their due within the discipline of health equity. In general, in the making of health policy, there is a need to distinguish between equality in health achievements (or corresponding

---

[7] On this, see Sen (1992). See also Mooney (1998) and, in the same volume, Schneider-Bunner (1998); Bleichrodt (1998); Hurley (1998); Rice (1998).

capabilities and freedoms) and equality in the distribution of what can be generally called health resources. While the latter has relevance, I have argued, through process considerations, it is the former that occupies a central territory of equity in general and health equity in particular.

2.3. GENERAL CONSIDERATIONS AND PARTICULAR PROPOSALS

I turn finally to questions and debates on substantive claims about the content of health equity. Since health equity has to be seen, as I have tried to argue, as a broad discipline, rather than as a narrow and formulaic criterion, there is room for many distinct approaches within the basic idea of health equity. But the breadth of the idea of health equity is itself in some need of defence. The problems and difficulties in taking a particularly confined interpretation of health equity do not typically lie in the relevance of what that interpretation *asserts* (this is, often enough, not in doubt), but rather in what it *denies*. It is possible to accept the significance of a perspective, without taking that perspective to be ground enough for rejecting other ways of looking at health equity, which too can be important.

Consider Alan Williams's powerful idea of a 'fair innings' (Williams 1997, 1998), which relates to—but substantially extends—the approach to health equity as developed by Anthony Culyer and Adam Wagstaff.[8] Williams develops the case for fair innings with great care, pointing to the ethics underlying the approach: 'the notion of a 'fair innings' is based on the view that we are each entitled to a certain level of achievement in the game of life, and that anyone failing to reach this level has been hard done by, while anyone exceeding it has no reason to complain when their time runs out' (Williams 1998: 319). Developing this insight, Williams arrives at the position that

if we think (as I do) that a fair innings should be defined in terms of *quality-adjusted life expectancy at birth*, and that we should be prepared to make some sacrifice to reduce that inequality, it is quite feasible to calculate a set of weights representing the differential social value of improvements in quality-adjusted life years delivered to different sorts of people in our current situation.

Through this procedure, Williams neatly captures the important equity issue related to the fact that the differences in prospects of a fair innings can be very large between different social classes.

There is no doubt that this approach has much to commend, and in particular it seems to deal with interclass inequality in a fulsome way. And yet the question can be asked whether this is all that needs to be captured in applying the idea of health equity. Just to raise an elementary question, let me return to the issue of fewer health hazards and greater survival chances that women have

---

[8] Culyer and Wagstaff (1993); Culyer (1995).

compared with men. Williams notes this fact, and notes that 'the difference in life expectancy at birth *between men and women* in the United Kingdom is even greater than that between social classes!' He goes on to point out that the gender difference in QALYs is comparatively less than in unadjusted life expectancy (women seem to have a tougher time than men while alive), but also notes that 'whereas nearly 80 per cent of women will survive long enough to enjoy a fair innings (which in this case I have taken to be 60 QALYs), less than 60 per cent of men will do so'.

Williams point out, using this line of reasoning, 'We males are not getting a fair innings!' (p. 327). The difficult issues arise after this has been acknowledged. What should we then do? If, as the fair innings approach presumes, this understanding should guide the allocation of health care, then there has to be inequality in health care, in favour of men, to redress the balance. Do we really want such inequality in care? Is there nothing in the perspective of process equality to resist that conclusion, which would militate against providing care on the basis of the gender of the person for an identical ailment suffered by a woman and a man?

The issue of gender difference illustrates a more general problem, namely that differences in quality-adjusted life expectancy need not give us ground enough to ignore the demands of nondiscrimination in certain vital fields of life, including the need for medical care for treatable ailments. Sometimes the differences are very systematic, as with gender contrasts, or for that matter with differences in age: indeed as Williams notes, 'whatever social group we belong to, the survivors will slowly improve their chances of achieving a fair innings, and as their prospects improve, the equity weights attached to them should decline' (pp. 326–7). Fair innings is a persuasive argument, but not the only persuasive one. We do not, for example, refuse to take *King Lear* to be a tragedy on the ground that Lear had, before Shakespeare starts his story, a long and good life, with many excellent 'quality-adjusted life years', adding up to more than a 'fair innings'.

This problem is not special only to Alan Williams's proposal, but applies generally to all approaches that insist on taking a single-dimensional view of health equity in terms of achievement of health (or, for that matter, the capability to achieve health). For example, it applies just as much to the policy conclusion arrived at by Tony Culyer and Adam Wagstaff in their justly celebrated paper on 'equity and equality in health and health care' (1993) that 'equity in health care should...entail distributing care in such a way as to get as close as is feasible to an equal distribution of health.' But should we really? A gender-check, followed by giving preference to male patients, and other such explicit discriminations 'to get as close as is feasible to an equal distribution of health' cannot but lack some quality that we would tend to associate with the process of health equity.

I should make it clear that I am not arguing for giving priority to process equity over all other considerations, including equity in health and the capability to achieve good health. Culyer and Wagstaff are right to resist that, and they would not have done better if instead they were to give absolute priority, in general, to equity in health delivery, irrespective of consequences. They take us not from the frying pan to fire, but rather from fire to the frying pan. But I want to be neither in the fire, nor in the frying pan. Health equity is a broad and inclusive discipline, and any unifocal criterion like 'fair innings' or 'equal distribution of health' cannot but leave out many relevant concerns.[9] The assertive features of what Williams, Culyer, Wagstaff, and others want deserve recognition and support, but that should not be taken to imply the denial of the relevance of other claims (as they seem to want, through giving unconditional priority to their unifocal criterion).

To conclude, health equity has many aspects, and is best seen as a multi-dimensional concept. It includes concerns about achievement of health and the capability to achieve good health, not just the distribution of health care. But it also includes the fairness of processes and thus must attach importance to nondiscrimination in the delivery of health care. Furthermore, an adequate engagement with health equity also requires that the considerations of health be integrated with broader issues of social justice and overall equity, paying adequate attention to the versatility of resources and the diverse reach and impact of different social arrangements.

Within this broad field of health equity, it is, of course, possible to propose particular criteria that put more focus on some concerns and less on others. I am not trying to propose here some unique and pre-eminent formula that would be exactly right and superior to all the other formulae that may be proposed (though it would have been, I suppose, rather magnificent to be able to obtain one canonical answer to this complex inquiry). My object, rather, has been to identify some disparately relevant considerations for health equity, and to argue against any arbitrary narrowing of the domain of that immensely rich concept. Health equity is a broad discipline, and this basic recognition has to precede the qualified acceptance of some narrow criterion or other for specific—and contingently functional—purposes. The special formulae have their uses, but the general and inclusive framework is not dispensable for that reason. We need both.

References

Anand, Paul and Allan Wailoo (2000). 'Utilities Versus Rights to Publicly Provided Goods: Arguments and Evidence from Health Care Rationing', *Economica*, 67: 543–77.

Anand, Sudhir and Kara Hanson (1997). 'Disability Adjusted Life Years: A Critical Review', *Journal of Health Economics*, 16(6): 685–702.

—— and —— (1998). 'DALYs: Efficiency versus Equity', *World Development*, 26(2): 307–10.

[9] See also Anand and Wailoo (2000).

Barer, Morris L., Thomas E. Getzen, and Gred L Stoddart (eds.) (1998). *Health, Health Care and Health Economics*. New York: Wiley.

Bleichrodt, Han (1998) 'Health Utility Indices and Equity Considerations', in M. L. Barer et al. (eds.), *Health, Health Care and Health Economics*. New York: Wiley.

Culyer, A. J. (1995). 'Equality of *What* in Health Policy? Conflicts between Contenders', Discussion Paper No. 142, Centre for Health Economics, University of York.

Culyer, Anthony J. and A. Wagstaff (1993). 'Equity and Equality in Health and Health Care', *Journal of Health Economics*, 12: 431–57.

Hurley, Jeremiah (1998). 'Welfarism, Extra-Welfarism and Evaluative Economic Analysis in the Health Sector', in M. L. Barer et al. (eds.), *Health, Health Care and Health Economics*. New York: Wiley.

Marmot M. G., M. Bobak, and G. Davey Smith (1995). 'Explorations for Social Inequalities in Health', in B. C. Amick, S. Levine, A. R. Tarlov, and D. Chapman (eds.), *Society and Health*. Oxford: Oxford University Press.

Marmot M., M. Shipley, and G. Rose (1984). 'Inequalities in Death—Specific Explanations of a General Pattern', *Lancet*, May 05: 1003–6.

——G. Davey Smith, S. Stansfeld, C. Patel, F. North, J. Head, I. White, E. Brunner, and A. Feeney (1991). 'Health Inequalities Among British Civil Servants: the Whitehall II Study', *Lancet*, 337: 1387–93.

Mooney, Gavin (1998). 'Economics, Communitarianism, and Health Care', in M. L. Barer et al. (eds.), *Health, Health Care and Health Economics*. New York: Wiley.

Murray C. J. L. and A. D. Lopez (1996). 'The Global Burden of Disease: A Comprehensive Assessment of Mortality and Disability From Disease, Injuries, and Risk Factors in 1990 and Projected to 2020', Geneva: World Health Organization.

——(1994). 'Quantifying the Burden of Disease: the Technical Basis for Disability-Adjusted Life Years', *Bulletin of the World Health Organization*, 72: 429–45.

Rawls, John (1971). *A Theory of Justice*. Cambridge, MA: Harvard University Press.

Rice, Thomas (1998). 'The Desirability of Market-Based Health Reforms: A Reconsideration of Economic Theory', in M. L. Barer et al. (eds.), *Health, Health Care and Health Economics*. New York: Wiley.

Ruger, Jennifer Prah (1998). 'Aristotelian Justice and Health Policy: Capability and Incompletely Theorized Agreements', Ph.D. thesis (Harvard University 1998).

Schneider-Bunner, Claude (1998). 'Equity in Managed Competition', in M. L. Barer et al. (eds.), *Health, Health Care and Health Economics*. New York: Wiley.

Sen A. (1970). *Collective Choice and Social Welfare*. San Francisco: Holden-Day 1970; republished Amsterdam: North-Holland, 1979.

——(1980). 'Equality of what?', in S. McMurrin (ed.), *Tanner Lectures on Human Values*, Vol 1. Cambridge: Cambridge University Press.

——(1985). 'Well-being, Agency and Freedom: The Dewey Lectures 1984', *Journal of Philosophy*, 82: 169–221.

——(1992). *Inequality Reexamined*. Cambridge, MA: Harvard University Press, and Oxford: Clarendon Press, 1992.

——(1997). 'Maximization and the Act of Choice', *Econometrica*, 65: 745–79.

——(2000). 'Consequential Evaluation and Practical Reason', *Journal of Philosophy*, 97: 477–502.

Wilkinson, R. (1996). *Unhealthy Societies: the Afflictions of Inequality*. London: Routledge.

Williams, Alan (1997). 'Intergenerational Equity: An Exploration of the "Fair Innings" Argument', *Health Economics*, 6: 117–32.

——(1998). 'If We Are Going to Get a Fair Innings, Someone Will Need to Keep the Score!', in M. L. Barer et al. (eds.), *Health, Health Care and Health Economics*. New York: Wiley.

WHO (2000). *World Health Report 2000*. Geneva: World Health Organization.

PART II

HEALTH, SOCIETY, AND JUSTICE

3

Social Causes of Social Inequalities in Health

MICHAEL MARMOT

The relation between society and health is challenging and important for two complementary reasons. For economists and those concerned with social policy, health may be a marker, a way of keeping score of how well the society is doing in delivering well-being. In public health, our concern is not with economic performance, of which mortality may be an indicator, but with health status of which economic and social performance may be determinants. That is to say, I am concerned with how to lower mortality rates and improve health, and am therefore interested in the major influences that shape it. In this context, I am concerned with economic performance only as a means to an end.

There is no conflict between the social policy and public health perspective and, for both of these purposes, health as an indicator and the determinants of health—social inequalities in health are important. In the public health case, these inequalities are a manifestation of the social influences on health. I must add that they do not represent the whole extent, and may overstate it as well. In theory, at least some of the social inequalities in health may not be caused by the effect of social forces on health. Two ways this could come about are selection (health determining social position, of which more below) or a common antecedent determining both health and social position, for example, genetic endowment. Nature/nurture is perhaps the oldest debate in biology. There is, however, no evidence to support a common genetic basis for social position and health risks and a great deal of evidence to suggest that this will not do as an explanation.

Some of the causes of social inequalities may of course lead to worse health across the social spectrum. Smoking, or low level of perceived control over work environments or life circumstance, may account for worse health of lower socio-economic groups but may account for worse health of smokers or

I would particularly like to thank Jim Smith who made helpful comments on the above manuscript. The Whitehall II study has been supported by grants from the Medical Research Council, British Heart Foundation, Health and Safety Executive, Department of Health, US National Heart Lung and Blood Institute (RO1-HL36310), US National Institutes on Aging (RO1-HS06516), and the John D. and Catherine T. MacArthur Foundation Research Networks on Successful Midlife Development and Socio-economic Status and Health. MM is supported by an MRC Research Professorship.

people with low control, wherever they are in the social spectrum. In other words, social inequalities in health are a fertile ground for discovering and testing hypotheses related to health of the whole population, as well as in themselves being socially and morally important. I shall endeavour to make the case, however, that we should not equate differences in health among individuals in society and inequalities between social groups.

In the other case, health as a guide to how the society is doing, there is a case to be made that wider inequalities in health represent wider inequalities in society—although the evidence on this is still problematic.

There is another way of looking at inequalities in health, and that is between societies. I shall say a little on the proposition that the causes of inequalities in health among societies may be similar to the differences among social groups within society, although not necessarily of the causes of variation among individuals.

This concern with 'outcomes', life and death, diseases, and health states, is in the British tradition of pragmatism and empiricism and what my sociological colleagues love to criticise as atheoretical ('positivist' seems to have gone out of style as a criticism—perhaps through the exhaustion of constant repetition rather than reform of our habits). In preparation for this meeting, I read for the first time, Amartya Sen's writing on Inequality (1992, 1997, 1998). I felt like the man who had discovered he had been talking prose. I was intrigued to discover that some of the conclusions towards which my colleagues and I had been struggling on the basis of our evidence, were elegantly laid out there—in particular the focus on capability rather than on primary resources alone. For example, as discussed later, a 'fair' distribution of educational resources such as equal expenditure per capita may benefit children from economically advantaged backgrounds more than it does less advantaged children. Because of deprived backgrounds these children have less capacity to benefit—less capability. To reduce inequality in educational outcome we should focus on capacity to benefit. This resonates with our concern to go beyond material circumstances of life to psychosocial factors and how they may be important determinants of health.

3.1. A CONCERN WITH OUTCOMES: THE SOCIAL GRADIENT

Figure 3.1 illustrates the problem I am seeking to understand, the policy implications of which I am seeking to explore. It comes from the twenty-five-year follow-up of British civil servants in the original Whitehall study, and shows the social gradient in all cause mortality (Marmot and Shipley 1996). These men were all in stable employment, in white collar occupations, in and around London, and none was in poverty in any absolute sense of that word, yet there is a gradient in mortality. Each grade in the civil service has higher mortality rates than the grade above it in the hierarchy. This figure shows the data for

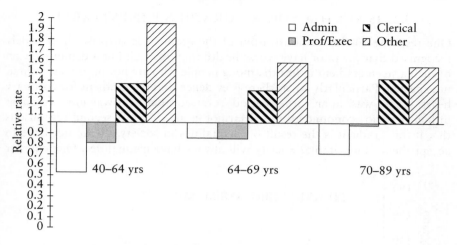

Figure 3.1. *All cause mortality by grade of employment Whitehall, men 25-year follow-up*

Source: Marmot and Shipley (1996).

all cause mortality, but there are similar gradients for all the major causes of death (Marmot et al. 1984; Von Rossum et al. 2000).

The observation that most major causes of death follow the social gradient is a challenge to understand. In comparing the slope of the social gradient for different causes of death, we could focus on similarities or on the differences. The gradient is steeper for lung cancer and respiratory disease which is in large part due to smoking. It is shallower for certain cancers not related to smoking (Davey Smith and Shipley 1991), and for breast cancer in women the gradient is reversed, that is, there is higher breast cancer mortality for high-status women. More striking than these exceptions, however, is that the direction of the social gradient does bring advantage to higher status people for most of the major causes of death. A major question of causation, therefore, relates to why position in the social hierarchy should be so intimately related to risk of a range of diseases which medical science suggests have different causes.

Is there one factor, that follows a social gradient, that renders people more likely to succumb to illness; the nature of the illness being caused by specific genetic or environmental factors? Or is being in lower social position linked to higher exposure to environmental pollution, tobacco, worse diet, and psychological stress which in turn are related to respiratory illness, lung cancer, heart disease, and mental illness and suicide? Below, I sketch out a causal model that incorporates elements of both of these types of explanation.

This social gradient in mortality is similar to that observed for morbidity. Our second study of civil servants, the Whitehall II study showed gradients in self-reported health, in diagnoses of a variety of diseases, and in sickness absence rates (Marmot et al. 1991; North et al. 1993).

3.2. IS SUCH A SOCIAL GRADIENT INEVITABLE?

One response to this demonstration of the gradient is surprise. It is widely recognised that the poor have worse health than the rich but a demonstration of such a steep gradient in health among people who are not poor was, at first, unexpected. Particularly so, as there is evidence that the gradient for coronary heart disease was, in an earlier period, reversed, that is, it was more frequent in higher socio-economic groups (Marmot et al. 1978). A second response is that if this gradient is the result of inequalities in society, do we not have to accept them as inevitable? Society will always have inequalities. One counter

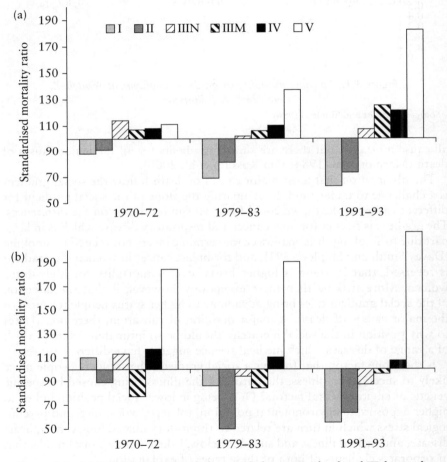

Figure 3.2. *(a) IHD and (b) Suicide by social class in England and Wales, males 1970–93*

Source: Drever et al. (1996).

Notes: 1970–72 does not include undetermined.

to this would be with recourse to the Sen type argument that it depends in which space you wish to measure inequalities (Sen 1992). If it were possible to break the link between income inequality and health inequality, one could achieve greater equality in the health space while still accepting inequality in the income space. This anticipates an understanding of the causes. If we understand the social causes of these inequalities in health, and could do something about them, this could inform debate as to whether we find the policies necessary to reduce inequalities in health acceptable for other reasons.

My starting position is that this gradient in ill health is a waste of human capital and is not inevitable. It varies over time within a society and the slope of the gradient varies between societies. Figure 3.2 shows national data for England and Wales over the time period 1970–93. Both for ischaemic heart disease and suicide the social gradient became considerably steeper over the last twenty years (Drever et al. 1996). There have been similar findings from the United States (Pappas et al. 1993). The magnitude of the gradient varies among countries as shown by the careful analyses of Kunst and Mackenbach (Mackenbach and Kunst 1992; Kunst 1997). If it can vary, presumably as the unintended consequence of government policies and other trends, it should be possible to vary it as an intended consequence. To do that, ideally, entails some understanding of causes.

3.3. IS THE GRADIENT IMPORTANT—INEQUALITY BETWEEN SOCIAL GROUPS OR AMONG INDIVIDUALS?

It was put to me by an economist, Jim Smith of RAND, that the social gradient in health was enormously important in being productive of scientific hypotheses, but we should be wary of promising too much in policy terms because it made little difference to overall inequalities in health. The first issue to be put aside is linguistic confusion: what I label individual differences he calls inequalities. In Britain, we had the experience in the early 1990s where social inequalities in health were officially labelled variations—the word inequality was not used in Department of Health-speak. What Jim Smith was discussing seemed to be going the other way: labelling individual variations in health states as inequalities. No doubt I am guilty of linguistic imprecision, but I use the term social inequality to apply to differences between social groups.[1]

The difference between us was not purely linguistic. Smith's argument is that the social gradient makes a marginal contribution to overall variation in mortality. In other words if one partialled out the variance into that due to variation between social groups and that due to variation among individuals, one would discover that the social variation made a marginal contribution. It is

---

[1] Inequality is also used to apply to gender, usually with the intention of drawing attention to the disadvantage of women. The problem with this usage is that in the developed world, for mortality, the advantage is with women.

Table 3.1. *Effects of grade of employment and smoking on 25 year mortality from coronary heart disease and lung cancer in the first Whitehall Study*

	Coronary heart disease	Lung cancer
No. of deaths	2,480	638
% of deviance explained by:		
age and employment grade	2.2%	3.7%
age, smoking and others	3.9%	7.4%
Rate ratio:		
lowest grade vs highest grade	1.7	4.1

swamped by individual variability. In so far as this is the appropriate way to analyse the data, he is correct. This is true not only for the contribution of social variation, but also for variation contributed by any single cause that we know about. I use the word cause in the public health usage of a potentially reversible influence that would change the incidence of disease. This is illustrated in Table 3.1 with mortality data from the twenty-five-year follow-up of the first Whitehall study. This shows that grade of employment, together with age, accounts for at most 2.2 per cent of the deviance (used instead of variance because mortality is a dichotomous variable here) in coronary heart disease mortality, despite the fact that the lowest grade has a 70 per cent increased risk compared to the highest.

Is this the right way to look at these data? I think not. Take lung cancer: smoking, age, respiratory function, and other risk factors accounted for 'only' 7.4 per cent of the deviance in lung cancer mortality. Following the individual variance approach, age and smoking make a trivial contribution to explaining variability in lung cancer mortality rates. This then becomes a variant of the argument that most smokers do not get lung cancer. Something must determine which individual smokers do and which do not get lung cancer. There is another way to look at this. There were 638 deaths from lung cancer in the twenty-five-year follow up from this first Whitehall cohort; fewer than 5 per cent of them occurred among non-smokers. If smoking had not occurred, 95 per cent of the lung cancer deaths would not have occurred in the same time period. In other words, for practical purposes, smoking is *the* cause of lung cancer. One could have a whole research endeavour to identify genetic or other susceptibility to smoking, to help understand which smokers do and which do not get lung cancer, but no matter how marginal its contribution to the total variance in lung cancer mortality, elimination of smoking would have a huge not a marginal public health impact.

Can we apply the same approach to social inequalities in health? Table 3.2 shows that life expectancy at age forty-five for this population differed by 4.4 years between the bottom two and the top two of the four employment grades in the first Whitehall cohort. Is this a lot? The second half of Table 3.2 shows that if the major cause of death in the whole population of civil servants,

Table 3.2. *Employment grade and coronary heart disease effects on life expectancy—25 year mortality follow up of the first Whitehall study*

	Expectancy of life at age 45 (yrs)
Employment grade:	
Administrative/Professional/Executive	34.70
Clerical/Other	30.32
difference in life expectancy	4.38
Coronary heart disease:	
Subjects dying from non-CHD causes	37.38
Subjects dying from all-causes	33.38
difference in life expectancy	4.00

coronary heart disease, were reduced to zero, it would add 4.0 years to life expectancy. Therefore, were it possible to identify the causes of social inequalities in health, to change them, and if changing them reversed their effect on mortality, we could, potentially, deliver a bigger benefit to the less advantaged group of the population than reducing their coronary rates to zero. It will, of course, be argued that we will never flatten the social gradient in mortality. But then, we will have difficulty in reducing the CHD rates to zero. In both cases it is a social and public health problem worth grappling with.

Social inequalities are important when looked at this way but why do we do so poorly in explaining individual differences in mortality? It is unlikely to be because we have left out one big risk factor. There are few associations with chronic disease that are stronger or more practically useful than smoking with lung cancer. We must assume that most associations will be a good deal weaker than that. Part of the unexplained variation will be measurement error, but part, in our ignorance, we may attribute to random fluctuation. To illustrate with the example of atheroma which is the underlying process that leads to coronary heart disease: if exposed for long enough to a high fat diet, smoking and other risk factors for coronary disease, a high proportion of the population will develop atheromatous plaques in the coronary arteries. Such build-up in the arteries may be 'silent', that is, accompanied by no symptoms. We think that a myocardial infarction, a catastrophic event, is precipitated by plaque rupture. The probability of having a plaque is altered by the presence or level of coronary risk factors. The mechanism of plaque rupture is moderately well understood but the predictors of its timing are not. We do not have the means to predict which asymptomatic individual will have a ruptured plaque tomorrow, which next week, and which in five or ten years' time. In our present state of ignorance we may say that it is a stochastic process. An individual with a high plasma cholesterol will have a greater probability of having a plaque than one with a low cholesterol. We can improve our predictive power by adding in other risk factors, but there will still be a great deal of individual variation unexplained.

Geoffrey Rose pointed out that the causes of individual differences in illness rates may be different from the causes of the population rate of disease (Rose 1992). I have argued that this has important implications for social causes (Marmot 1998). It may be the wrong level of analysis to search for individual differences in risk factors, if the aim is to reduce the social gradient in mortality. This is even more the case when we examine geographic differences. In the United States, the county with the longest life expectancy is in Utah (Cache, Rich), and life expectancy at birth is, for men, 77.5 years (Murray et al. 1998). The nation's capital, District of Columbia, is the county with the second worst life expectancy for men at 62.2 years. We could, of course, treat the citizens of the United States as one large group of individuals and take county as a variable and show that it makes a trivial contribution to 'explaining' individual differences in life expectancy. Given how little we know of what does explain individual differences, and given the magnitude of the geographic differences perhaps a scientific strategy that would, potentially, have a bigger public health payoff is to ask why there should be a fifteen-year gap in life expectancy between the best and the worst and what the appropriate policy response should be.

In the nature/nurture debate let us make a simplifying assumption. Suppose that all the individual level variance in susceptibility were genetic and all the geographic and socio-economic differences were environmental. Then following the partition of variance argument above, the majority of the variance would be genetic. The gains to public health from such knowledge, however, might well be trivial. On the other hand if we could add 4.4 years to life expectancy by bringing the level of health of the lower half of the civil service hierarchy up to that of the better-off half, the gain to public health would be substantial. This is, of course, a likely overstatement of the contribution of genetic variability as the evidence that the individual level variance is genetic, by and large, does not exist. Similarly, the evidence that the group level difference is not genetic is circumstantial, but the evidence that there are important social environmental causes is strong. Before considering these, we should consider an alternate to a social environmental explanation.

3.4. SOCIAL CAUSATION OR HEALTH SELECTION (ENDOGENEITY)?

There is evidence that the relation between health and socio-economic status at the individual level may be two way: health may determine socio-economic position as well as social circumstances affecting health (Smith 1999). Where the link is between individual social status and health outcome, this possibility must be considered. Health could be a major determinant of life chances. This has been termed health selection, and is I understand, what is labelled in economics as endogeneity. The implication being that health 'selects' people into different social strata.

Perhaps one way of judging the social causation hypothesis is to consider the merits of the alternate, health selection hypothesis. For the purpose of argument let us consider what the extreme case would look like, that is, if *all* the observed relations between social conditions and health (Marmot and Wilkinson 1999) were the result of health selection. This would lead to the argument that ill health led to: lower position in the social hierarchy, social exclusion, having a job that offered less opportunities for control and imbalance between efforts and rewards, increased risk of unemployment and job insecurity, living in a deprived neighbourhood, having less participation in social networks, eating worse food, indulging in addictive behaviour, and breathing in polluted air as well as being sedentary.

These have varying degrees of plausibility. Plausibility, however, is no guarantee that selection is actually operating. Apart from judging the relative plausibility of the causation and selection arguments, there have been a number of other research strategies, of which three are worth highlighting. The first deals with the question head on. Longitudinal studies allow a judgement to be made as to which came first, health or social circumstances. This has been examined in considerable depth by a number of studies (Goldblatt 1990). Perhaps the clearest answers come from the birth cohort studies in the United Kingdom, the 1946 and 1958 birth cohorts (Wadsworth 1986; Power et al. 1991). In the 1946 birth cohort, children who showed evidence of illness were less likely to be upwardly mobile than healthy children and more likely to be downwardly mobile (Wadsworth 1986). The effect was small however and could not account for the relation between social position and ill health in adulthood (Blane et al. 1993).

Second, we have changing social class differences over time (Marmot and McDowall 1986; Drever et al. 1996). The increase in social class differences in mortality rates over time in England & Wales cannot easily be explained by selection. It has been argued that as social class V (unskilled manual) shrinks in size, those in better health are upwardly mobile, hence those left behind have higher mortality rates. Perhaps. If this were the explanation, however, one might have expected the mortality of the higher classes to go up as their ranks are swollen with the less healthy recruits from lower down. This is not the case. At the same time as mortality rates of social class V have failed to decline, there has been improvement in that of the higher social classes.

The third approach to dealing with selection is to examine the effect of social circumstances that could not have plausibly been affected by health status of individuals. For example, it is plausible that sick individuals may be more likely to lose their jobs and remain unemployed than healthy people. Where unemployment is imposed from the outside, as in large-scale factory closures, individual illness is unlikely to be a determinant of unemployment status (Bartley and Owen 1996). Similarly, geographic and population differences in disease rates could not all be attributed to selective migration of healthy people to 'good' areas or of unhealthy people to 'bad' areas. More plausibly these area differences in disease rates relate to characteristics of the social environment (Wilkinson 1996). The causal direction, therefore, is likely to be from social environment to illness, not the other way.

3.5. COUNTRY DIFFERENCES IN HEALTH: SOCIAL CAUSES?

The fact that rich countries in general have better mortality records than poor countries bears on both the previous questions. Country level differences cannot be explained by health selection (or endogeneity). Nor is it particularly relevant to policy to ponder why there is individual level variation in infant mortality if the overall country level is, for example, 50/1000 live births compared to perhaps 6 or 7/1000 in Europe. The clear policy implication is to relieve poverty in order to lessen the diseases of poverty. This is not the whole story. There has been much interest in routes to low mortality in poor countries that are plausibly related to aspects of society other than gross national product (GNP) per capita (Caldwell 1986; United Nations Development Programme 1994). Education, particularly of women, seems to be an important predictor of having a better mortality record than predicted by GNP. This in turn may be marker of social capital.

The obverse may be happening in Europe (Bobak and Marmot 1996) as Figure 3.3 illustrates. It shows life expectancy at age fifteen, thereby removing the effect of infant and child mortality. In 1970 the differences in life expectancy between the Nordic and European Union countries on the one hand and the communist countries of Central and Eastern Europe on the other, was relatively small. The Soviet Union lagged behind the other countries and the difference in life expectancy for men at age fifteen was four years compared with the European Union. Over the next twenty-five years, life expectancy improved steadily in the Nordic and EU countries and stagnated or declined in the countries of Central and Eastern Europe. By 1994 the gap in life expectancy at age fifteen between Russia and the European Union was about ten years—a dramatic widening of inequalities across Europe in a relatively short time. The causes of death that contribute most to the East–West difference in mortality are cardiovascular disease and external causes of death (Bobak and Marmot 1996). Interestingly, these particular causes make a major contribution to inequalities in mortality within the United Kingdom and the United States. This has led us to speculate that the causes of inequalities in health within countries may be similar to the causes of international differences (Bobak and Marmot 1996).

The worsening mortality pattern has not affected all groups equally within Central and Eastern European countries. In general, there has been a widening social gradient within those countries (Marmot and Bobak 2000).

The fact that, in addition to poverty, other more general social factors may also be operating is illustrated by the comparison of three countries that all had an equivalent GNP in the early 1990s of around $2,000 (Table 3.3). The

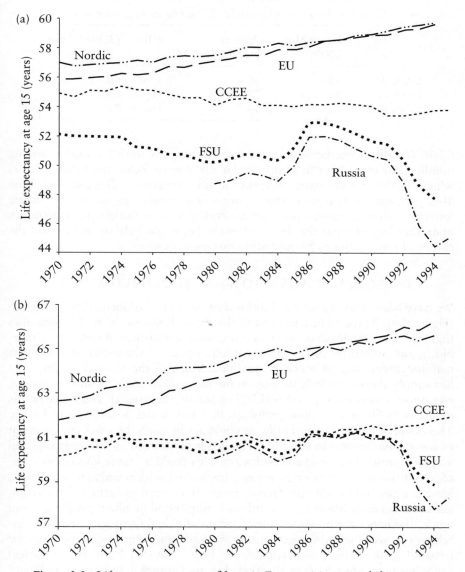

Figure 3.3. *Life expectancy at age fifteen in Europe, (a) men and (b) women*

high infant mortality in South Africa is related to poverty as is the high probability of death between the ages of fifteen and sixty, given that ischaemic heart disease mortality is low. The relatively favourable infant mortality in Hungary and Costa Rica is, in a sense, better than one would have predicted from their

Table 3.3. *Structure of mortality in middle income countries*

	Infant Mort/ 1000	Prob of Death 15–60 M	IHD	LE Birth Males
South Africa	53	30.8	Low	60
Hungary	15	27.7	High	65
Costa Rica	14	14.5	Low	74

GNP. The difference between these two countries is in the mortality among middle-aged men, high in Hungary, largely due to ischaemic heart disease, which results in a dramatic difference in life expectancy. There is something about society in Hungary, that cannot be summed up under the rubric 'poverty', that relates to the high mortality among middle-aged men. An understanding of what this factor(s) might be, might help us understand the causes of inequalities in health within our own societies.

3.6. SOCIAL CAUSATION—A SIMPLIFIED MODEL

We have been working with a simplified causal model of inequalities in health (Figure 3.4). At the right-hand end of this figure it shows the health outcomes that have been the focus of much of our research: measures of well-being, morbidity, and mortality; and at the upper left, aspects of the social structure that manifest themselves as social inequalities. Much of the research in this area has simply shown the link between some measure of social position, income, education or occupation, and health. The aim of our research and hence of this model is to fill in the causal pathways that link social position to ill health. This could operate from early life; or could act through the work environment or social environment in adult life. The boxes in between are an oversimplified way of representing the causal pathways. This could be made impossibly complex, but this simple version provides a framework within which to study how, for example, individual risk factors might have been influenced by circumstances from early life or the conditions in adulthood in which people live and work, and hence the potential role of these individual factors in mediating the relation between social factors and disease outcome. Our research endeavour is to fill in the boxes, in particular to show how social and psychological processes may affect biology to cause disease. Culture may have an influence on health separate from narrowly defined socio-economic status. These social and cultural influences act as a genetic substrate.

3.6.1. *Medical care?*

This is not the place to discuss the role of medical care in producing these social inequalities. In the Whitehall II study, we showed no evidence of

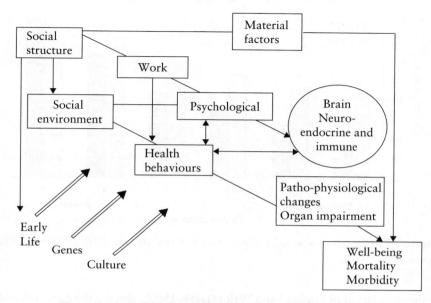

Figure 3.4. *Model of pathways of social influences on health*

under-treatment for cardiovascular disease according to socio-economic status and clear differences in CHD incidence (Marmot et al. 1997). This, and a variety of other evidence lead us to conclude that the social gradient in disease in Britain is not the result of unequal access to health care.

3.6.2. *Individual lifestyle?*

An approach to explanation that emphasises individual lifestyle is inadequate. In the first Whitehall study, a combination of the major coronary risk factors accounted for approximately a quarter of the social gradient in mortality (Marmot et al. 1984). These included smoking, lack of physical activity, obesity, high plasma cholesterol level, and high blood pressure. This can be illustrated with smoking. Smoking rates show a social gradient in the Whitehall II study (Marmot et al. 1991), as in many countries, and differences in smoking make an important contribution to explaining the social gradient; but the social differences in CHD mortality rates in Whitehall were as big in nonsmokers as in smokers (Marmot et al. 1984). This means that we have to have two approaches, first to ask why there is a social gradient in smoking—examine the causes of the causes; and second to ask what else may account for the social gradient in disease other than smoking or other behaviours usually thought of as lifestyle.

Figure 3.5 shows the relation between deprivation and smoking in 1973 and 1996 in data from the General Household Survey (GHS)—representative samples

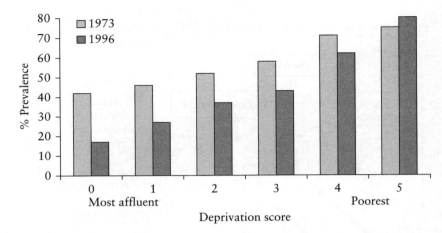

Figure 3.5. *Cigarette smoking by deprivation in Great Britain: GHS 1973 and 1996*
Source: Jarvis (1997).

of the population of England and Wales (Jarvis 1997). Among the most affluent, smoking rates went from higher than 40 per cent to less than 20 per cent over the twenty-three-year period represented here. Among the poorest, prevalence remained at over 70 per cent. How does this contribute to our understanding of the social causes of inequalities in health? One response to this might be that smoking is a freely chosen behaviour, if poorer people choose to kill themselves in this way, the only concern of society is to ensure that they do it in full knowledge of the consequences, that is, guarantee that the information is available. In this way individual freedom is preserved. Such an individualistic approach is ignoring the fact that there are persistent social gradients. These are not panel surveys. The individual people in successive surveys are not the same. If the individuals change but the social gradient persists, surely we have to look beyond particular individuals for the causes of smoking: both uptake and cessation (Jarvis and Wardle 1999).

3.7. ISSUES IN SOCIAL CAUSATION OF INEQUALITIES IN HEALTH

3.7.1. *Poverty or inequality?*

The relation between poverty and poor health is most clearly seen in developing countries. The high infant and middle-age mortality in South Africa, shown in Table 3.3, is an example. The situation in Central and Eastern Europe with rising rates of coronary heart disease in the period up to 1989, cannot easily be attributed to poverty, as seen by the relatively low infant mortality rates. Nor can the Whitehall gradient. There are undoubted pockets of poverty in rich countries that are associated with worse health. The life expectancy of 62.2 years for men in the District of Columbia, cited above, may well be an example of this. But clerical officers in the British Civil Service are not deprived in the same sense and are in stable, albeit relatively low paid jobs. And executive officers are better off than them but still have worse health than the administrators above them in the hierarchy. The evidence from Whitehall suggests that inequality is important: place in the hierarchy appears to predict risk of death and disease.

This gives rise to the notion of relative deprivation. Anticipating the comments below, material deprivation is related to illness. Poverty may also be a relative concept and relate to where someone is in relation to society's norms.

This conclusion is *related to, but slightly different* from Wilkinson's (Wilkinson 1996). He observed that for the rich countries, above a GNP per capita of around $5,000, there is little relation between average GNP and life expectancy. There is a strong relation with income inequality. This relation between income inequality and mortality has also been shown for states of the United States (Kaplan et al. 1996; Kennedy et al. 1996). Wilkinson's conclusion is that income inequality is a reflection of the social environment. Areas with greater income inequality are likely to have more fragmented social environments. Therefore inequality may be bad not only for those individuals who are relatively deprived but it may be a feature that harms the whole of society.

3.7.2. *Psychosocial or Material Causes of Inequalities*[2]

In Britain, there has been lively debate as to how much of the causes of inequalities in health are material or psychosocial. There is a good case to be made that material deprivation in one way or another accounts for the link between poverty and ill health. Even here, material deprivation may have an important psychosocial component. The ways of doing without in Britain, at least, have changed (Alan Marsh, personal communication). Whereas in the past, material deprivation meant inadequate housing, undernutrition, inadequate clothing, risky work places, now the definition of what it means to be on the 'bread line' has broadened. It also means inability to entertain children's friends, buy children new clothes, go on holiday, pursue a hobby or leisure activity. In other words material deprivation in a modern context may mean inability to participate fully in society and to control one's life.

Thus, there is a link with the concept of relative deprivation that may underlie the social gradient. The mechanisms linking social position to health, across the whole social gradient, are likely to involve psychosocial factors. Among the psychosocial factors with the strongest evidence to support their role in generating inequalities in health are: social supports/social integration,

---

[2] This section of the chapter draws on my lecture to the Kansas Conference on 'Health and its Determinants', Kansas Health Institute, 20–1 April, 1998.

the psychosocial work environment, control/mastery, and hostility. The influence of early life will be touched on below.

Social supports/integration

Lisa Berkman has reviewed the evidence for the strong and consistent protective effect of participation in social networks and of social supports (Berkman 1985). Evidence from the Whitehall II study shows that the lower the position in the hierarchy, the less participation in social networks outside the family, and the more negative the degree of social support (Stansfeld and Marmot 1992).

Data from Central and Eastern European countries show that the adverse trend in mortality has affected particularly men who were single, widowed or divorced (Hajdu et al. 1995; Watson 1995). The adverse effect was not seen in women. One possible explanation for this is that marriage provided the main source of support for men in societies where other forms of social participation were weak (Rose 1995). Women on the other hand were more likely to participate in informal social networks, at least in part, because barter and other forms of informal exchange were mechanisms that allowed families to function.

Psychosocial work environment

The two dominant models in the field of the psychosocial work environment are the demand/control model (Karasek and Theorell 1990) and that of effort reward imbalance (Siegrist 1996). The demand/control posits, with evidence to support it, that it is not too much work pressure alone that causes stress-related illness, but too much psychological demand in the face of low control over circumstances at work. Control, in turn, is measured by degree of authority over decisions and appropriate use of skills.

In the Whitehall II study, along with a number of other studies (Hemingway and Marmot 1999) the demand dimension did not predict coronary heart disease. Low control in the workplace was an important predictor of CHD incidence rates (Bosma et al. 1997). Figure 3.6, from the Whitehall II study shows the social gradient in the occurrence of incident CHD events (Marmot et al. 1997) and the contribution of three sets of factors, taken one at a time to explaining this social gradient. Short height, as a measure of early life effects is a predictor of coronary heart disease incidence and makes a small contribution to explaining the social gradient. As in Whitehall I, the standard coronary risk factors, serum cholesterol, blood pressure, smoking, body mass index, physical activity accounted for between a quarter and a third of the social gradient. More than half the gradient appeared to be accounted for by low control in the workplace. Figure 3.7 shows that, in multivariate analysis, the combination of height, coronary risk factors, and low control in the workplace appear to provide a complete explanation for the social gradient in occurrence of CHD.

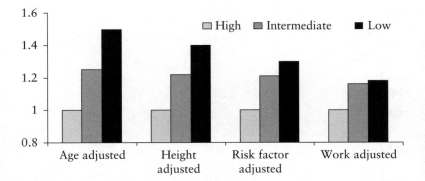

Figure 3.6. *Odds ratio for new CHD in Whitehall II by employment grade—men*
Source: Marmot et al. (1997).

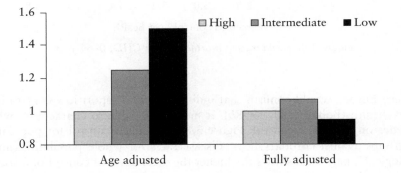

Figure 3.7. *Odds ratio for new CHD in Whitehall II by employment grade—men.*
Fully adjusted: adjusted for height, coronary risk factors, low control at work
Source: Marmot et al. (1997).

Using the same methods, but in a very different population in the Czech Republic, we had remarkably similar findings. A combination of coronary risk factors and low control in the workplace provided an explanation for the association between low education and risk of myocardial infarction (Bobak et al. 1998*a*).

In discussing these findings we noted that there are, of course, social gradients in the occurrence of coronary heart disease among people who are not working. This does not negate the importance of low control. It does not derive only from the workplace. Low control may be a feature of the social conditions under which people live, as well as work.

Control/mastery

There is a large literature on this subject (Skinner 1996). It tends to view low control as a characteristic of individuals. Indeed, our work from Central and

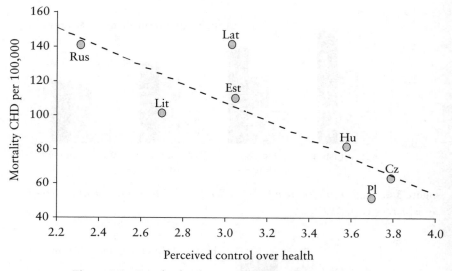

Figure 3.8. *Standardised mortality from CHD, 0–64 years*

Eastern Europe would confirm that individuals who report low control have worse health (Bobak et al. 1998*b*). It may be possible to characterise whole societies on degree of control. Figure 3.8 plots mean control for population subgroups against coronary heart disease rates for whole populations in an 'ecological' analysis. It shows the higher the mean level of control of a society the lower the coronary heart disease rates.

Hostility

Redford Williams has produced similar findings for hostility (Williams et al. 1980). He and others have shown that hostile people have higher risk of coronary heart disease than those that are not hostile. If hostility is viewed as a stable trait of individuals, there is no particular reason why it should be related to the environment. Williams did a Gallup survey of ten American cities and showed that they differed in mean hostility levels. He showed further that there was a direct correlation between mean hostility of a city and that city's mortality from coronary heart disease (Williams 1991).

3.8. EARLY LIFE OR CURRENT CIRCUMSTANCES?

There is ample evidence that factors in the current environment of adults affects their disease rates. Change these and disease rates change. Evidence on giving up smoking or lowering cholesterol or blood pressure show that coronary heart disease rates can change within five years. The changing social class distribution of disease does not show a birth cohort pattern, suggesting that is likely to be the result of change in adult circumstances.

Barker's group in the United Kingdom have provided strong evidence for the programming hypothesis (Barker 1990). The *in utero* environment programmes organ systems of the developing foetus that change the individuals likelihood of developing chronic disease later in life. There is good evidence that early life experiences, beyond birth, affect mental illness later in life (Fonagy 1996; Maughan and McCarthy 1997). It seems likely that there will be effects on physical illness as well. This is confirmed by the British Birth Cohorts Studies: there are substantial effects of early life that continue to influence disease risk later in life (Wadsworth 1991, 1997; Power et al. 1991). Working with data from the 1958 Birth Cohort, Power shows that it is accumulation of advantage and disadvantage throughout the lifecourse that accounts for inequalities in health in adulthood (Power et al. 1998). This has led to an interest in the life course approach to chronic disease (Kuh and Ben-Shlomo 1997).

One particular feature of early life that has been the focus of much attention is education. Education, as a marker of socio-economic status has been shown in a large variety of studies to be related to morbidity and mortality. One feature of these results is that, to some extent, it deals with the health selection argument, in that educational status is determined long before the major killing diseases of middle and later life have started to become manifest. This does not necessarily mean that education per se is the determinant of socio-economic differences in health outcomes. There is a strong link between social deprivation and outcome of education, measured as exam results (Blane et al. 1996). Education may therefore be a marker of relative degree of deprivation. There is some evidence that equal expenditure on education will benefit more children from advantaged backgrounds (Mortimore and Whitty 1997), that is, it could lead to greater inequality in the outcome of educational achievement. One conclusion from the link between social deprivation and educational outcome has been to recommend that attention be paid to children's ability to benefit from school, in particular pre-school education.

3.9. WHERE YOU ARE OR WHO YOU ARE?

Examples of marked geographic differences in the occurrence of disease were given above. A question that has exercised researchers is whether this is due to composition of the areas, that is, the characteristics of individuals who live there, or whether context, social characteristics of the area itself, exerts an influence on health over and above the characteristics of the individuals who live there. Where the focus is pollution of the air or water, there would be no doubt that there are area effects. Can the social environment be thought of in the same way? For example, crime rates tend to be high in deprived areas. Can worse health in those areas be ascribed to this area effect, or is it because there are more deprived individuals in those areas? The evidence adduced by Wilkinson (1997); Kawachi (Kawachi et al. 1997); Haan and Kaplan (Haan et al. 1987); and Macintyre (Macintyre et al. 1993) suggest that there is indeed an area effect that applies to the social as well as the physical environment.

The data cited above for hostility and low control suggest that these characteristics can be used not only to characterise individuals, but whole populations (Marmot 1998).

3.10. BIOLOGICAL PATHWAYS

It could be argued, that we did not need to know what the biological effects were of smoking to reach conclusions about its health effects. However, the criteria for assessing causation developed by Bradford-Hill and the US Surgeon General had much to do with the controversy around smoking and health. One of these criteria is biological plausibility. The argument was that without a biologically plausible mechanism, the causal nature of epidemiological association remains suspect.

When we reported our findings suggesting that low control in the workplace was an important contributor to the social gradient in coronary heart disease, we asked ourselves why pick on low control in the workplace? (Marmot et al. 1997) After all, a number of factors showed a social gradient, why incriminate this particular feature of the workplace? Part of our answer was that low control was related to levels of plasma fibrinogen (Brunner et al. 1996) and that plasma fibrinogen in turn is a predictor of coronary heart disease. We do not think that plasma fibrinogen is necessarily 'the answer' to the question of biological mechanisms. Plasma fibrinogen is an acute phase protein and is correlated with the metabolic syndrome of insulin resistance (Brunner et al. 1997). This is an active area of research and it is important for those of us concerned with social and psychological causes of illness not to be ignorant of modern biology (Brunner and Marmot 1999).

Insights as to biological pathways linking social status to cardiovascular risk come from animal work. Low status non-human primates have higher rates of lipid and endocrine disturbance (Sapolsky and Mott 1987), psychological disturbance (Suomi 1991), and atherosclerosis (Shively and Clarkson 1994; Shively et al. 1996). Reviews of this work on non-human primates show the importance of the hypothalamic pituitary and sympatho-adrenal medullary axis.

3.11. IMPLICATIONS FOR POLICY

At this workshop on health equity, there has been much discussion about theories of justice and the extent to which distributive justice should be the central criterion. To caricature a complex discussion: which is more important, a fair process or a fair outcome? Sen has argued that we need to recognise that there may be inequality in a variety of different spaces (Sen 1992). My starting point is unashamedly with outcomes, mortality, and morbidity. The effort is to trace the causal chain back into society to understand how these social inequalities in health and disease are generated. The implications for policy might lead us into different spaces. My aim, however, would be that those libertarians who consider equality of rights to be paramount should at least recognise that these might have consequences in terms of generating inequalities in health. Similarly, utilitarians who wish to maximise utility in society (might that include health?) regardless of its distribution should acknowledge that they may not be addressing social inequalities in health. The general point is that particular economic and social policies are likely to have health implications if we can but understand the causal links.

3.12. POSTSCRIPT

This chapter was prepared for a conference in 1998. In the years between this conference and the publication of this book much has happened in Britain on inequalities in health. The Government set up an inquiry into inequalities in health (chaired by former Chief Medical Officer, Sir Donald Acheson) of which I was a member. It made thirty-nine recommendations to Government as to what it could do to reduce inequalities in health. After a latent period, Her Majesty's Treasury chaired a Cross Cutting Spending Review on Health Inequalities. This brought together officials from Government departments and agencies with a view to coordinating their activities in order to reduce health inequalities. There are now a number of processes in place to try and take some action. The important point is that the action the Government is seeking to take is consistent with its general view about inequalities in society. It has clearly not gone as far as some would like in reducing these inequalities; while at the same time having taken steps to retard the growth of inequalities that occurred over the previous two decades. We now wait with active interest to see if the various policies that have been put in place produce the desired effects.

References

Barker, D. J. (1990). 'The Fetal and Infant Origins of Adult Disease', *British Medical Journal*, 301: 1111.

Bartley, M. and C. Owen (1996). 'Relation between Socio-Economic Status, Employment, and Health during Economic Change, 1973–93', *British Medical Journal*, 313: 445–9.

Berkman, L. F. (1985). 'The Relationship of Social Networks and Social Support to Morbidity and Mortality', in S. Cohen and S. L. Syme (eds.), *Social Support and Health*. San Diego: Academic Press, Inc., pp. 241–6.

Blane, D., G. Davey Smith, and M. Bartley (1993). 'Social Selection: What Does it Contribute to Social Class Differences in Health?' *Sociology of Health and Illness*, 15: 1–15.

Blane, D., J. N. Morris, and I. R. White (1996). 'Education, Social Circumstances and Mortality', in D. Blane, E. Brunner, and R. Wilkinson (eds.), *Health and Social Organisation: Towards a Health Policy for the 21st Century.* London: Routledge, pp. 171–87.

Bobak, M. and M. Marmot (1996). 'East-West Mortality Divide and its Potential Explanations: Proposed Research Agenda', *British Medical Journal*, 312: 421–5.

——, C. Hertzman, Z. Skodova, and M. Marmot (1998*a*). 'Association Between Psychosocial Factors at Work and Non-Fatal Myocardial Infarction in a Population Based Case-Control Study in Czech Men', *Epidemiology*, 9: 43–7.

——, H. Pikhart, C. Hertzman, R. Rose, and M. Marmot (1998*b*). 'Socio-Economic Factors, Perceived Control and Self-Reported Health in Russia. A Cross-Sectional Survey', *Social Science and Medicine*, 47: 269–79.

Bosma, H., M. Marmot, H. Hemingway, A. Nicholson, E. Brunner, and S. Stansfeld (1997). 'Low Job Control and Risk of Coronary Heart Disease in the Whitehall II (Prospective Cohort) Study', *British Medical Journal*, 314: 558–65.

Brunner, E., G. Davey Smith, M. Marmot, R. Canner, M. Beksinska, and J. O'Brien (1996). 'Childhood Social Circumstances and Psychosocial and Behavioural Factors as Determinants of Plasma Fibrinogen', *Lancet*, 347: 1008–13.

——, M. Marmot. K. Nanchahal, M. Shipley, S. Stansfeld, M. Juneja, and K. G. M. M. Alberti (1997). 'Social Inequality in Coronary Risk: Central Obesity and the Metabolic Syndrome. Evidence from The Whitehall II Study', *Diabetologia*, 40: 1341–9.

——and M. Marmot (1999). 'Social Organization, Stress and Health', in M. Marmot and R. Wilkinson (eds.), *Social Determinants of Health*. Oxford: Oxford University Press, pp. 17–43.

Caldwell, J. C. (1986). 'Routes to Low Mortality in Poor Countries', *Population and Development Review*, 2: 171–220.

Davey Smith, G. and M. Shipley (1991). 'Confounding of Occupation and Smoking: its Magnitude and Consequences', *Social Science and Medicine*, 32: 1297–300.

Drever, F., M. Whitehead, and M. Roden (1996). 'Current Patterns and Trends in Male Mortality by Social Class (Based on Occupation)', *Population Trends*, 86: 15–20.

Fonagy, P. (1996). 'Patterns of Attachment, Interpersonal Relationships and Health', in D. Blane, E. Brunner and R. Wilkinson (eds.), *Social Organization and Health*. London: Routledge, pp. 125–51.

Goldblatt, P. (1990). *1971–1981 Longitudinal Study. Mortality and Social Organisation*. London: HMSO.

Haan, M., G. A. Kaplan, and T. Camacho (1987). 'Poverty and Health: Prospective Evidence from the Alameda County Study', *American Journal of Epidemiology*, 125: 989–98.

Hajdu, P., M. McKee, and F. Bojan (1995). 'Changes in Premature Mortality Differentials by Marital Status in Hungary and in England and Wales', *European Journal of Public Health*, 5: 259–64.

Hemingway, H. and M. Marmot (1999). 'Psychosocial Factors in the Aetiology and Prognosis of Coronary Heart Disease: A Systematic Review of Prospective Cohort Studies', *British Medical Journal*, 318: 1460–7.

Jarvis, M. J. (1997). 'Patterns and Prediction of Unaided Smoking Cessation in the General Population', in C. T. Bollinger and K. O. Fagerstrom (eds.), *The Tobacco Epidemic. Progress in Respiratory Research*, Vol. 28. Basel: Karger, pp. 151–64.

—— and J. Wardle (1999). 'Social Patterning of Individual Health Behaviour: the Case of Cigarette Smoking', in M. Marmot and R. Wilkinson (eds.), *The Social Determinants of Health*. Oxford: Oxford University Press, pp. 240–55.

Kaplan, G. A., E. R. Pamuk, J. W. Lynch, R. D. Cohen, and J. L. Balfour (1996). 'Inequality in Income and Mortality in the United States: Analysis of Mortality and Potential Pathways', *British Medical Journal*, 312: 999–1003.

Karasek, R. and T. Theorell (1990). *Healthy Work: Stress, Productivity, and the Reconstruction of Working Life*. New York: Basic Books.

Kawachi, I., B. P. Kennedy, K. Lochner, and D. Prothrow-Stith (1997). 'Social Capital, Income Inequality, and Mortality', *American Journal of Public Health*, 87: 1491–8.

Kennedy, B. P., I. Kawachi, and D. Prothrow-Stith (1996). 'Income Distribution and Mortality: Cross Sectional Ecological Study of the Robin Hood Index in the United States', *British Medical Journal*, 312: 1004–7.

Kuh, D. and Y. Ben-Shlomo (1997). *A Life Course Approach to Chronic Disease Epidemiology*. Oxford: Oxford University Press.

Kunst, A. (1997). *Cross-National Comparisons of Socioeconomic Differences in Mortality*. Rotterdam: Erasmus University Rotterdam.

MacIntyre, S., S. MacIver, and A. Sooman (1993). 'Area, Class and Health: Should We Be Focusing on Places or People?' *Journal of Social Policy*, 22: 213–34.

Mackenbach, J. P. and A. E. Kunst (1992). *An International Comparison of Socio-Economic Inequalities in Mortality*. Rotterdam: Erasmus University Rotterdam.

Marmot, M., A. M. Adelstein, N. Robinson, and G. Rose (1978). 'The Changing Social Class Distribution of Heart Disease', *British Medical Journal*, 2: 1109–12.

——, M. Shipley, and G. Rose (1984). 'Inequalities in Death—Specific Explanations of a General Pattern', *Lancet*, i: 1003–6.

—— and M. McDowall (1986). 'Mortality Decline and Widening Social Inequalities', *Lancet*, ii: 274–6.

——, G. Davey Smith, S. Stansfeld, C. Patel, F. North, J. Head, I. White, E. Brunner, and A. Feeney (1991). 'Health Inequalities Among British Civil Servants: the Whitehall II Study', *Lancet*, 337: 1387–93.

—— and M. Shipley (1996). 'Do Socio-Economic Differences in Mortality Persist after Retirement? 25 Year Follow up of Civil Servants from the First Whitehall Study', *British Medical Journal*, 313: 1177–80.

——, H. Bosma, H. Hemingway, E. Brunner, and S. Stansfeld (1997). 'Contribution of Job Control and Other Risk Factors to Social Variations in Coronary Heart Disease', *Lancet*, 350: 235–40.

——(1998). 'Improvement of Social Environment to Improve Health', *Lancet*, 351: 57–60.

—— and R. Wilkinson (eds.) (1999). *Social Determinants of Health*. New York: Oxford University Press.

—— and M. Bobak (2000). 'Psychosocial and Biological Mechanisms Behind the Recent Mortality Crisis in Central and Eastern Europe', in G. A. Cornia and R. Pannacia (eds.), *The Mortality Crisis in Transitional Economies*. Oxford: Oxford University Press.

Maughan, B. and G. McCarthy (1997). 'Childhood Adversities and Psychosocial Disorders', *British Medical Bulletin*, 53: 156–69.

Mortimore, P. and G. Whitty (1997). *Can School Improvement Overcome the Effects of Disadvantage?* London: Institute of Education.

Murray, C. J. L., C. M. Michaud, M .T. McKenna, and J. S. Marks (1998*). US Patterns of Mortality by County and Race: 1965–94.* Cambridge, MA: Harvard Center for Population and Development Studies, pp. 1–97.

North, F., S. L. Syme, A. Feeney, J. Head, M. Shipley, and M. Marmot (1993). 'Explaining Socio-Economic Differences in Sickness Absence: the Whitehall II Study', *British Medical Journal*, 306: 361–6.

Pappas, G., S. Queen, W. Hadden, and G. Fisher (1993). 'The Increasing Disparity in Mortality Between Socio-Economic Groups in the United States, 1960 and 1986', *New England Journal of Medicine*, 329: 103–9.

Power, C., O. Manor, and J. Fox (1991). *Health and Class: The Early Years.* London: Chapman & Hall.

——, S. Matthews, and O. Manor (1998). 'Inequalities in Self-Rated Health: Explanations from Different Stages of Life', *Lancet*, 351: 1009–14.

Rose, G. (1992). *Strategy of Preventive Medicine.* Oxford: Oxford University Press.

Rose, R. (1995). 'Russia as an Hour-Glass Society: a Constitution Without Citizens', *East European Constitutional Review*, 4: 34–42.

Sapolsky, R. M. and G. E. Mott (1987). 'Social Subordinance in Wild Baboons is Associated with Suppressed High Density Lipoprotein-Cholesterol Concentrations: the Possible Role of Chronic Social Stress', *Endocrinology*, 121: 1605–10.

Sen, A. (1992). *Inequalities Re-examined.* Oxford: Oxford University Press.

—— (1998). 'Mortality as an Indicator of Success and Failure', *The Economic Journal*, 108(446): 1 25.

—— (1997). 'Development Thinking at the Beginning of the 21st Century', in L. Emmerij (ed.) Economic and Social Development in the XXI century. Washington D.C.: Inter-American Development Bank and Johns Hopkins University Press.

Shively, C. A. and T. B. Clarkson (1994). 'Social Status and Coronary Artery Atherosclerosis in Female Monkeys', *Arteriosclerosis, Thrombosis, and Vascular Biology*, 14: 721–6.

——, K. Laber Laird, and R. F. Anton (1996). 'The Behaviour and Physiology of Social Stress and Depression in Female Cynomolgus Monkeys', *Biological Psychiatry*, 3: 2–43.

Siegrist, J. (1996). 'Adverse Health Effects of High-Effort/Low-Reward Conditions', *Journal of Occupational Health and Psychology*, 1: 27–41.

Skinner, E. A. (1996). 'A Guide to Constructs of Control', *Journal of Personality and Social Psychology*, 71: 549–70.

Smith, J. P. (1999). 'Healthy Bodies and Thick Wallets: The Dual Relationship between Health and Socioeconomic Status.' *Journal of Economic Perspectives*, 13(2): 145–66.

Stansfeld, S. and M. Marmot (1992). 'Deriving a Survey Measure of Social Support: the Reliability and Validity of the Close Persons Questionnaire', *Social Science and Medicine*, 35: 1027–35.

Suomi, S. J. (1991). Early Stress and Adult Emotional Reactivity in Rhesus Monkeys, in Ciba Foundation Symposium (ed.), *The Childhood Environment and Adult Disease—Symposium No. 156.* Etobicoke (Ontario): Wiley, pp. 171–85.

United Nations Development Programme (UNDP) (1994). *Human Development Report.* New York: Oxford University Press.

Von Rossum, C. T. M., M. Shipley, H. van de Mheen, D. E. Grobbee, and M. Marmot (2000). 'Employment Grade Differences in Cause Specific Mortality. A 25-year

Follow Up of Civil Servants from the Whitehall II Study', *Journal of Epidemiology and Community Health*, 54: 178–84.

Wadsworth, M. E. J. (1986). 'Serious Illness in Childhood and its Association with Later-Life Achievement', in R. G. Wilkinson (ed.), *Class and Health*. London: Tavistock Publications Ltd., pp. 50–74.

——(1991). *The Imprint of Time: Childhood, History and Adult Life*. Oxford: Clarendon Press.

——(1997). 'Changing Social Factors and their Long Term Implications for Health', in M. Marmot and M. E. J. Wadsworth (eds.), 'Fetal and Early Childhood Environment: Long-term Health Implications', *British Medical Bulletin*, 53: 198–209.

Watson, P. (1995). 'Explaining Rising Mortality among Men in Eastern Europe', *Social Science and Medicine*, 41: 923–34.

Wilkinson, R. (1996). *Unhealthy Societies: the Afflictions of Inequality*. London: Routledge.

——(1997). 'Health Inequalities: Relative or Absolute Material Standards', *British Medical Journal*, 314: 591–5.

Williams, R., T. Haney, K. Lee, Y. Kong, J. Blumenthal, and R. Whalen (1980). 'Type A Behavior, Hostility and Coronary Heart Disease', *Psychosomatic Medicine*, 42: 539–49.

Williams, R. B. (1991). 'A Relook at Personality Types and Coronary Heart Disease', *Progress in Cardiology*, 4: 91–7.

4

Health and Inequality, or, Why Justice is Good for Our Health

NORMAN DANIELS, BRUCE KENNEDY,
AND ICHIRO KAWACHI

4.1. JUSTICE AND HEALTH INEQUALITIES

We have known for over 150 years that an individual's chances of life and death are patterned according to social class: the more affluent and better educated people are, the longer and healthier their lives (Villerme 1840; cited in Link et al. 1998).[1] These patterns persist even when there is universal access to health care—a finding quite surprising to those who think financial access to medical services is the primary determinant of health status. In fact, recent cross-national evidence suggests that the greater the degree of socio-economic inequality that exists within a society, the steeper the *gradient* of health inequality. As a result, middle-income groups in a more unequal society will have worse health than comparable or even poorer groups in a society with greater equality. Of course, we cannot infer *causation* from *correlation*, but there are plausible hypotheses about pathways which link social inequalities to health, and, even if more work remains to be done to clarify the exact mechanisms, it is not unreasonable to talk here about the social 'determinants' of health (Marmot 1999).

When is an inequality in health status between different socio-economic groups unjust?[2] An account of justice should help us determine which inequalities are unjust and which acceptable. Many who are untroubled by some kinds of inequality are particularly troubled by health inequalities. They believe that a socio-economic inequality that otherwise seems just becomes unjust if it contributes to health inequalities. Is every health inequality that

Norman Daniels, Bruce P. Kennedy, and Ichiro Kawachi are recipients of Robert Wood Johnson Foundation Investigator Awards in health policy research. Another version of this paper appeared in *Daedalus* 128(4) (Winter 1999): 215–51, and we thank the publisher for permission to draw on that paper here.

[1] Throughout we view disease and disability as departures from (species-typical) normal functioning and view health and normal functioning as equivalent.

[2] To avoid additional complexity, we concentrate in this paper on class or socio-economic inequalities, though many of our points generalize to race and gender inequalities in health as well.

results from unequally distributed social goods unjust? If there is an irreducible health gradient across socio-economic groups, does that make the very existence of those inequalities unjust?

Alternatively, are some health inequalities the result of acceptable trade-offs? Perhaps they are simply an unfortunate byproduct of inequalities that work in other ways to help worse-off groups. For example, it is often claimed that permitting inequality provides incentives to work harder, thereby stimulating growth that will ultimately benefit the poorest groups. To whom must these trade-offs be acceptable if we are to consider them just? Are they acceptable only if they are part of a strategy aimed at moving the situation toward a more just arrangement? Does it matter in our judgements about justice exactly how social determinants produce inequalities in health status?

These are hard questions. Unfortunately, they have been almost totally ignored within the field of bioethics, as well as within ethics and political philosophy more generally. Bioethics has been quick to focus on exotic new medical technologies and how they might affect our lives. It has paid considerable attention to the doctor–patient relationship and how changes in the health care system affect it. With some significant exceptions, it has not looked 'upstream' from the point of delivery of medical services to the role of the health care system in delivering improved population health. It has even more rarely looked further upstream to social arrangements that determine the health achievement of societies (Dahlgren and Whitehead 1991; Benzeval et al. 1995; Marchand et al. 1998).

This omission is quite striking, since a concern about 'health equity' and its social determinants has emerged as an important consideration in the policies of several European countries over the last two decades (Benzeval et al. 1995). The World Health Organization (WHO) has devoted growing attention to inequalities in health status and the policies that cause or mitigate them. So have research initiatives, such as the Global Health Equity Initiative, funded by the Swedish International Development Agency and the Rockefeller Foundation.

In what follows, we shall attempt to fill this bioethical gap by addressing some of these questions about justice and health inequalities. We explore the conjecture Rawls's theory of 'justice as fairness' and the extension one of us has made of it to health care (Rawls 1971; Daniels 1981, 1985) provides a defensible account of how to distribute the social determinants of health fairly. We focus on Rawls's theory for several reasons. By providing philosophical justification for a principle protecting fair equality of opportunity, it also provides the basis for answering the question, 'Why is health care of special moral importance and what is objectionable about avoidable health disparities?' At the same time, it is a theory that justifies some socio-economic inequalities, and thus leaves room for exploring the tension between protecting health and opportunity and allowing for otherwise just inequalities. We do not suggest that Rawls's theory is the only fruitful way to address these matters, and we later argue that Sen's (1999) account of freedom converges in practice, and to some extent in theory, with the account we defend here.

If we are right, this unexpected application to a novel problem demonstrates a fruitful generalisability of Rawls's theory, analogous to the extension in scope or power of a non-moral theory, and permits us to think more systematically across the disciplines of public health, medicine, and political philosophy. This surprising result is not just serendipity, however. Justice as fairness was formulated to specify terms of social cooperation that free and equal citizens can accept as fair. Specifically, it assures people of equal basic liberties, including the value of political participation, guarantees a robust form of equal opportunity, and imposes significant constraints on inequalities. Together, these principles aim at meeting the 'needs of free and equal citizens', a form of egalitarianism Rawls calls 'democratic equality'. (Rawls 1971; Daniels 2003) A crucial component of democratic equality is providing all with the social bases of self-respect and a conviction that prospects in life are fair. As the empirical literature demonstrates, institutions conforming to these principles together focus on several crucial pathways through which many researchers believe inequality works to produce health inequality. As a result, conformance with Rawls's principles significantly reduces health disparities, and we shall have to consider when any remaining inequalities are unjust. Of course, this theory does not answer all of our questions about justice and health inequality, since there are some crucial points on which it is silent, but it does provide considerable guidance on central issues.

Before developing our central philosophical claims in Section 4.4, in Section 4.2 we very briefly review some of the key findings about the social determinants of health inequalities, sharpening the questions posed earlier about justice and inequality. In Section 4.3 we examine an analysis of health 'inequities' prominent in the public health policy literature. The need to deepen that analysis is what drives us in Section 4.4 to examine the implications of Rawls's theory for these issues. We conclude with some remarks about alternative approaches, noting the convergence of Rawls's approach with Sen's, and we briefly note some policy implications of this analysis.

4.2. SOCIAL DETERMINANTS OF HEALTH: SOME BASIC FINDINGS

We highlight five central findings in the literature on the social determinants of health, each of which has implications for an account of justice and health inequalities. First, the income/health gradients we observe are not the result of some fixed or determinate laws of economic development but are influenced by policy choices. Second, the income/health gradients are not just the result of the deprivation of the poorest groups. Rather, a gradient in health operates across the whole socio-economic spectrum within societies. Third, the slope or steepness of the income/health gradient is affected by the degree of inequality in a society. Fourth, as a corollary to three, relative income or socio-economic status is as important as, and may be more important than, the absolute level of income in determining health status, at least once societies have passed a certain threshold of economic development. Fifth, there are identifiable social and psychosocial pathways through which inequality produces its effects on health and little support for 'health selection'—the claim that health status determines economic position (Marmot 1999, 1994). As indicated in the first thesis, these causal pathways are amenable to specific policy choices that should be guided by considerations of justice.

4.2.1. Cross-national evidence on health inequalities

The pervasive finding that prosperity is related to health, whether measured at the level of nations or individuals, might lead one to the conclusion that these 'income/health gradients' are inevitable. They might seem to reflect the natural ordering of societies along some fixed, idealised teleology of economic development. At the individual level, the gradient might appear to be the result of the natural selection of the most 'fit' members within a society who are thus better able to garner socio-economic advantage.

Despite the appeal and power of these ideas, they run counter to the confirmation. Figure 4.1 shows the relationship between the wealth and health of nations as measured by per capita gross domestic product (GDPpc) and life expectancy. There is a clear association between GDPpc and life expectancy, but only up to a point. The relationship levels off beyond about $8,000–10,000 GDPpc, with virtually no further gains in life expectancy.

This levelling effect is most apparent among the advanced industrial economies (Fig. 4.2) which largely account for the upper tail of the curve in

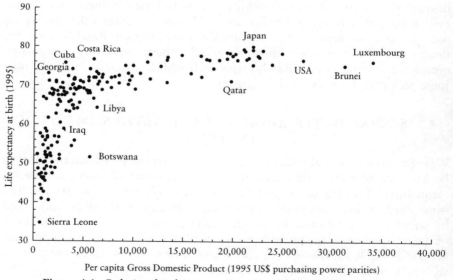

Figure 4.1. *Relationship between country wealth and life expectancy*
Source: United Nations Human Development Report Statistics (1998).

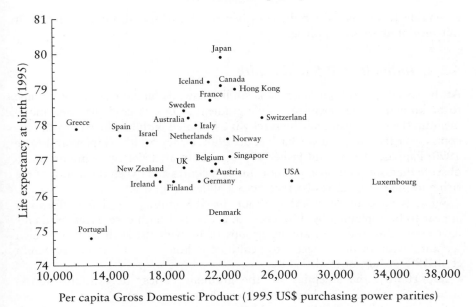

Figure 4.2. *Relationship between country wealth and life expectancy among advanced industrial economies*

Notes: r = 0.0500; *p* = 0.809.

Source: United Nations Human Development Report Statistics (1998).

Fig. 4.1. The lack of relationship between wealth and health is true *within* individual countries as well.

Closer inspection of these two figures points up some startling discrepancies. Though Cuba and Iraq are equally poor (GDPpcs about $3,100), life expectancy in Cuba exceeds that in Iraq by 17.2 years. The difference between the GDPpc for Costa Rica and the United States, for example, is enormous (about $21,000), yet Costa Rica's life expectancy exceeds that of the United States (76.6 versus, 76.4). In fact, despite being the richest nation on the globe, the United States performs rather poorly on health indicators.

Taken together, these observations support the notion that the relationship between economic development and health is not fixed, and that the health achievement of nations is mediated by processes other than wealth. To account for the cross–national variations in health, it is apparent that other factors such as culture, social organization, and government policies are significantly involved in the determination of population health, and that variations in these factors may go some distance in explaining the differences in health outcomes among nations.

If we are right that the health of nations does not reflect some inevitable natural order, but that it reflects policy choices—or features of society that are amenable to change via policies—then we must ask about the justice or injustice of alternative policies.

4.2.2. *Individual SES and health*

At the social group level, numerous studies have documented what has come to be known as the 'socio-economic gradient'. On this gradient, each increment up the socio-economic hierarchy is associated with improved health outcomes over the rung below (Black et al. 1988; Davey-Smith, Shipley, and Rose 1990; Pappas, Queen, and Fisher 1993; Adler et al. 1994). It is important to observe that this relationship is not simply a contrast between the health of the rich and the poor, but is observed across all levels of SES.

What is particularly notable about the SES gradient is that it does not appear to be explained by differences in access to health care. Steep gradients have been observed even among groups of individuals, such as British civil servants, with adequate access to health care, housing, and transport (Smith et al. 1990; Marmot et al. 1998).

Importantly, the steepness of the gradient varies substantially across societies. Some societies show a relatively shallow gradient in mortality across SES groups. Others, with comparable or even higher levels of economic development, show much steeper gradients in mortality rates across the socio-economic hierarchy. The determining factor in the steepness of the gradient appears to be the extent of income inequality in a society. Thus middle-income groups in a country with high income inequality may have lower health status than comparable or even poorer groups in a society with less income inequality. We find the same pattern within the United States when we examine state and metropolitan area variations in inequality and health outcomes (Kennedy et al. 1998a; Lynch et al. 1998).

These results lead to the question: To what extent do social inequalities lead to health inequalities and in which cases may these be considered just or unjust?

4.2.3. *Relative income and health*

A lively debate exists in the empirical literature about whether income inequality is a determining factor in the steepness of the gradient. Were this true, we might find that middle income groups in a country with high income inequality might have lower health status than comparable or even poorer groups in a society with less income inequality. There is some evidence for this pattern within the United States if variations in inequality among states are examined (Kennedy et al. 1998a; Lynch et al. 1998). This effect is apparent in Fig. 4.3, where the prevalence of self-reported fair/poor health is higher for almost every income group (and the gradient steeper) for those living in the highest income inequality states (Kennedy et al. 1998a). This effect of shifting the

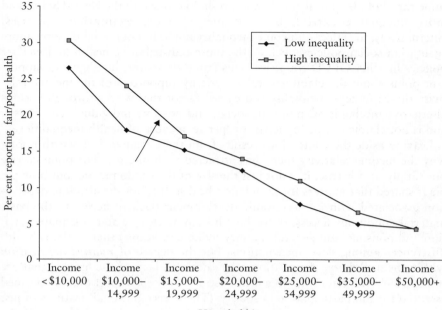

Figure 4.3. *Self-rated health and individual household income*

Notes: The income-poor health curve is shifted up in the states with the highest income inequality for almost the entire population as shown by the arrow.

curve, if it is supported by further empirical findings, would suggest that there is an effect of income inequality over and above what is implied by the concavity of the SES gradient itself.

Sparked by Wilkinson's (1992) paper showing a correlation between national measures of income inequality and the gradient of health inequality among a select groups of OECD countries, researchers in the United States and elsewhere have found conflicting results during the subsequent decade. The initial positive results from the OECD countries disappear when a full rather than selected set of them is studied. Negative results are also found primarily in countries more egalitarian than the United States (Sweden, Japan, Canada, Denmark, New Zealand), as noted by Subramanian et al. (2003); Subramanian and Kawachi (2003). Some negative results are also found in the United States, especially if units of aggregation are smaller, such as municipalities rather than states. A significant number of US studies support the claim, especially at the state level. Positive results are also found in a recent study in Chile (Subramanian and Kawachi 2003), a country with more income inequality than exists in the United States.

One hypothesis that would explain this pattern of seemingly conflicting results is that income inequality has its effect on health inequalities only above some threshold level of inequality, a threshold crossed in the United States and more unequal countries, but not met in more egalitarian countries. Alternatively, the effect of income inequality might be countered by some more egalitarian social policies, such as the more redistributive health and welfare policies in other OECD countries. This latter alternative highlights an important point about the claim generally made by supporters of the income relativity thesis: income inequality is a causal factor that works through various alternative mechanisms, political, social, and possibly individual (e.g. stress), and is not claimed to be 'by itself' or 'per se' a cause of health inequalities.

Leaving aside the contentious results from these studies, it is worth noting why the income relativity thesis has attracted such interest. The point can be put simply: if it is true, it is not just the size of the economic pie, but how the pie is shared that matters for population health. It is not the absolute deprivation associated with low economic development (lack of access to the basic material conditions necessary for health such as clean water, adequate nutrition and housing, and general sanitary living conditions) that explains health differences among developed nations, but the degree of *relative deprivation* within them. Relative deprivation refers not to a lack of the 'goods' that are basic to survival, but rather to a lack of sources of self-respect that are deemed essential for full participation in society. (These 'recognitional' features of just arrangements are emphasised in Rawls's account, as we note later). If the income relativity thesis can be established, it would then require elaboration of the causal mechanisms that underlie it.

In the United States, in those studies that support the thesis, the size of this relationship between social inequality and health inequality is not trivial. A recent study across US metropolitan areas, rather than states, found that areas with high income inequality had an excess of death compared to areas of low inequality that was equivalent in magnitude to all deaths due to heart disease (Lynch et al. 1998).

While most of the evidence so far has been accumulated from cross-sectional data, time trend data support similar conclusions. Widening income differentials in the United States and United Kingdom appear to be related to a slowing down of life-expectancy improvements. In many of the poorest areas of the United Kingdom, mortality for younger age cohorts has actually increased during the same period that income inequality widened (Wilkinson 1996). In the United States, states with the highest income inequality showed slower rates of life-expectancy improvement compared to states with more equitable income distributions between 1980 and 1990 (Kaplan et al. 1996; Kawachi et al. 1999).

The income relativity thesis is worth further investigation, but whether or not it is true, the claim we make later about the positive effect of Rawls's Difference Principle on aggregate health and the improved health of worst off groups is supported. As we shall see, there is strong evidence supporting the fact that health inequalities are reduced if we concentrate first on making those who are in the worst off groups socially and economically as well off as possible, paying special attention to improvements in human capital and investments in public health. If true, the income relativity thesis would strengthen support for giving priority to making the worst off as well off as possible, for it would make an even stronger claim for the result that it works to the advantage of all. In addition, it might point us more specifically to additional mechanisms that we may have to address.

Pathways linking social inequalities to health inequalities

Our final contention is that there are plausible and identifiable pathways through which social inequalities produce inequalities in health. Some of these occur at the societal level, where income inequality patterns the distribution of social goods, such as public education, thereby affecting patterns the access to life opportunities which are in turn strong determinants of health.

The evidence for these associations, while fairly new, is quite striking. In the United States, the most inegalitarian states with respect to income distribution invest less in public education, have larger uninsured populations, and spend less on social safety nets (Kaplan et al. 1996; Kawachi and Kennedy 1997). Differences in human capital investment are particularly striking. These are demonstrated for educational spending and more importantly for outcomes, where even when controlling for median income, income inequality explains about 40 per cent of the between state variation in the percentage of children in the 4th grade who are below the basic reading level. Similarly strong associations are seen for the percentage of high school drop out rates. It is quite evident from these data, that educational opportunities for children in high income inequality states are quite different from those in states with more egalitarian distributions. Furthermore, these early effects not only have an immediate impact on health, increasing the likelihood of premature death during childhood and adolescence (as evidenced by the much higher death rates for infants and children in the high inequality states), but also have lasting effects showing up later in life as part of the SES gradient in health (Bartley et al. 1997; Barker 1998; Davey Smith et al. 1998).

Differential investment in human capital is also a strong predictor of health across nations. Indeed, one of the strongest predictors of life expectancy among developing countries is adult literacy, particularly the disparity between male and female adult literacy, which explains much of the variation in health achievement among these countries after accounting for GDPpc. For example, among the 125 developing countries with GDPpcs less than $10,000 the difference between male and female literacy accounts for 40 per cent of the variance in life expectancy after factoring out the effect of GDPpc. The fact that gender disparities in access to basic education drives the level of health achievement further emphasises the role of broader social inequalities in patterning health inequalities. Indeed, in the United States, differences between the states in women's status—measured in terms of their economic autonomy and political participation—are more strongly correlated with higher female mortality rates (Kawachi et al. 1999; Wilkinson, Kennedy and Kawachi, forthcoming).

These societal mechanisms are tightly linked to the political processes that influence government policy. One way that income inequality affects health, appears to be through its role in undermining civil society. Income inequality erodes social cohesion, as measured by higher levels of social mistrust and reduced participation in civic organizations, both of which are central features of civil society (Kawachi and Kennedy 1997; Kawachi et al. 1997). Lack of social cohesion is in turn reflected in significantly lower participation in political activity (for example, voting, serving in local government, volunteering for political campaigns, etc.), thus undermining the responsiveness of government institutions in addressing the needs of the worst off in society. This is demonstrated by the human capital investment data presented earlier, but it is also reflected by the lack of investment in human security. States with the highest income inequality, and thus lowest levels of social capital and political participation, are far less generous in the provision of social safety nets. For example, the correlation between social capital, as measured by low interpersonal trust, and the maximum welfare grant as a percent of state per capita income is 0.76 (Kawachi and Kennedy 1999).

How can these five theses we have highlighted from scientific literature on social determinants be integrated into our views about the moral acceptability of health inequalities? Historically, disciplinary boundaries have stood as an obstacle to an integrated perspective. The social science and public health literature sharpens our understanding of the causes of health inequalities, but it contains no systematic way to evaluate the overall fairness of those inequalities and the socio-economic inequalities that produce them. The philosophical literature has produced theories aimed at evaluating socio-economic inequalities, but it has tended to ignore health inequalities and their causes. To produce an integrated view, we shall need the resources of a more general theory of justice. We can better see the need for such a theory if we first examine an analysis of 'health inequities' that has been developed within a policy-based public health literature.

4.3. HEALTH INEQUALITIES AND INEQUITIES

When is a health inequality between two groups 'inequitable'?

This version of our earlier question about health inequalities and justice has been the focus of European and WHO efforts, as noted above. One initially useful answer to it that has been influential in the WHO programmes is the claim that health inequalities count as inequities when they are *avoidable, unnecessary,* and *unfair* (Dahlgren and Whitehead 1991; Whitehead 1992; Braveman 1999). If we can agree on what is avoidable, unnecessary, and unfair, and this analysis is correct, then we can agree on which inequalities are inequitable.

The Whitehead–Dahlgren analysis is deliberately broader than our central question about differences in socio-economic status. Age, gender, race, and ethnic differences in health status exist that are independent of socio-economic differences, and they raise distinct questions about equity or justice. For example, should we view the lower life expectancy of men compared to women in developed countries as an inequity? If it is rooted in biological differences that we do not know how to overcome, then, according to this analysis, it is not avoidable and therefore not an inequity. This is not an idle controversy: taking average, rather than gender-differentiated life expectancy in developed countries as a benchmark or goal will yield different estimates of the degree of inequity women face in some developing countries. In any case, the analysis of inequity is here only as good as our understanding of what is avoidable or unnecessary.

The same point applies to judgements about fairness. Is the poorer health status of some social class or ethnic groups that engage in heavy alcohol use unfair? We may be inclined to say it is not unfair provided that participation in the risky behaviors or their avoidance is truly voluntary. But if many people in a cultural group or class behave similarly, there may also be factors at work that reduce how voluntary their behaviour is and how much responsibility we should ascribe to them for it (Wikler 1978; Roemer 1998). The analysis thus leaves us with the unresolved complexity of these judgements about responsibility, and, as a result, with disagreements about fairness (or avoidability).

The poor in many countries lack access to clean water, sanitation, adequate shelter, basic education, vaccinations, and prenatal and maternal care. As a result of some or all of these factors, there are infant mortality differences between them and richer groups. Since social policies could supply the missing determinants of infant health, then the inequalities are avoidable.

Are these inequalities also unfair? Most of us would immediately think they are, perhaps because we believe that policies that create and sustain poverty are unjust, and we also believe that social policies that compound poverty with lack of access to the determinants of health are doubly unfair. Of course, libertarians would disagree. They would insist that what is merely unfortunate is not unfair; on their view, we have no obligation of justice, as opposed to charity, to provide the poor with what they are missing. Many of us might be inclined to reject the libertarian view as itself unjust because of this dramatic conflict with our beliefs about poverty and our social obligations to meet people's basic needs.

The problem becomes more complicated, however, when we remember one of the basic findings from the literature on social determinants: we cannot eliminate health inequalities simply by eliminating poverty. Health inequalities persist even in societies that provide the poor with access to all of the determinants of health noted above, and they persist as a gradient of health throughout the social hierarchy, not just between the very poorest groups and those above them.

At this point, many of us would have to reexamine what we believe about the justice of the remaining socio-economic inequalities. Unless we believe that *all* socio-economic inequalities (or at least all inequalities we did not choose) are unjust—and very few embrace such a radical egalitarian view—then we must consider more carefully the problem created by the health gradient and the fact that it is made steeper under more unequal social arrangements. Our judgements about fairness, to which we, rightly or wrongly, felt confident in appealing when rejecting the libertarian position, give us less guidance in thinking about the broader issue of the social determinants of health inequalities. Indeed, we may even believe that some degree of socio-economic inequality is unavoidable or even necessary, and therefore not unjust.

4.4. JUSTICE AS FAIRNESS AND HEALTH INEQUALITIES

In this section, we explain in more detail how Rawls's theory, originally idealized to assume no one is ill, can be extended, through its opportunity principle, to explain the moral importance we ascribe to health care and the objections we have to avoidable health disparities. Yet, the theory also allows for other inequalities that can produce health disparities. We must therefore explain the rationale for allowing these inequalities, and give an account of the proper way to measure them. We can then state just how far Rawls's principles take us toward reducing health disparities and consider what to do about those that remain.

4.4.1. *Justice when no one is ill*

One reason we develop general ethical theories, including theories of justice, is to provide a framework within which to resolve important disputes about conflicting moral beliefs or intuitions of the sort we have raised in the previous section. For example, in *A Theory of Justice* (1971), Rawls sought to leverage our relatively broad liberal agreement on principles guaranteeing certain equal basic liberties into an agreement on a principle limiting socio-economic inequalities, a matter on which liberals have considerable disagreement (Cohen 1989). His strategy was to show that a social contract that was designed to be fair to free and equal people ('justice as [procedural] fairness') would not only justify the choice of those equal basic liberties but would also justify the choice of principles guaranteeing equal opportunity and limiting inequalities to those that work to make the worst off groups fare as well as possible.

Our contention is that Rawls's account, though developed to answer this general question about social justice, turns out to provide principles for the just distribution of the social determinants of health, unexpectedly adding to its scope and power as a theory. The extra power of the theory is a surprise, since Rawls deliberately avoided talking about disease or health in his original account. To simplify the construction of his theory, Rawls assumed his contractors were be fully functional over a normal life span, that is, no one becomes ill or dies prematurely.

4.4.2. *Extending Rawls's Theory*

This idealization itself provides a clue about how to extend this theory to the real world of illness and premature death. The goal of public health and medicine is to keep people as close as possible to the idealization of normal functioning, under reasonable resource constraints. (Resources are necessarily limited since maintaining health cannot be our only social good or goal.) Since maintaining normal functioning makes a limited but significant contribution to protecting the range of opportunities open to individuals, it is plausible to see the principle guaranteeing fair equality of opportunity as the appropriate principle to govern the distribution of health care, broadly construed to include primary and secondary preventive health as well as medical services (Daniels 1985; Rawls 1993). This way of extending Rawls's theory also suggests that health status should be incorporated through its effects on opportunity into the index of primary goods, which is used to evaluate the well-being of contractors and citizens. (We return to issues about the index of primary goods shortly.)

It will help to describe more fully the relationship between normal functioning and opportunity, one of the primary social goods. Impairments of normal functioning reduce the range of opportunity open to an individual in which he may construct or pursue a 'plan of life'. Life plans for which we are otherwise suited are rendered unreasonable by impairments of normal functioning, including early death. In a given society, with a given level of wealth, technology, and social organization, the *normal opportunity range* is the array of life plans that people in it find it reasonable to choose, given their talents and skills. Individuals' fair shares of that societal normal opportunity range are the arrays of life plans it is reasonable for them to choose, given their talents and skills, assuming normal functioning.

Disease and disability thus diminish individual fair shares of the normal opportunity range. The seriousness of the impact on the opportunity range is a crude measure of the relative importance of meeting the health needs that create the problem as compared to others. By promoting normal functioning for a population, comprehensive health care—and social structures aimed at maintaining population health—thus make a significant, but limited, contribution to the protection of fair equality of opportunity.[3] This approach is not just concerned with inequalities in health status, but with improvements in population health because of the importance of normal function to the capabilities of citizens in a democracy. Judged from the perspective of Rawlsian contractors, this way of extending the theory seems both reasonable and rational. Contractors will judge that they have a fundamental interest in

---

[3] This extension of Rawls's theory expands the notion of opportunity beyond just access to jobs and offices, since participation in other aspects of a plan of life also are affected by departures from normal functioning. Rawls endorses the overall approach in PL (184 n.14).

preserving the opportunity to revise their conceptions of the good through time. They will thus have a pressing interest in maintaining normal functioning by establishing institutions, such as health care systems, that do just that.

Institutionally, an opportunity-based account of health care will require universal access to a system of public health, preventive, acute and chronic care services—that is, access that meets needs other than by ability to pay for the services. In general, this requires a universal, mandatory national insurance system (but details of organization and financing can vary considerably). Given real resource limits, services will have to be allocated in ways that meet people's needs fairly, since not all health needs can be met. A key principle in the design of such systems is that they do not arbitrarily omit certain kinds of beneficial services but adopt limits to care based on reasons that all can accept as relevant to meeting needs fairly under resource constraints (Daniels and Sabin 1997). What emerges, then, is that inequalities in health status among individuals are addressed in part by designing *health care* institutions that aim in a reasonable and fair way at protecting normal functioning for the whole population.

4.4.3. *Justifying Inequality in Rawls's Theory*

What is particularly appealing about examining the social determinants of health inequalities from the perspective of Rawls's theory is that the theory is at once egalitarian in orientation and yet justifies certain inequalities that might contribute to health inequalities. In addition, Daniels's extension of Rawls links the protection of health to the protection of equality of opportunity, again setting up the potential for internal conflict. To see whether this combination of features simply leads to contradictions in the theory or to insight into the problem, we must examine the issue in more detail.

How does Rawls justify socio-economic inequalities? Why would free and equal contractors met simply insist on strictly egalitarian distributions of all social goods, just as they insist on equal basic liberties and equal opportunity?

Rawls's answer is that it is irrational for contractors to insist on equality if doing so would make them worse off. Specifically, he argues that contractors would choose his Difference Principle, which permits inequalities provided that they work to make the worst off groups in society as well off as possible.[4] The argument for the Difference Principle appears to suggest that relative

---

[4] A careful discussion of Rawls's argument for the difference principle and the extensive critical literature it has generated is beyond the scope of this chapter. It is important, however, to distinguish Rawls's own social contract argument from the many informal and intuitive reformulations of it. See Brian Barry (1989). *Theories of Justice* London: Harvester Wheatsheaf, 213–34; G.A. Cohen (1995). 'The Pareto Argument for Inequality', *Social Philosophy and Policy*, 12 (Winter): 160–85; Joshua Cohen (1989). 'Democratic Equality', *Ethics*, 99 (July): 727–51; Norman Daniels (2003). 'Democratic Equality: Rawls's Complex Egalitarianism', in Samuel Freeman (ed.), *Cambridge Companion to Rawls*. Cambridge: Cambridge University Press, 241–77.

inequality is less important than absolute well-being, a suggestion that is in tension with other aspects of Rawls's view. Thus he also insists that inequalities allowed by the Difference Principle should not undermine the value of political liberty and the requirements of fair equality of opportunity. The priority given these other principles over the Difference Principle thus limits the inference that Rawls has no concern about relative inequality. Specifically, as we shall see, these principles work together to constrain inequality and to preserve the social bases of self-respect for all.

Two points will help avoid misunderstanding of the Difference Principle and its justification. First, it is not a mere 'trickle-down' principle, but one that requires maximal flow in the direction of helping the worst off groups. The worst off, and then the next worst off, and so on (Rawls [1971] calls this 'chain connectedness') must be made as well off as possible, not merely just somewhat better off, as a trickle-down principle implies. The Difference Principle is thus much more demanding than a principle that would permit any degree of inequality provided there was some 'trickle' of benefits to the worst off. Indeed, it is more egalitarian than alternative principles that merely assure the worse off a 'decent' or 'adequate' minimum. Part of the rationale for the more demanding principle is that it would produce less strain of commitment, less sense of being unfairly left out, at least for those who are worst off, than principles that allow more inequality (Cohen 1989). Indeed, from what we have learned about the social determinants of health, the more demanding Difference Principle would also produce less health inequality than any proposed alternative principles that allow inequalities. By flattening the health gradient, it also benefits middle-income groups and not simply the poorest. In this regard, its benefits are important beyond the level where we have helped the worst off to achieve 'sufficiency'. This point provides a reply to those who suggest that the Difference Principle has no appeal once the worst off are sufficiently provided for (Gutmann and Thompson 1995).

Second, when contractors evaluate how well off the principles they choose will make them, they are to judge their well-being by an index of 'primary social goods'. The primary social goods, which Rawls thinks of as the 'needs of citizens', include liberty, powers, opportunities, income, and wealth, and the social bases of self-respect. Including the social bases of self-respect might seem surprising here. Without self-respect, however, it is difficult for individuals to use their capabilities as individuals and citizens; since social structures critically support or undermine self-respect, Rawls includes the social basis of it on the index. (All of these objective measures of well-being should be contrasted with measures of happiness or desire satisfaction that are familiar from utilitarian and welfare economic perspectives). In his exposition of the Difference Principle, Rawls illustrates how it will work by asking us to consider only the simpler case of income inequalities. In doing so, he assumes that the level of income will correlate with the level of other social goods on the index (Rawls 1971: 62, 1993: chapter 5).

This simplification should not mislead us, for, in crucial cases, the correlation may not obtain. For example, let us suppose that having 'democratic' control over one's workplace is crucial to self-realization and the promotion of self-respect. Suppose further that hierarchical workplaces are more efficient than democratic ones, so that a system with hierarchical workplaces would have resources to redistribute that meant higher incomes for worst off workers than democratic workplaces would permit (Cohen: unpublished ms). Then the Difference Principle does not clearly tell us whether the hierarchical workplace contains allowable inequalities since the worst off are better off in some ways but worse off in others. Without knowing the weighting of items in the index, we cannot use it to say clearly what inequalities are permitted. When we are evaluating which income inequalities are allowable, by asking which ones work to make the worst off groups as well off as possible, we must, in any case, judge how well off groups are by reference to the *whole* index of primary goods and not simply the resulting income.

This point is of particular importance in the current discussion. Daniels's extension of Rawls treats health status as a determinant of the opportunity range open to individuals. Since opportunity is included in the index, the effects of health inequalities are thereby included in the index.

Unfortunately, Rawls says very little about how items in the index are to be weighted. This is one of the crucial points on which the theory says less than we might have wished. Therefore we have little guidance about how these primary goods are to be traded off against each other in its construction. This silence pertains not only to the use of the index in the contract situation, but also to its use by a legislature trying to apply the principles of justice in a context where many specific features of a society are known. We return to this point shortly.

4.4.4. *How conformance with Rawls's principles promotes population health and reduces health disparities*

We can now say more directly why justice, as described by Rawls's principles, is good for our health. To understand this claim, let us start with the ideal case, a society governed by Rawls's principles of justice that seeks to achieve 'democratic equality' (Daniels 2003). Consider what it requires with regard to the distribution of the social determinants of health. In such a society, all are guaranteed equal basic liberties, including the liberty of political participation. In addition, there are institutional safeguards aimed at assuring all, richer and poorer alike, the worth or value of political participation rights. Without such assurance, basic capabilities of citizens cannot develop. The recognition that all citizens have these capabilities protected is critical to preserving self-esteem, in Rawls's view. In requiring institutional support for political participation rights, Rawls rejects the claim that freedom of speech of the rich is unfairly restricted by limiting their personal expenditures on their own campaigns, a limitation the Supreme Court ruled unconstitutional in *Buckley* v. *Valeo* (Rawls 1993). After all, the limitation does not unduly burden the rich compared to others. Since there is evidence that political participation is itself a social determinant of health (see above), the Rawlsian ideal assures institutional protections that counter the usual effects of socio-economic inequalities on participation and thus on health.

The Rawlsian ideal of democratic equality also involves conformity with a principle guaranteeing fair equality of opportunity. Not only are discriminatory barriers prohibited by the principle, but also it requires robust measures aimed at mitigating the effects of socio-economic inequalities and other social contingencies on opportunity. In addition to equitable public education, such measures would include the provision of developmentally appropriate day care and early childhood interventions intended to promote the development of capabilities independently of the advantages of family background. Such measures match or go beyond the best models of such interventions we see in European efforts at day care and early childhood education. We also note that the strategic importance of education for protecting equal opportunity has implications for all levels of education, including access to graduate and professional education.

The equal opportunity principle also requires extensive public health, medical, and social support services aimed at promoting normal functioning for all (Daniels 1985; Daniels et al. 1996). It even provides a rationale for the social costs of reasonable accommodation to incurable disabilities, as required by the Americans with Disabilities Act (Daniels 1996*a*, *b*). Because the principle aims at promoting normal functioning for *all* as a way of protecting opportunity for all, it at once aims at improving population health and the reduction of health inequalities. Obviously, this focus requires provision of universal access to comprehensive health care, including public health, primary health care, and medical and social support services.

To act justly in health policy, we must have knowledge about the causal pathways through which socio-economic (and other) inequalities work to produce differential health outcomes. Suppose we learn, for example, that structural and organizational features of the workplace that induce stress and a loss of control tend to promote health inequalities. We should then view modifying those features of work place organization in order to mitigate their negative effects on health as a public health requirement of the equal opportunity approach; it is thus on a par with the requirement that we reduce exposures to toxins in the work place (Daniels 1985).

Finally, in the ideal Rawlsian society, the Difference Principle places significant restrictions on allowable inequalities in income and wealth.[5] The inequalities

---

[5] G. A. Cohen has argued that a *strict* interpretation of the Difference Principle would allow few incentive-based inequalities; for a more permissive view, see Daniels, 'Democratic Equality: Rawls's Complex Egalitarianism' (ibid.).

allowed by this principle (in conjunction with the principles assuring equal opportunity and the value of political participation) are probably more constrained than those we observe in even the most industrialised societies. If so, then the inequalities that conform to the Difference Principle would produce a flatter gradient of health inequality than we currently observe in even the more extensive welfare systems of Northern Europe.

In short, Rawls's principles of justice regulate the distribution of the key social determinants of health, including the social bases of self-respect. There is nothing about the theory, or Daniels's extension of it, that should make us focus narrowly on medical services. Properly understood, justice as fairness tells us what justice requires in the distribution of all socially controllable determinants of health.

4.4.5 *The problem of residual gradients*

We still face a theoretical issue of some interest. Even if the Rawlsian distribution of the determinants of health flattens health gradients further than what we observe in the most egalitarian, developed countries, we must still expect a residue of health inequalities. In part, this may happen because we may not have adequate knowledge of all the relevant causal pathways or interventions that are effective in modifying them. The theoretical issue is whether the theory requires us to reduce *further* those otherwise justifiable inequalities because of the inequalities in health status they create.

We should not further reduce those socio-economic inequalities if doing so reduces productivity to the extent that we can no longer support the institutional measures we already employ to promote health and reduce health inequalities. Our commitment to reducing health inequality should not require steps that threaten to make health worse off for those with less-than-equal health status. So the theoretical issue reduces to this: would it ever be reasonable and rational for contractors to accept a trade-off in which some health inequality is allowed in order to produce some non-health benefits for those with the worst health prospects?

4.4.6. *Can contractors trade health for other goods?*

We know that in real life people routinely trade health risks for other benefits. They do so when they commute longer distances for a better job, or take a ski vacation. Some such trades raise questions of fairness. For example, when is hazard pay a benefit workers gain only because their opportunities are unfairly restricted, and when is it an appropriate exercise of their autonomy (Daniels 1985)? Many such trades are ones we think it unjustifiably paternalistic to restrict; others we see as unfair.

Rawlsian contractors, however, cannot make such trades on the basis of any specific knowledge of their own values. They cannot decide that their enjoyment of skiing makes it worth the risks to their knees or necks. To make the contract fair to all participants, and to achieve impartiality, Rawls imposes a thick 'veil of ignorance' that blinds them to all knowledge about themselves, including their specific views of the good life. Instead, they must judge their well-being by reference to an index of primary social goods (noted earlier) that includes a weighted measure of rights, opportunities, powers, income and wealth, and the social bases of self-respect. When Kenneth Arrow (1973) first reviewed Rawls's theory, he argued that this index was inadequate because it failed to tell us how to compare the ill rich with the well poor; Sen (1980, 1992) argues that the index is insensitive to the way in which disease, disability, or other individual variations would create inequalities in the capabilities of people who had the same primary social goods. By extending Rawls's theory to include health care through the equal opportunity account, some of Arrow's (and Sen's) criticism is undercut (Daniels 1990). But our theoretical question about residual health inequalities reminds us that the theory says too little about the construction of the index to provide us with a clear answer to it.

One of Rawls's central arguments for singling out a principle protecting equal basic liberties and giving it (lexical) priority over his other principles of justice is his claim that once people achieve some threshold level of material well-being, they would not trade away the fundamental importance of liberty for other goods (Rawls 1971). Making such a trade might deny them the liberty to pursue their most cherished ideals, including their religious beliefs, whatever they turn out to be. Can we make the same argument about trading health for other goods?

There is some plausibility to the claim that rational people should refrain from similar trades of health for other goods. Loss of health may preclude us from pursuing what we most value in life. We do, after all, see people willing to trade almost anything to regain health once they lose it.

If we take this argument seriously, we might conclude that Rawls should give opportunity, including the effects of health status, a heavier weighting in the construction of the index than income alone.[6] Such a weighting would mean that absolute increases in income for that might otherwise have justified increasing relative income inequality, according to the Difference Principle, now fail to justify those inequalities because of the negative effects on opportunity. Although income of the worst off would increase, they are not better off according to the whole (weighted) index of primary social goods, and so the greater inequality is not permitted. Rawls's simplifying assumption about income correlating with other goods fails in this case (as it did in the hypothetical example about workplace democracy cited earlier).

---

[6] Rawls does suggest that since fair equality of opportunity is given priority over the Difference Principle, that within the index, we can assume opportunity has a heavier weighting: Rawls (1971), *Theory of Justice*. Cambridge, MA: Harvard University Press, 93.

Nevertheless, there is also strong reason to think the priority given to health and thus opportunity is not as clear-cut as the previous argument implies, especially where the trade is between a *risk* to health and other goods that people highly value. Refusing to allow any (*ex ante*) trades of health risks for other goods, even when the background conditions on choice are otherwise fair, may seem unjustifiably paternalistic, perhaps in a way that refusals to allow trades of basic liberties is not.

We propose a pragmatic route around this problem, one that has a precedent elsewhere in Rawls. Fair equality opportunity, Rawls admits, is only approximated even in an ideally just system, because we can only mitigate, not eliminate, the effects of family and other social contingencies (Fishkin 1983). For example, only if we were willing to violate widely respected parental liberties could we intrude into family life and 'rescue' children from parental values that arguably interfere with equal opportunity. Similarly, though we give a general priority to equal opportunity over the Difference Principle, we cannot achieve complete equality in health any more than we can achieve completely equal opportunity. Even ideal theory does not produce perfect justice. Justice is always rough around the edges. Specifically, if we had good reason to think that 'democratic equality' had flattened inequalities in accord with the principles of justice, then we might be inclined to think we had done as much as was reasonable to make health inequalities fair to all. The residual inequalities that emerge with conformance to the principles are not a 'compromise' with what justice ideally requires; they are acceptable as just.

4.4.7. *Can legislators trade health for other goods?*

So far, we have been considering whether the theoretical question can be resolved from the perspective of individual contractors. Instead, suppose that the decision about such a trade-off is to be made through the legislature in a society that conforms to Rawls's principles. Because those principles require effective political participation across all socio-economic groups, we can suppose that groups most directly affected by any trade-off decision have a voice in the decision. Since there is a residual health *gradient*, groups affected by the trade-off include not only the worst off, but those in the middle as well. A democratic process that involved deliberation about the trade-off and its effects might be the best we could do to provide a resolution of the unanswered theoretical question (Daniels and Sabin 1997).

In contrast, where the fair value of political participation is not adequately assured—and we doubt it is so assured in even our most democratic societies—we have much less confidence in the fairness of a democratic decision about how to trade health against other goods. It is much more likely under actual conditions that those who benefit most from the inequalities, that is, those who are better off, also wield disproportionate political power and will influence decisions about trade-offs to serve their interests. It may still be that the use of a democratic process in non-ideal conditions is the fairest resolution we can practically achieve, but it still falls well short of what an ideally just democratic process involves.

4.4.8. *An objection to our approach and a remark about generalizability*

Does our approach involve redundancy in the following way? Daniels's extension of Rawls's equal opportunity principle to cover health care implies that we should view as 'health care needs' whatever is involved in the promotion of normal functioning. This implies that an appropriate distribution of the social determinants is already captured as a prerequisite for fair equality of opportunity. Why invoke the rest of Rawls's principles? Are they needed?

If we used the equal opportunity principle alone to force the proper distribution of social determinants, our theory would be narrowly based on the importance of health care to well-being. What is particularly interesting about seeing *all* of Rawls's principles as *together* requiring a fair distribution of the social determinants is that they do so somewhat independently of what we think about health and its impact on well-being. They are focused on well-being much more broadly construed, and the rationale for them does not depend so directly on a special view about the importance of health care. What we have is an important convergence, not a mere redundancy.

To see that this convergence is empirically and philosophically interesting, consider what would happen if the social determinants of health had the opposite effect to the one we document in this discussion. Suppose—what is empirically possible—that conformance with the principles of justice made our health worse. There would then be true tension between the fair equality of opportunity principle account of the importance of health and health care and the way in which Rawls's principles distribute the social determinants of (poor) health. Two aspects of well-being would have pulled in opposite directions. That they pull together in this world makes the convergence interesting and not a mere redundancy.

The answer to the objection about redundancy is thus connected to a suggestion we made in Section 4.1, namely that extension of Rawls theory to address questions about fair distribution of the social determinants of health shows the theory is generalizable in fruitful ways, and that this generalizability is analogous to the increase in scope and power of a non-moral theory we discover can explain phenomena beyond the domain for which its laws were initially developed. What exactly is the analogy?

When an empirical theory turns out to explain new phenomena that were not part of the evidentiary base for its laws, we tend to conclude that the concepts incorporated in it are 'projectable' in a desired way. We may think of them as better confirmed as a way of dividing up or describing the world. In Rawls's case, he began with certain political concepts thought crucial to our well-being—to meeting our needs as free and equal citizens of a democracy. Using these ideas, the goal was to select terms of cooperation that all free and equal citizens could agree are fair and reasonable. It then turns out, given the social science literature, that the aspects of well-being captured by these ideas expand to include the health of the population as well. Whatever controversy might have been thought to surround some of these political components of well-being, they do connect—albeit empirically—to some incontrovertibly objective components of our social well-being, namely, the health of the population. If this were an empirical rather than normative theory, we would think the evidence of projectibility counted in its favor and constituted support for the theory. Is there additional 'support' for Rawls's theory?

One view is that there is not. If the facts about population health turned out to be different, so that socio-economic inequality did not produce the health gradients we observe, then we would not be inclined to say there was less support for Rawls political theory. We would, properly on this view, say that these kinds of facts should not matter in this way to the support given the theory. The proponent of this view might still say that the theory has the resources to respond to the actual facts, and it can answer questions it was not originally designed to answer. But there is no extra support here because if the facts were different we would not have subtracted support from the theory.

There is another way to view the situation. True, we might not subtract from the support we now give the theory if the facts were different about the relationship between socio-economic inequality and health. But that does not mean we should not add to the support we think the theory has if it turns out to have the projectibility described earlier. A lack of evidence of greater projectibility is not evidence against a theory; it is and should be a neutral finding. If, however, we found that population health were undermined by greater political well-being of the sort the original theory talked about (before its extension), then we would have a puzzle to address. Why is one aspect of our well-being working in opposition to other elements of it?

This discussion is admittedly too brief to establish a firm conclusion, but we are inclined to think there is some corroborative support for Rawls's theory from the fact that it generalizes to the phenomena of population health in this way.

4.5. RAWLS VERSUS ALTERNATIVES

We have focused on Rawlsian theory because it provides, however fortuitously, a developed account of how to distributive the social determinants of health. Since the publication of *Theory of Justice*, there has been an extensive literature on egalitarianism proposing alternatives to Rawls's view. A number of the philosophers responding to Rawls have suggested that a basic question in distributive justice is, equality of what? Rawls's answer—equality with respect to primary social goods—focuses on the wrong space. We should instead focus on other answers, such as equal opportunity for welfare or advantage (Arneson 1988; G.A. Cohen 1989), or equality of capabilities or positive freedom (Sen 1980, 1992). We offer only a few brief remarks on these alternatives here and refer the reader to a more detailed discussion by one of us (Daniels 2003).

One alternative view to Rawls's picks up on an intuitive line of argument Rawls offers for his Fair Equality of Opportunity and Difference Principles. Rawls argues that we view certain social and natural contingencies as morally arbitrary and seek principles of justice that nullify their effect. The alternative view takes Rawls' idea to an extreme, which may go beyond what Rawls would accept. In this view, we are owed compensation for any inequality of opportunity for welfare or advantage that derives through no fault or choice of our own. Theories that focus, as these do, on a distinction between 'brute' luck (results of the social and natural lottery that do not depend in any way on our choices) and 'option' luck (the consequences of things we choose or are responsible for choosing) need a developed account of just when we are responsible for things that happen (Roemer 1998).

One important difference between these accounts and Rawls's is that Rawls's principles provide for our 'needs' as free and equal citizens regardless of the reasons for the deficit we suffer (Anderson 1999). We can imagine very bad 'option luck' leaving us without adequate opportunity or worth of political liberty, but these theories fail to meet our needs as citizens if we are 'responsible' for having these needs. A further problem with these theories is that they focus primarily on issues of equality in the distribution of some domain of goods without attending to the full scope of what is involved in a theory of justice, namely the need to integrate concerns about equality, liberty, and efficiency (Buchanan et al. 2000). They purport to give us an answer to the question 'what does justice require with regard to equality?' that stands independently, perhaps as an ideal that can then be compromised, from whatever happens when we integrate our concerns about equality with those about liberty and efficiency. In contrast, Rawls is content to mitigate the moral arbitrariness of natural and social contingencies through the operation of his principles without viewing the result as a compromise with what justice ideally requires.

Sen has also argued that Rawls's theory, with its proposal that we measure inequalities by reference to an index of primary social goods, is operating in the wrong 'space'. Sen, who agrees with Rawls (and disagrees with Arneson 1988 and Cohen 1989) in avoiding measures of well-being that are focused on experience, such as welfare or satisfaction, claimed (in his early papers on this topic) that Rawls's index is 'fetishist' because it ignores the ways in which such variations as disease, disability, and nutritional needs might lead, with the same inputs of primary social goods, to the development of very different *capabilities* or 'positive freedom', the freedom to do or be what we wish.

There is much more convergence between Sen's approach and Rawls's than there might seem to be given the debate about 'equality of what?' First, Sen is aware that concerns about equality with regard to positive freedom must be integrated with considerations of liberty and equality, though he does not say much about how that is to be done. Second, if we actually take the cases where we can agree that the capabilities of some people are clearly worse than those of others, we are likely to find ourselves talking about clear instances of disease and disability. In that case, the extension we have made of Rawls's theory, incorporating normal functioning within opportunity, captures the most important points of divergence between Sen's view and Rawls's view as originally stated.[7] Many other differences in capabilities between people will be 'incommensurable' on Sen's view because people will disagree about how to rank those differences. Third, if we focus Sen's account on the capabilities needed for democratic citizenship, as Anderson (1999) has done in an imaginative discussion, then the convergence between Rawls and Sen is quite apparent. Both talk about 'democratic equality' and the capabilities needed for free and equal citizenship. Rawls has provided more of the principles and institutional framework for thinking about it; Sen has focused on the importance of the capabilities of such citizens.[8]

4.6. IMPLICATIONS FOR A JUST DISTRIBUTION OF THE SOCIAL DETERMINANTS OF HEALTH

We earlier suggested that the Whitehead/Dahlgren analysis of health inequities (inequalities that are avoidable and unfair) is useful, provided that we can agree on what counts as avoidable and unfair. We then suggested that the Rawlsian account of justice as fairness provides a fuller account of what is fair and unfair in the distribution of the social determinants of health. The theory provides a more systematic way to think about which health inequalities are inequities.

Compared to that ideal, most health inequalities that we now observe world wide among socio-economic and racial or ethnic groups are 'inequities' that should be remedied. Even some countries with the shallowest health gradients, such as Sweden and England, have viewed their own health inequalities as unacceptable and initiated policy measures to mitigate them. Clearly, the broader World Health Organization efforts in this direction are, probably without exception, also aimed at true inequities.

[7] Norman Daniels (1990). 'Equality of What? Welfare, Resources, or Capabilities?' *Philosophy and Phenomenological Research* 50 (Fall) Suppl.: 273–96, reprinted in Norman Daniels (1996b). *Justice and Justification: Reflective Equilibrium in Theory and Practice*, chapter 10. New York: Cambridge University Press. See also Allen Buchanan, Dan Brock, Norman Daniels, Daniel Wikler (2000). *From Chance to Choice: Genetics and Justice*, chapter 4. Cambridge: Cambridge University Press.

[8] Sen has stated in a seminar at Harvard Center for Population Studies that there is more overlap between his views and Rawls's than he at first emphasised. See also, Norman Daniels (2003). 'Democratic Equality: Rawls's Complex Egalitarianism', in Samuel Freeman (ed.), *Cambridge Companion to Rawls*. Cambridge: Cambridge University Press.

A central policy implication of our discussion is that reform efforts to improve health inequalities must be intersectoral and not just focused on the traditional health sector. Health is produced not just by having access to medical prevention and treatment but, to a measurably greater extent, by the cumulative experience of social conditions across the life course. In other words, by the time a 60-year-old patient presents to the emergency room with a heart attack to receive medical treatment, that encounter represents the result of bodily insults that accumulated over a lifetime. Medical care is, figuratively speaking, 'the ambulance waiting at the bottom of the cliff'. Much of the contemporary discussion about increasing access to medical care as a means of reducing health inequalities misses this point. An emphasis on intersectoral reform will recognize the primacy of social conditions, such as access to basic education, levels of material deprivation, a healthy workplace environment, and equality of political participation in determining the health achievement of societies (Lavis and Stoddart 1994).

A focus on intersectoral reform does not imply that we should ignore medical services and health sector reform because other steps have a bigger pay-off. Even if we had a highly just distribution of the social determinants of health and of public health measures, people will still become ill and need medical services. The fair design of a health system arguably should give some extra weight to meeting actual medical needs. Even if some moral theories would require that we be 'impartial' between identified victims, who are already sick, and 'statistical' victims, who may become sick, there are still 'agent-relative' considerations that give providers, family members, friends, and even current fellow citizens obligations to help those they are in a position to help, even if that sacrifices some impartiality.

What sorts of social policies should governments pursue in order to reduce health inequalities? Certainly, the menu of options should include equalising access to medical care, but it should also include a broader set of policies aimed at equalising individual life opportunities, such as investment in basic education, affordable housing, income security, and other forms of antipoverty policy. Though the connection between these broad social policies and health may seem somewhat remote, and they are rarely linked to issues of health in our public policy discussions, growing evidence suggests that they should be so linked. The kinds of policies suggested by a social determinants perspective encompasses a much broader range of instruments than would be ordinarily considered for improving the health of the population.

Our discussion also has implications for international development theory, as well as for economic choices confronted by industrialised countries. To the extent that the income distribution matters for population health status, it is not obvious that giving strict priority to economic growth is the optimal strategy for maximising social welfare. Raising everyone's income will improve the health status of the poor (the trickle-down approach), but not as much as by paying attention to the *distribution* of the social product. Within the developing world, a comparison of the province of Kerala in India with more unequal countries like Brazil and South Africa illustrates this point. Despite having only one-third to a quarter of the income of Brazil or South Africa (and thereby having a higher prevalence of poverty in the absolute sense), the citizens of Kerala nonetheless live longer, most likely as a result of the higher priority that the government of Kerala accords to a fair distribution of economic gains (Sen 1998).

The real issue for developing countries is what *kind* of economic growth is salutary. Hence, Dreze and Sen (1989) distinguish between two types of successes in the rapid reduction of mortality, which they term 'growth mediated' and 'support-led' processes. The former works mainly *through* fast economic growth, exemplified by mortality reductions in countries like South Korea or Hong Kong. Their successes depended on the growth process being wide-based and participatory (e.g. full employment policies), and on the gains from economic growth being utilised to expand relevant social services in the public sector, particularly health care and education. Their experience stands in stark contrast to the example of countries like Brazil, which have similarly achieved rapid economic growth, but lagged behind in health improvements.

In contrast to growth-mediated processes, 'support-led' processes operate not through fast economic growth, but through governments giving high priority to the provision of social services that reduce mortality and enhance the quality of life. Examples of such countries include China, Costa Rica, and the Indian state of Kerala already mentioned above.

A similar choice between policies emphasising growth versus more equality applies to developed nations as well. Application of the Rawlsian difference principle suggests that a society like the United States has much room to move towards a more equitable (perhaps a more European) distribution of its national income without suffering a loss in productivity or growth. At the same time it would benefit from a gain in the health status of its citizens.

References

Acheson, D. et al. (1998). *Report of the Independent Inquiry into Inequalities in Health*. London: Stationery Office.

Adler N. E., T. Boyce, M. A. Chesney, S. Cohen, S. Folkman, R. I. Kahn, and S. L. Syme (1994). 'Socio-Economic Status and Health: The Challenge of the Gradient', *American Psychologist*, 49: 15–24.

Anderson E. (1999). 'What is the Point of Equality?', *Ethics*, 109: 287–337.

Arneson R. J. (1988). 'Equality and Equal Opportunity for Welfare', *Philosophical Studies*, 54: 79–95.

Arrow K. (1973). 'Some Ordinalist-Utilitarian Notes on Rawls's Theory of Justice', *Journal of Philosophy*, 70: 253 ff.

Barker D. (1998). *Mothers, Babies and Health in Later Life*. Edinburgh: Churchill Livingstone.

Bartley M., D. Blane, and S. Montgomery (1997). 'Socio-Economic Determinants of Health: Health and the Life Course: Why Safety Nets Matter?', *British Medical Journal*, 314: 1194.

Benzeval M., K. Judge, and M. Whitehead (eds.) (1995). *Tackling Inequalities in Health: An Agenda for Action*. London: Kings Fund.

Black D., J. N. Morris, C. Smith, P. Townsend, and M. Whitehead (1988). *Inequalities in Health: The Black Report; The Health Divide*. London: Penguin Group.

Braveman P. (1999). *Monitoring Equity In Health: A Policy-Oriented Approach in Low- and Middle-Income Countries*. Geneva: World Health Organization.

Buchanan A., D. Brock, N. Daniels, and D. Wikler (2000). *From Chance to Choice: Genetics and the Just Society*. New York: Cambridge University Press.

Cohen G. A. (1989). 'On the Currency of Egalitarian Justice', *Ethics*. 99: 906–44.

Cohen J. (1989). 'Democratic Equality', *Ethics*, 99: 727–51.

—— 'The Pareto Argument' unpublished ms, ND.

Dahlgren G. and M. Whitehead (1991). *Policies and Strategies to Promote Social Equity in Health*. Stockholm: Institute of Future Studies.

Daniels N. (1979). 'Wide Reflective Equilibrium and Theory Acceptance in Ethics', *Journal of Philosophy*, 76: 256–82.

—— (1981). 'Health-Care Needs and Distributive Justice', *Philosophy and Public Affairs*, 10: 146–79.

—— (1985). *Just Health Care*. New York: Cambridge University Press.

—— (1990). 'Equality of What: Welfare, Resources, or Capabilities?', *Philosophy and Phenomenological Research*, 50 (Suppl.): 273–96.

—— (1996a). 'Mental Disabilities, Equal Opportunity and the ADA', in R. J. Bonnie, and J. Monahan (eds.), *Mental Disorder, Work Disability, and the Law*. Chicago: University of Chicago Press, 282–97.

—— (1996b). *Justice and Justification: Reflective Equilibrium in Theory and Practice*. New York: Cambridge University Press.

—— (2003). 'Democratic Equality: Rawls's Complex Egalitarianism', in Samuel Freeman (ed.), *Cambridge Companion to Rawls*. Cambridge: Cambridge University Press, 241–77.

—— D. Light, and R. Caplan (1996). *Benchmarks of Fairness for Health Care Reform*. New York: Oxford University Press.

—— and J. E. Sabin (1997). 'Limits to Health Care: Fair Procedures, Democratic Deliberation, and the Legitimacy Problem for Insurers', *Philosophy and Public Affairs*, 26: 303–50.

Davey Smith G., M. J. Shipley, and G. Rose (1990). 'Magnitude and Causes of Socioeconomic Differentials in Mortality: Further Evidence from the Whitehall Study', *Journal of Epidemiology and Community Health*, 44: 265–70.

—— C. Hart, D. Blane, and D. Hole (1998). 'Adverse Socio-Economic Conditions in Childhood and Cause Specific Adult Mortality: A Prospective Observational Study?', *British Medical Journal*, 316: 1631–5.

Deaton A. and D. Lubotsky (2003). 'Mortality, inequality and race in American cities and states'. *Social Science and Medicine*, 56: 1139–53.

Dreze J. and A. K. Sen (1989). *Hunger and Public Action*. Oxford: Clarendon Press.

Fishkin J. (1983). *Justice, Equal Opportunity, and the Family*. New Haven, CT: Yale University Press.

Gutmann A. and D. Thompson (1995). *Democratic Disagreement*. Cambridge: Harvard University Press.

Kaplan G. A., E. R. Pamuk, J. W. Lynch, R. D. Cohen, and J. L. Balfour (1996). 'Inequality in Income and Mortality in the United States: Analysis of Mortality and Potential Pathways', *British Medical Journal*, 312: 999–1003.

Kawachi I. and B. P. Kennedy (1997). 'Health and Social Cohesion: Why Care about Income Inequality?', *British Medical Journal*, 314: 1037–40.

——, ——, K. Lochner, and D. Prothrow-Stith (1997). 'Social Capital, Income Inequality and Mortality', *American Journal of Public Health*, 87: 1491–8.

——, ——, D. Prothrow-Stith, and V. Gupta (1999). 'Women's Status and the Health of Women: A View from the States', *Social Science and Medicine*, 48: 21–32.

—— and —— (1999). 'Income Inequality and Health: Pathways and Mechanisms', *Health Services Research*, 34: 215–27.

Kawachi I., B. P. Kennedy, and R. Wilkinson (eds.) (1999). *Income Inequality and Health: A Reader*. New York: The New Press.

Kennedy B. P., I. Kawachi, R. Glass, and D. Prothrow-Stith (1998a). 'Income distribution, Socio-Economic Status, and Self-Rated Health: A US Multi-Level Analysis', *British Medical Journal*, 317: 917–21.

——, ——, D. Prothrow-Stith, and V. Gupta (1998b). 'Income Inequality, Social Capital and Firearm-Related Violent Crime', *Social Science and Medicine*, 47: 7–17.

Lavis J. N. and G. L. Stoddart (1994). 'Can We Have too Much Health Care?' *Daedalus*, 123: 43–60.

Link B. G., M. E. Northridge, J. C. Phelan, and M. L. Ganz (1998). 'Social Epidemiology and the Fundamental Cause Concept: On the Structuring of Effective Cancer Screens by Socio-economic Status', *Milbank Quarterly*, 76: 375–402.

Lochner K. (1999). *State Income Inequality And Individual Mortality Risk: A Prospective Multilevel Study*. Ph.D. thesis, Harvard University 1999.

Lynch, J. W., G. A. Kaplan, E. R. Pamuk, R. D. Cohen, J. L. Balfour, and I. H. Yen (1998). 'Income Inequality and Mortality in Metropolitan Areas of the United States', *American Journal of Public Health*, 88: 1074–80.

Marchand S., D. Wikler, and B. Landesman (1998). 'Class, Health, and Justice', *Milbank Quarterly*, 76: 449–68.

Marmot M. (1994). 'Social Differentials in Health Within and Between Populations', *Daedalus*, 123: 197–216.

—— (1999). 'Social Causes of Social Inequalities in Health', Harvard Center for Population and Development Studies, Working Paper Series 99.01, January.

Marmot M. G., H. Bosma, H. Hemingway, E. Brunner, and S. Stansfield (1997). 'Contributions of Job Control and other Risk Factors to Social Variations in Coronary Heart Disease Incidence', *Lancet*, 350: 235–9.

Mellor J, and J. Milyo (2002) 'Is Exposure to Income Inequality a Public Health Concern? Lagged Effects of Income Inequality in Individual and Population Health', *Health Services Research*, 38(1): 137–51.

Pappas G., S. Queen, and G. Fisher (1993). 'The Increasing Disparity in Mortality Between Socioeconomic Groups in the United States', 1960 and 1986', *New England Journal of Medicine*, 329: 103–9.

Rawls J. (1971). *A Theory of Justice*. Cambridge MA: Harvard University Press.

—— (1993). *Political Liberalism*. New York: Columbia University Press.

Roemer J. (1998). *Equality of Opportunity*. Cambridge, MA: Harvard University Press.

Sen A. K. (1980). 'Equality of what?', in S. McMurrin (ed.), *Tanner Lectures on Human Values*, Vol 1. Cambridge: Cambridge University Press.

—— (1992). *Inequality Re-examined*. Cambridge MA: Harvard University Press.

—— (1998). 'Mortality as an Indicator of Economic Success and Failure', *The Economic Journal*, 108: 1–25.

—— (1999). *Development as Freedom*. New York: Alfred A. Knopf.

Subramanian, S. V., and I. Kawachi (2003). 'The association between state income inequality and worse health is not confounded by race', *International Journal of Epidemiology*, 32: 1022–8.

——, I. Delgado, L. Jadue, J. Vega, and I. Kawachi (2003). 'Income inequality and health: multilevel analysis of Chilean communities', *Journal of Epidemiology and Community Health*, 57: 844–8.

Villerme L. (1840). *Tableau d'Etat Physique et Moral des Ouvriers*, Vol 2. Paris: Renourard.

Whitehead M. (1992). 'The Concepts and Principles of Equity and Health', *International Journal of Health Services*, 22: 429–45.

Wikler D. (1978). 'Persuasion and Coercion for Health: Issues in Government Efforts to Change Life Style', *Milbank Quarterly*, 56: 303–38.

Wilkinson R. G. (1992). 'Income Distribution and Life Expectancy', *British Medical Journal*, 304: 165–8.

—— (1994). 'The Epidemiological Transition: From Material Scarcity to Social Disadvantage?' *Daedalus*, 123: 61–77.

—— (1996). *Unhealthy Societies: The Afflictions of Inequality*. London: Routledge.

—— I. Kawachi, and B. Kennedy (1998). 'Mortality, the Social Environment, Crime and Violence', *Sociology of Health and Illness*, 20(5): 578–97.

—— B. P. Kennedy, and I. Kawachi (1999). 'Women's Status and Men's Health in a Culture of Inequality', *Sociology of Health and Illness*, forthcoming.

5

Health Equity and Social Justice

FABIENNE PETER

5.1. INTRODUCTION

There is consistent and strong empirical evidence for social inequalities in health, as a vast and fast growing literature shows. Social inequalities in health are significant variations in health outcomes (as measured by life expectancy at birth, infant mortality, morbidity, etc.) across different social groups. Typically, the lower a group's social position, the worse the average health status of its members (e.g. Marmot et al. 1978; Black et al. 1990; Krieger et al. 1993; Gwatkin and Guillot 2000). Gender, race, social class, occupational status, and socio-geographic location are examples of social categories that define social groups. More recently, a new set of studies has emerged that focuses on the relationship between income inequality and population health. Though still contested, the findings suggest that the more unequal a society, the worse its achievements in (aggregate) health (Wilkinson 1996; Kawachi et al. 1999).

Explanations for the occurrence of social inequalities in health are manifold and often difficult to establish.[1] The principal upshot of these studies is that one explanation that seems at first plausible, namely differences in access to health care, does not get us very far. Access to health care is only one social factor among others that influences people's health. The goal of empirical studies of social inequalities in health is to understand *social determinants* of health, and, increasingly, to explain the *mechanisms* or *pathways* that lead to the observed social differences in health outcomes. The latter is accompanied by a renewed interest in the social sciences and a move towards more inter-disciplinary analysis of the social processes underlying inequalities in health (e.g. Berkman et al. 2000).

This development is often labelled a 'new public health', but, as for example Ann Robertson (1998: 1419) stresses, '[m]any would argue that this is not so much a new public health as a return to the historical commitments of public

I have benefited from so many people, that it is impossible to acknowledge everybody. But I would like to thank the people in the Global Health Equity Initiative which have made me start thinking about these issues; I am particularly grateful to Ben Amick, Sudhir Anand, and Tim Evans. I would also like to thank Sissela Bok, Norman Daniels, and Dan Wikler for very helpful comments.

[1] For a good review, see Marmot et al. (1995).

health to social justice'.[2] In the public health field, the concern with health equity and social justice is recognised as having a normative dimension, that is, as involving value judgements in an explicit way. According to the frequently quoted definition by Margaret Whitehead, health inequities are 'differences [in health] which are unnecessary and unavoidable but, in addition, are also considered unfair and unjust' (Whitehead 1990: 5). While it points in the right direction, this definition leaves open how we should go about making judgements of unfairness and injustice. The problem a theory of health equity faces is, therefore, how to go from the *empirical* identification of *social inequalities* in health to a *normative* judgement about *health inequities*. What is needed is a framework within which the ethical issues raised by the empirical literature can be addressed and which helps determining which inequalities in health outcomes are unjust.

Until recently, there has been little work in ethics and political philosophy that deals with these issues. General theories of justice, such as John Rawls' theory of justice as fairness (Rawls 1971), often do not address health specifically. In bioethics, efforts have tended to concentrate on access to *health care*.[3] There are, of course, good reasons for focusing on health care. The premise for any theory of justice is that there is some good that can be (re)distributed, that something can be changed about the situation that is considered unjust. If, in the context of health, the allocation of health care is perceived to be the instrument that is best suited to correct health outcomes, then conceptions of equity will concentrate on health care—not health. Furthermore, we may regard people's access to health care as being important in and of itself, independently of its contribution to an equitable distribution of health outcomes.[4] If, however, we are concerned not just with health care but also with health outcomes, and if there are serious social inequalities in health outcomes that cannot be traced back to differential access to health care, then conceptions of health equity have to go beyond health care.

The situation has started to change and a literature on public health ethics is emerging (Pereira 1993; Marchand et al. 1998; Beauchamp and Steinbock 1999; Daniels et al., in Chapter 4, this volume). This chapter seeks to contribute to this literature by putting forward a theoretical framework for making health equity judgements.

The paper defends what I call an *indirect* approach. I call an approach *direct* if it isolates health from other social spheres and is defined with respect to particular distributions of health outcomes—most existing approaches to health equity, as I shall explain later, are direct. An indirect approach, in contrast, is based on the premise that social inequalities in health are wrong not simply because actual health outcomes deviate from some pattern of health outcomes

---

[2] On this, see also Krieger and Birn (1998).

[3] An authoritative work on justice in health care is Daniels (1985).

[4] As Poland et al. (1998) have stressed, the population health perspective should not be read as implying that health care is not important.

that is considered ideal, but rather because, and insofar as, they are the expression and product of unjust economic, social, and political institutions. It thus embeds the pursuit of health equity in the pursuit of social justice in general. In addition, the approach I shall present also stresses the reverse relationship between inequalities in health and social justice: an understanding of social inequalities in health and the mechanisms by which they are produced, may reveal something important about how the institutions of society work and may hence inform our assessment of the justice of these institutions. The emphasis placed on the larger social processes that bring about social inequalities in health is in line with the development in public health research to focus more on the 'upstream' influences on people's possibilities to be healthy.[5]

The approach I shall present is based on Rawls' theory of justice as fairness (Rawls 1971), in particular as it is presented in his later book *Political Liberalism* (1993). Although Rawls has not himself addressed the topic of health, I shall argue that the conception of justice as fairness provides a useful framework for evaluating social inequalities in health.

I shall elaborate on the distinction between direct and indirect approaches to health equity in Section 5.3 and will highlight some important concepts of Rawls' theory of justice as fairness in Section 5.4. Section 5.5 synthesizes the previous two sections to a framework for health equity analysis. Before pursuing further the question of how to make health equity judgements, it will be important to discuss the notion of health itself—this is the subject of the next section.

5.2. HEALTH

What makes thinking about health equity difficult from the outset is that the concept of health itself is not easy to grasp and varies considerably across places and times. Although general observations can be made with respect to the meaningfulness of different definitions of health, it is likely that their adequacy will vary with the context in which we refer to it.

As, for example, the authors of the Black Report stress, a relationship between health and society is present not only at the level of social inequalities in health but already at the level of health itself (Black et al. 1990: chapter 3). They argue that the medical profession's approach to health is only one among others, and its partiality may impede finding solutions to pressing health problems. Instead of the 'medical model', they advocate a 'social model' of health—grounded in the social sciences. They suggest that the role of social studies of health problems should be 'in part, to increase understanding of the social and socio-economic factors which play a part in the promotion of health and

---

[5] An editorial in *The Lancet* (1994: 429), for example, stresses that '[t]here is a need to move away from the almost exclusive focus of research on individual risk, towards the social structures and processes within which ill health originates, and which will often be more amenable to modification.' See also the contributions in Amick et al. (1995).

the causation of disease and in part to take the natural next step and relate these factors themselves to the broader social structure' (Black et al. 1990: 36). A general criticism of the medical model is that it directs too much attention to diseases and their remedy. There is thus a danger of losing sight of such issues as why good health is important for people, what good health means to them, and what the broader social context is in which the pursuit of health and the response to disease are shaped.[6] In some sense, the WHO definition, according to which 'health is a state of complete physical, mental and social well-being and not merely the absence of disease or infirmity' (WHO 1976: 1), and quality-of-life approaches to health can be read as a reaction against this paradigm.[7] A definition of health as extensive as the one by WHO runs into problems of its own, however. It is not clear in what ways health is distinct from other components of well-being. The definition thus does not allow for the possibility that (some) well-being might be achieved while health is bad, or that health might be good yet well-being low. It is also not clear how well-being can be defined in a way that is consistent with a plurality of conceptions of the good life—a characteristic of modern democratic societies. A further objection to the WHO definition is that such a broad conception of health bears the danger of overly medicalising social problems.[8] As Vincanne Adams (1998: 6) writes in a related context, it may treat the social pursuit of health 'as a technical problem with technical solutions, rather than a political problem with a political solution'.[9]

Amartya Sen's capability approach offers a fruitful alternative for assessing health problems in society.[10] The idea underlying the capability approach is that in policy evaluation, the appropriate information is not individual utility or well-being, nor the resources people have access to (e.g. medical care), but something in between. Sen argues that what matters is what people can *do* with the resources they have access to—a notion of freedom. A person's capability tries to capture that. Capability is the set of 'functionings'—the various 'doings and beings'—that a person can achieve (but may decide not to). Examples of functionings are being adequately nourished, being able to read, or, more complex, achieving self-respect. Sen often cites good health

[6] René Lériche (1937) wrote: 'in disease, when all is said and done, the least important thing is man' (quoted in Canguilhem 1991: 92). Critical medical anthropology in particular examines the meaning of illness for people. See, for example, Kleinman (1988); Corin (1995); Frank (1995). See also Foucault (1973) for an account of the development of the biomedical model and its political context.

[7] Brock (1993) discusses the switch that has taken place in the public policy context from the biomedical model to a quality-of-life approach for evaluating health and the implications thereof for social evaluation in general.

[8] Engelhardt (1986: 157) writes: 'Medicine medicalizes reality. It translates sets of problems into its own terms. Medicine molds the ways in which the world of experience takes shape; it conditions reality for us'. A few pages below he adds (ibid. 163): 'Seeing an element of life as a medical problem raises more than issues of scientific medicine. The medicalization of reality raises issues of public policy and of ethics.'   [9] Das (n.d.) makes a similar point.

[10] Sen (1993) provides a good overview of the capability approach.

as an example of a functioning (e.g. Sen 1993: 31). It may, however, be more promising to see health as a capability of its own, or, more precisely, as a subset of a person's capability. The idea is that health itself is composed of several functionings—such as, for example, being able to move around, not being tired, etc.

Sen leaves it largely open which functionings should be included when assessing a particular social situation. What is more, he stresses that in each case, this will require a process of selecting the relevant functionings and weighing their relative importance.[11] Seeing health as a capability (subset) in this way thus accommodates the insight that defining a concept of health is a process that involves value judgements and which is potentially subject to political contestation—an issue that has just recently been stressed by Robertson in her paper on the 'politics of need' and its implications for public health (Robertson 1998). It recognises that defining health and determining what counts as a health problem and what as another type of social problem is not a task that can be resolved by health specialists alone, but depends on other aspects of social institutions, and may change over time. Medicine and public health can contribute to the resolution of certain social problems, but they cannot, by themselves, determine goals and priorities for individuals and for society as a whole.

5.3. FOR WHAT SAKE HEALTH EQUITY?

Returning to the main subject of this paper, namely to the question of how to assess the justice or injustice of social inequalities in health, let me start by discussing the distinction between direct and indirect approaches to health equity. A direct approach sees health equity as an end in itself.[12] This is to say that the goal is to achieve justice with respect to the distribution of health outcomes, independently of, but in parallel with, justice in other spheres, such as, for example, income or education.

To give an example of a direct approach, it is sometimes assumed that what is disturbing about social inequalities in health is that the health of the population *overall* is lower than it could be. The 'Black Report', for example, uses this language.[13] Such an approach is informed by the utilitarian principle of maximising overall well-being—in our case the health of the population. Utilitarianism is, however, often criticised for being blind to distributive considerations.[14] In the case of population health, a maximising approach implies that we are indifferent between health benefits to, say, the poor and to the rich, as long as these benefits have the same impact on overall population health.

---

[11] In contrast to Sen, Nussbaum (1992) argues for a specific set of capabilities.

[12] For a good review of such approaches, see Marchand et al. (1998).

[13] I owe this point to Marchand et al. (1998).

[14] A critique of utilitarianism can be found in Rawls (1971: 22–33); Rawls formulated his theory of justice as fairness as an alternative to utilitarianism. See also Williams (1973a).

More explicitly concerned with equity are principles of *specific egalitarianism*—another family of direct approaches to health equity.[15] Egalitarian principles recognise that equality of health outcomes is hardly obtainable, but postulate it as a goal that we should strive for insofar as possible. For the bioethicist Robert Veatch (1991: 83), for example, egalitarianism in the context of health encompasses "any number of closely related positions that among other things include the moral rule that justice requires that persons be given an opportunity to have equal net welfare insofar as possible and that, applied to health care, *justice requires that persons be given an opportunity to have equal health status insofar as possible*" (emphasis added).

Whitehead seems to be defending an approach of that kind when she writes that health equity is 'concerned with creating equal opportunities for health and with bringing health differentials down to the lowest level possible' (Whitehead 1990: 9). Davidson Gwatkin (2000), finally, articulates a third possible approach to health equity by suggesting that we should focus primarily on the health of the poor. This view is akin to what is known as the 'priority view' in moral philosophy. It is articulated by Derek Parfit (1997) and put forward as an alternative to egalitarianism. Parfit argues that our moral concern should not be with differences in and of themselves, but rather with absolute deprivation. Improving the lot of those who suffer most will yield the greatest gain in social utility or well-being. The priority view is thus a variant of utilitarianism. Adapted to health equity—and given the premise that there is a link between health and poverty—this approach would imply giving priority to improving the health of the poor.[16]

In spite of the many differences, what characterises such direct approaches is that a situation is judged inequitable if the health status of the population differs from what is perceived to be the ideal—whether judged by a measure of aggregate population health or by a measure that is sensitive to the distribution of health outcomes (or a combined measure).

An indirect approach, in contrast, treats the pursuit of health equity as embedded in and interlinked with the pursuit of social justice. Let me explain the idea in more detail.

There are two forms of potential interlinkage between social inequalities in health and justice. First, an indirect approach sees differences in health outcomes as inequitable if they are the result of unjust social arrangements. The emphasis thus lies not on the pattern of distribution of health outcomes, but on the broader social processes underlying health inequalities. An indirect

---

[15] I borrowed the term 'specific egalitarianism' from Marchand et al. (1998). On various forms of specific egalitarianism in health, see, for example, Williams (1973b); Walzer (1983); Veatch (1991); Nussbaum (1992). Dworkin (1993) has argued against what he calls the 'insulation thesis'—the tendency to single out health as a special good.

[16] If there is no such empirical link, the priority view would require focusing on the sickest, independently of their social situation, and one would have to distinguish from that view one that focuses on the health of the poor. On this, see Marchand et al. (1998).

approach can thus make sense of the intuition that there is more reason to be concerned if we find that whites have significantly higher life expectancy than blacks in similar socio-economic positions, than if we find that women have higher life expectancy than men.

The second form of interlinkage stresses the opposite direction. It is based on the premise that a society's achievements and failures in health may contain important information about the injustice of particular social arrangements and thus supplement our assessment of these arrangements in general. A couple of recent publications have explored this line of reasoning (Sen 1998; Kim et al. 2000). At this level, even in an indirect approach, there is a role for examining distributive patterns of health outcomes. They can provide a starting point for an in-depth analysis of how social institutions work and the injustices they may embody.

One advantage of the indirect approach is that it provides a basis for choosing relevant social groups in the assessment and explanation of social inequalities in health. What the above example underlines is that even if a direct approach is adopted prima facie, the choice of relevant social groups is based on an implicit judgement about unjust social arrangements that disadvantage certain groups. An indirect approach makes such judgements explicit.

Moreover, by stressing interlinkages between the health sphere and other social spheres, the indirect approach avoids elevating health to an organising principle of society, nor does it strictly privilege another social sector over health. It was argued above that health is not a static concept and that an approach to health equity should be able to accommodate this. A conception of health equity that builds exclusively on the medical model of health tends to downplay the inevitable biases and value judgements inherent in the disciplines of medicine and public health. An indirect approach to health equity is more compatible with a social model of health, which takes into account the influence of a variety of social factors on health.

It should be noted, however, that the direct and indirect approaches to health equity overlap. For it is clear that an indirect approach will need some justification for why health is considered a relevant indicator and such a justification will draw upon the nature of the good of health.[17] In other words, both need some account of why health is an important good. But they differ with respect to the context in which such an account is given and to the type of account given. While there is a tendency implicit in direct approaches to take health as an unambiguous, objective social goal, the indirect approach can better deal with the inherent complexity of health, which makes it difficult to confine health to a sphere of its own, independent of all other social spheres.

---

[17] What I am concerned with here is not so much the *empirical* correlation between health outcomes and some indicator of general performance. The issue is, rather, the *theoretical* question whether performance in the health space might tell us something important about social arrangements. I thank Sudhir Anand for pointing this difference out to me.

5.4. A THEORETICAL FRAMEWORK FOR SOCIAL JUSTICE

Rawls' theory of justice as fairness has been the most influential theory of social justice put forward in the twentieth-century.[18] As mentioned, however, it does not specifically address the issue of health. What is more, Rawls explicitly rules out situations such as those we are interested in here. He assumes the healthy and able-bodied person as the norm. Rawls concedes that because accidents and illness have the potential to induce great suffering, and to hinder a person from pursuing his or her goals in life, they may require social action. But in Rawls' view, social action takes the form of restoring people to good health—of providing health care.[19]

In spite of this I shall argue that the conceptions of justice as fairness and of political liberalism that Rawls has developed can provide guidelines for how to assess social inequalities in health. This section provides some necessary background. What a theory of justice must do, according to Rawls, is provide principles for the regulation of 'the inequalities in life prospects between citizens that arise from social starting positions, natural advantages, and historical contingencies' (Rawls 1993: 271). A key premise of Rawls' theory of justice as fairness is that of society as a *fair system of cooperation*—to be understood in contrast with society as a loose association of individuals.[20] The idea of cooperation stresses a functional relation between the social division of labour in the production and distribution of social goods and the social roles and positions into which individuals are slotted. According to this view, the social conditions into which somebody is born have a profound impact on what she or he can achieve and aspires to achieve. From the point of view of justice, there is thus a limit on the claims people who do well have on their achievements. By the same token, people who do not do well may have a claim on social goods.

The principles of justice aim at regulating the terms of social cooperation. However, their scope is limited to what Rawls calls the *basic structure* of society—society's main political, social, and economic institutions. There are several reasons why Rawls focuses on the basic structure.[21] In *A Theory of Justice* Rawls explains it as follows (Rawls 1971: 7):

The basic structure is the primary subject of justice because its effects are so profound and present from the start. The intuitive notion here is that this structure contains various

---

[18] See in particular Rawls (1971, 1993).

[19] '[W]e assume that persons as citizens have all the capacities that enable them to be cooperating members of society.... [W]e do not mean to say, or course, that no one ever suffers from illness and accident; such misfortunes are to be expected in the ordinary course of life, and provision for these contingencies must be made'. (Rawls 1993: 20).

[20] See, for example, Rawls (1993: 15).

[21] I cannot discuss this issue in full here, but see in particular Rawls (1993: 257–88).

social positions and that men [*sic!*] born into different positions have different expectations of life determined, in part, by the political system as well as by economic and
social circumstances. In this way the institutions of society favour certain starting
places over others. These are especially deep inequalities. Not only are they pervasive,
but they affect men's initial chances in life; yet they cannot possibly be justified by an
appeal to the notions of merit or desert. It is these inequalities, presumably inevitable
in the basic structure of any society, to which the principles of social justice must in the
first instance apply.[22]

The basic structure of society affects not only the distribution of material
resources and through this people's chances to carry out different life plans,
but also, as Rawls emphasises, the talents and abilities people have.[23]
Moreover, what Rawls does not mention but what the literature on social
inequalities in health suggests, is how social arrangements affect people's life
expectancy and general possibilities of being healthy. I shall come back to this
issue in the next section.

The main idea expressed in the principles of justice as fairness is that social
and economic inequalities are tolerated in the basic structure of society insofar
as they do not jeopardise the fundamental equality of all members of society.
More precisely, justice is seen as undermined if society's main economic, social,
and political institutions require sacrifices from the worse-off groups purely to
the benefit of the better-off groups. Such a social division of labour would not
be compatible with the idea of society as a 'fair system of cooperation'.

5.5. HEALTH EQUITY AND THE JUSTICE OF
SOCIETY'S BASIC INSTITUTIONS

What does this interpretation of justice imply for an approach to health
equity? First, I will argue that it would be incompatible with what I called a
direct approach to health equity. The principal reason is related to taking as a
starting point for a theory of justice the premise that societies are characterised
by a pluralism of religious, philosophical, and moral doctrines (Rawls 1993:
3*f*). This implies that justice cannot be based on some notion of the common
good, or some shared notion of individual well-being. Rawls explicitly rejects
assessing justice on the grounds of some account of well-being (Rawls 1982).
In consequence, an interpretation of health that stresses well-being, such as the

[22] Just to avoid confusion, when Rawls speaks of 'expectations of life', he is not alluding to
mortality, but to the chances people have to carry out different life plans.

[23] '[W]e cannot view the talents and abilities of individuals as fixed natural gifts. To be sure,
even as realized there is presumably a significant genetic component. However, these abilities and
talents cannot come to fruition apart from social conditions, and as realized they always take but
one of many possible forms. . . . So not only our final ends and hopes for ourselves but also our
realized abilities and talents reflect, to a large degree, our personal history, opportunities, and
social position' (Rawls 1993: 270).

WHO definition, would not be compatible with Rawlsian justice. Similarly, a notion of health that claims to be objective and value-free, but that in fact is not, would not be appropriate.

Moreover—and again in respect of pluralism—justice as fairness refrains from specifying a particular distributive pattern for certain goods:

[T]he two principles of justice do not insist that the actual distribution conform at any given time...to any observable pattern, say equality, or that the degree of inequality computed from the distribution fall within a certain range, say of values of the Gini coefficient.[24]

For this reason, a Rawlsian approach to health equity is necessarily an indirect approach.[25] In the passage just quoted, Rawls continues: 'What is enjoined is that (permissible) inequalities should make a certain functional contribution to the expectations of the least favoured, where this functional contribution results form the working of the system of entitlements set up in public institutions.' The idea here is that how basic social institutions work is more important than the resulting outcomes—as characterised by distributive patterns—that are observed. In Rawlsian justice, the focus is thus shifted from health outcomes to the mechanisms implicit in basic social institutions that produce social inequalities in health.

Above, I introduced two forms of interlinkage between social inequalities in health and justice. How do they relate to Rawlsian justice? On the one hand, justice as fairness offers a framework for evaluating social inequalities in health—for making health equity judgements. It points to the particular weight of inequalities that can be traced back to society's principal social and economic institutions. And it identifies as unjust those class, race, gender or socio-geographical inequalities in health that originate in the basic structure of society and are the result of a social division of labour that benefits the better-off groups at the expense of the worse off. Again, the goal is not to achieve a specific pattern of health outcomes, but a just basic structure of society. If the basic structure is just, then all outcomes these institutions produce can be considered just.[26]

On the other hand, research on social inequalities in health and their causes may tell us something about whether basic social arrangements have the effect

---

[24] Rawls (1993: 283).

[25] Justice as fairness is often called a *procedural* conception of justice—in contrast to consequentialist theories. Consequentialism requires us to assess different social arrangements with respect to the goodness of the consequences in which they result. Given that the approach to health equity sketched here builds on Rawls' theory of justice, one may call it a procedural approach to health equity. I decided against using this term, and called my approach 'indirect' instead, to underline the need to include considerations of goodness in assessing health equity.

[26] It may be added that justice as fairness does not translate into a right to health. In general, it can be said that the interpretation of justice as fairness presented here is less threatened by the 'bottomless pit' problem that is sometimes discussed in relation to the maximin principle—a reductionist version of Rawls' difference principle.

of undermining the fundamental equality of all members of society—whether these arrangements do or do not constitute a 'fair system of social cooperation'. Because of the links the empirical literature on social inequalities in health demonstrates between cultural, social, and economic parameters and health outcomes, such information can supplement economic and sociological information about the achievements of different social arrangements in the basic structure of society and their changes over time.

At this stage, it will be important to discuss a possible objection to this approach. It may be argued that the correct way to apply Rawlsian justice is to say that since health does not enjoy special status in justice as fairness, all social inequalities in health must be regarded as just, provided that the basic structure of society is just. In other words, this argument perceives only a one-way relationship between justice as fairness and social inequalities in health and fails to recognise how information about social inequalities in health may help assessing the justice of the basic structure. This particular link between justice as fairness and social inequalities in health requires further justification, therefore. In principle, justice as fairness suggests that the basic structure of society should be evaluated on the basis of 'primary goods'.[27] The list of primary goods includes basic rights and liberties, and income and wealth, among other things, but not health. The most important primary good, according to Rawls, is the social basis for self-respect (Rawls 1971: 440). This stems again from the idea of society as a fair system of cooperation, which requires that nobody is excluded a priori. If inequalities in the basic social arrangements which shape individual lives express a disvaluation of certain social positions and occupations in such a way that people cannot gain a sense of self-respect, then these structures are unjust.

The notion of 'social bases of self-respect' is of course very ambiguous and needs specification. In general, it can be said that the *implementation* of Rawlsian justice cannot avoid taking into account information that reaches beyond the primary goods framework that Rawls has laid out. Health information—in particular research that attempts to uncover the more 'upstream' causes of social inequalities in health—may play an important role for gaining understanding about how the organization of the basic structure of society affects people and groups of people. To illustrate, discrimination and lack of social respect seem to show in health outcomes (among other variables), as recent studies on inequalities between blacks and whites in the United States demonstrate (Krieger and Sidney 1996; Kennedy et al. 1997).

5.6. CONCLUDING REMARKS

This paper outlined an approach to health equity that proceeds indirectly and embeds health equity within the general pursuit of social justice. Building on

[27] For a list of primary goods, see Rawls (1993: 181).

Rawls' theory of justice as fairness, it was argued that social inequalities in health are unjust or inequitable if they result from an unjust basic structure of society—that is, a basic structure that imposes sacrifices on the worse off only to benefit the already better-off groups. This entails that to be able to pass a judgement on social inequalities in health, we need an understanding of the underlying causes. At the same time, information about the health status of people may give us important information to assess the justice of social arrangements. Understanding the effects the basic structure has on people's possibilities to be healthy may help us decide whether these institutions ensure the social bases for self-respect for everybody. While justice as fairness cannot offer a complete blueprint of what a just society would look like, it certainly provides a framework for thinking about issues related to social justice.

References

Adams, Vincanne (1998). *Doctors for Democracy: Health Professionals in the Nepal Revolution.* Cambridge, UK: Cambridge University Press.

Amick, Benjamin C. III, Sol Levine, Alvin R. Tarlov, and Diana Chapman Walsh (eds.) (1995). *Society and Health.* New York and Oxford: Oxford University Press.

Beauchamp, Dan and Bonnie Steinbock (1999). *New Ethics for the Public's Health.* New York: Oxford University Press.

Berkman, Lisa F., Thomas Glass, Ian Brissette, and Teresa E. Seeman (2000). 'From Social Integration to Health: Durkheim in the New Millenium', *Social Science and Medicine*, 51: 843–57.

Black, Douglas Sir, J. N. Morris, Cyril Smith, and Peter Townsend (1990). 'The Black Report', in Peter Townsend and Nick Davidson (eds.), *Inequalities in Health.* London: Penguin.

Brock, Dan (1993). 'Quality of Life Measures in Health Care and Medical Ethics', in Martha Nussbaum and Amartya Sen (eds.), *Quality of Life.* Oxford: Clarendon, pp. 95–132.

Canguilhem, Georges (1991). *The Normal and the Pathological*, New York: Zone Books.

Corin, Ellen (1995). 'The Cultural Frame: Context and Meaning in the Construction of Health', in Amick, B. III et al. (eds.), *Society and Health.* New York and Oxford: Oxford University Press, pp. 272–304.

Daniels, Norman (1985). *Just Health Care.* Cambridge: Cambridge University Press.

Das, Veena. n.d. 'What Do We Mean by Health?', *mimeo.*

Dworkin, Ronald (1993). 'Justice in the Distribution of Health Care', *McGill Law Journal*, 38(4): 883–98.

Engelhardt, H. Tristram Jr. (1986). *Foundations of Bioethics.* Oxford and New York: Oxford University Press.

Foucault, Michel (1973). *The Birth of the Clinic.* New York: Pantheon Books.

Frank, Arthur W. (1995). *The Wounded Storyteller: Body, Illness, and Ethics.* Chicago: University of Chicago Press.

Gwatkin, D. R. (2000). 'Health Inequalities and the Health of the Poor: What Do We Know? What Can We Do?' *Bulletin of the World Health Organization*, 78(1): 3–17.

Gwatkin Davidson R. and Michel Guillot (2000). *The Burden of Disease among the Global Poor: Current Situation, Future Trends, and Implications for Strategy.* Washington, DC: International Bank for Development and Reconstruction and World Bank.

Kawachi, Ichiro, Bruce P. Kennedy, and Richard G. Wilkinson (1999). *Income Inequality and Health.* New York: New Press.

Kennedy, Bruce P., Ichiro Kawachi, Kimberly Lochner, C. Jones, and Deborah Prothrow-Stith (1997). '(Dis)respect and Black Mortality', *Ethnicity and Disease,* 7(3): 207–14.

Kim, Jim Yong, Joyce V. Millen, Alec Irwin, and John Gershman (2000). *Dying for Growth.* Monroe: Common Courage Press.

Kleinman, Arthur (1988). *The Illness Narratives: Suffering, Healing, and the Human Condition.* New York: Basic Books.

Krieger, Nancy, D. L. Rowley, A. A. Herman, B. Avery, and M. T. Phillips (1993). 'Racism, Sexism, and Social Class: Implications for Studies of Health, Disease, and Well Being', *American Journal of Preventive Medicine,* 9(Supplement): 82–122.

—— and S. Sidney (1996). 'Racial Discrimination and Blood Pressure: The CARDIA Study of Young Black and White Woman and Men', *American Journal of Public Health,* 86: 1370–78.

—— and Anne-Emanuelle Birn (1998) 'A Vision of Social Justice as the Foundation of Public Health: Commemorating 150 years of the spirit of 1848', *American Journal of Public Health,* 88(11): 1603–6.

Lériche, René (1937). 'Introduction Générale', 'De la Santé à la Maladie', 'La Douleur dans les Maladies', 'Où Va la Médecine?' in *Encyclopédie Française volume 6.* Paris: Societé de Géstion de l'Encyclopédie Française.

Marchand, Sarah, Daniel Wikler, and Bruce Landesman (1998). 'Class, Health, and Justice', *The Milbank Quarterly,* 76(3): 449–68.

Marmot, Michael, G. Rose, M. Shipley and P. Hamilton (1978). 'Employment Grade and Coronary Heart Disease in British civil servants', *Journal of Epidemiology and Community Health,* 32: 244–9.

——, Martin Bobak, and George Davey Smith (1995). 'Explanations for Social Inequalities in Health', in Amick, B. III et al. (eds.), *Society and Health.* New York and Oxford: Oxford University Press, pp. 172–210.

Nussbaum, Martha C. (1992). 'Morality, Politics, and Human Beings: II. Human Functioning and Social Justice: In Defence of Aristotelian Essentialism', *Political Theory,* 20(2): 202–46.

Parfit, Derek (1997). 'Equality or Priority', *Ratio,* 10: 202–21.

Pereira, João (1993). 'What Does Equity in Health Mean?' *Journal of Social Policy,* 22(1): 19–48.

Poland, Blake, David Coburn, Ann Robertson, and Joan Eakin (1998). 'Wealth, Equity and Health Care: A Critique of a "Population Health" Perspective on the Determinants of Health', *Social Science and Medicine,* 46(7): 785–98.

Rawls, John (1971). *A Theory of Justice.* Cambridge, MA: Harvard University Press.

—— (1982). 'Social Unity and Primary Goods', in Amartya Sen and Bernard Williams (eds.), *Utilitarianism and Beyond.* Cambridge: Cambridge University Press, 159–185.

—— (1993). *Political Liberalism.* New York: Columbia University Press.

Robertson, Ann (1998). 'Critical Reflections on the Politics of Need: Implications for Public Health', *Social Science and Medicine,* 47(10): 1419–30.

Sen, Amartya (1985). 'Well-being, Agency and Freedom', *Journal of Philosophy*, 82: 169–221.

—— (1993). 'Capability and Well-being', in Martha Nussbaum and Amartya Sen (eds.), *Quality of Life*. Oxford: Clarendon Press. pp. 30–61.

—— (1998). 'Mortality as an Indicator of Economic Success and Failure', *The Economic Journal*, 108: 1–25.

Veatch, Robert M. (1991). 'Justice and the Right to Health Care: An Egalitarian Account', in T. J. Bole and W. B. Bondeson (eds.), *Rights to Health Care*. Dordrecht: Kluwer, pp. 83–102.

Walzer, Michael (1983). *Spheres of Justice*. Oxford: Blackwell.

Whitehead, Margaret (1990). *The Concepts and Principles of Equity and Health*, Copenhagen: World Health Organization.

WHO (World Health Organization) (1976). *World Health Organization: Basic Documents*, 26th edn. Geneva: WHO.

Wilkinson, Richard (1996). *Unhealthy Societies: The Afflictions of Inequality*. London and New York: Routledge.

Williams, Bernard (1973a). 'A Critique of Utilitarianism', in J. J. C. Smart and Bernard Williams (eds.), *Utilitarianism: For and Against*. Cambridge, UK: Cambridge University Press.

—— (1973b). 'The Idea of Equality', in B. Williams, *Problems of the Self*. Cambridge, UK: Cambridge University Press.

PART III

RESPONSIBILITY FOR HEALTH AND HEALTH CARE

6

Personal and Social Responsibility for Health

DANIEL WIKLER

6.1. INTRODUCTION

In many cases, illness is not something that just happens to a person. We are more likely to remain healthy if we take care of ourselves. People who live prudently tend to live longer and to avoid disability. The best hope for many people who are seeking to maintain or improve health is to adopt healthier lifestyles.

These facts suggest a division of labour in the pursuit of health. In addition to maintaining a health system for prevention and therapy, society can try to create a healthy social and physical environment, and can also provide information on risk factors. For their part, individuals can use this information, along with their own knowledge and common sense, to maintain their health as best they can to reduce the need for care.

In the ordinary public health perspective, avoiding diseases and disabilities that stem from personal choices is no less important as a goal than the avoidance of any other maladies. They may require different strategies for prevention, management, or cure, and the individual's liberties must be respected. Otherwise, however, a health need is a health need, equally deserving of concern and attention.

But this is not the only perspective from which to view the potential contribution of individual behaviour to health. Some would wish to respond differently to health needs depending on who is responsible for creating and maintaining them. In this view, what we can do for ourselves, we should not look to others to do for us. If we become sick or disabled as a result of neglecting to take care of ourselves, or by having taken undue risks, then dealing with these health needs should be seen as personal rather than social responsibilities and as such should not be considered on a par with other, unavoidable health needs.

Thanks are due to Sarah Marchand for help and ideas, to Robert Beaglehole, Dan Brock, Onora O'Neill, Fabienne Peter, and John Roemer for valuable criticism, and to Paul Dolan, Samia Hurst, Paula Lantz, Erik Nord, Aki Tsuchiya, and Peter Ubel for guidance in the social science literature.

The theme of personal responsibility has increased in prominence in health policy during the last twenty-five years. Initially, its principal use was to argue for policies that took account of externalities: burdens imposed on others when individuals gambled with health. These were debates over the financing and operation of the personal health care system. The solutions offered to the problem required that those who took risks with health assumed more of the burdens of the consequences: they might receive lower priority for treatment, or be made to pay fees for supplementary insurance. More recently, however, it has begun to figure in debates in public and international health. For example, it has been argued that any response in public health policy to the correlations between socio-economic status and health that have received much attention in recent years must take into account the degree to which the differences in health between social classes is due to differences in how well people in different strata take care of themselves. To the extent that class differences in health and longevity simply reflect how well or how badly people in different circumstances protect their health, in this view, these correlations are not a social responsibility and hence should not have priority over other health concerns.

More broadly still, the concept of personal responsibility for health has figured in efforts to delimit the sphere of public health, both national and international. In this view, public health should not address itself to 'risk factors' without first determining whether these risks are voluntarily assumed. If people know what risks they are taking, but accept them as the price of pursuing goals that they hold in higher priority, then it is not the business of public health to re-order these priorities and insist that the risk factors be avoided so that health is valued above all. For example, international efforts to curb the use of tobacco has been criticised on the grounds that the gamble one takes in smoking is a personal matter, and that scarce resources should be directed toward involuntary risks, focusing on those infectious diseases that afflict populations regardless of personal initiative.

Though it has been mentioned in these varied contexts, the claim that personal responsibility for health should be taken into account in health and public health policy is not one that has figured prominently in current debates. In my view, it is worth a more careful examination than its peripheral role in public health policy to date might indicate. This is not because this theme should figure more prominently in public health, for I argue that it deserves its place on the periphery. But to do this we must first acknowledge that the notion of personal responsibility for health may have considerable appeal. It seems to comport with basic intuitions about fairness, and also with a prominent strain in contemporary work in the theory of justice. Its implications for public health policy are striking and extensive. If, as I believe, the moral claims about personal responsibility for health should make at most a minor appearance in our public health debates, it is worth taking careful aim at arguments to the contrary and thereby to disarm potential opposition to what I believe are important and justifiable public health interventions.

In what follows, I will briefly describe the uses to which notions of personal responsibility have been put in health policy debates. To stay focused, but at some cost to clarity, I will rely on context to fix the sense of 'responsible' that figures in these debates. In Section 6.3, I connect these uses of the notion of personal responsibility for health to recent work in the theory of justice. The last section of the chapter attempts to point out some limitations on these arguments. I conclude that though individuals should be encouraged and enabled to remain healthy through informed and prudent habits of living, the misery that results from illness and injury should remain a burden that is shared.

6.2. THE POTENTIAL SIGNIFICANCE OF PERSONAL RESPONSIBILITY FOR HEALTH

Though concern for the individual's role in maintaining health is not at all new—such themes can be found in Galen (AD 180) and in other ancient medical traditions (Reiser 1985)—its prominence has increased in the wake of the epidemiological transition. With infectious diseases giving way in wealthier countries to non-communicable diseases as leading causes of illness and premature death, the scope for state intervention in reducing the transmission of infectious agents has declined in importance. For many of these maladies, the most effective actor is the individual, not the state, and thus the way a person lives—one's 'life style'—becomes the key to improvement in health. Emphasis on lifestyle in health policy was fuelled in the 1960s by the accumulation of evidence of the health effects of smoking and other behavioural risk factors. Not long afterward, a flurry of governmental white papers led to announcements that national health strategies would be retargeted. An emphasis on behavioural change would, according to the new policies of Canada (Lalonde 1974), the United Kingdom (DHSS 1976), and the United States (Surgeon General 1979), broaden the scope of national health policies beyond traditional medical and surgical interventions. The role of behaviour as a key to health was not limited to non-communicable disease, for within a decade some of the same strategies seemed to offer the most effective front-line defence against AIDS.

Though the governmental reports and proposals generally steered clear of moral judgements about those who would not take proper care of themselves, a few individuals did not. The most widely noted was John Knowles, then president of the Rockefeller Foundation, who wrote that 'one man's freedom in health is another man's shackle in taxes and insurance premiums', and urged that 'the idea of a "right" to health should be replaced by the idea of an individual moral obligation to preserve one's own health—a public duty if you will'. (Knowles 1977).

Knowles offered this observation as an argument in favour of prudent self-management, but offered little elaboration. A small literature that accumulated in the ensuing years, some supporting Knowles, others opposed, brought out some of its implications (Wikler 1978, 1985, 1987; Veatch 1980; Dworkin 1981; Leichter 1991; Wikler and Beauchamp 1995). A health policy that would take Knowles's proposal seriously would include several elements: prohibitions and other curbs on risk taking, lower priority for treatment in case of injury or illness and compulsory insurance payments, either as such or in the form of excise taxes.

The first way to ensure that people do not burden others with the costs of care stemming from imprudence is to enforce rules requiring healthy choices, such as requirements that drivers wear seatbelts and that motorcyclists use safety helmets. In such cases it may be difficult to separate out the motive of protecting others from avoidable costs from paternalist concern to protect the individual against his or her own reckless impulses. These goals offer separate and potentially reinforcing support for protective measures. Insofar as the weight of the law is used to ensure that individuals make healthy choices, however, it may not be right to say that these measures support the idea of personal responsibility.

The second element of health policy assigning responsibility for health to the individual would be the prospect that treatment for avoidable illness and injury would have lower priority, or perhaps would be left untreated, at least at public expense. Transplant surgeons, for example, conducted a long debate over whether alcoholics should have the same priority as others when needing new livers. Much of this discussion turned on medical suitability rather than any moral (or moralistic) notions, and the trend has been to accept alcoholics on a par with others (Starzl et al. 1988; Schenker et al. 1990; Knechtle et al. 1992). But the fact that this class of patients would be singled out on the basis of their (possibly) poor prognosis might also betray a sense that their role in ruining their livers weakened their claims. Similar conclusions might hold concerning a debate within the NHS over provision of *in vitro* fertilization to women who smoke (Sylvester 1999). While the head of the Royal College of Obstetricians and Gynaecologists formulated its principle as 'you do your bit and we will treat you'—a moral principle of reciprocity—the evidence given in support of its position referred to the lower probability of conception among smokers. Other manifestations in this vein which have been booted around occasionally in health policy debates include proposals to eliminate dentures from national health plans (on the ground that people who took proper care of their teeth throughout their lives would not need them) and arguments against long-term care for the aged (both because people should make arrangements with family or others to care for them in time of need and also because people who keep fit are less likely to need extended long-term care). A variation on this theme would involve withholding an expensive medical intervention unless and until the patient had tried first to achieve health through lifestyle modification, such as reduction of dietary salt intake versus anti-hypertension drugs.

A third way of assigning personal responsibility for health, or for the costs of treatment, would be to insist that the potential risk taker pay in advance for insurance against added risk, either in the form of a user fee or a specific tax. One example is the user fee for dangerous sports, intended to cover the added costs of paying for care in case of accident. The high cost of evacuation and treatment of alpinists injured on Mt. Ranier, near Seattle, prompted calls for higher fees for permits. Again, the motivation behind such steps may be complex. The principal motive for cigarette taxes, for example, may be to add to state revenue, or it may be paternalist. If the goal is to assign responsibility for costs to the individual, the appropriate taxation level is difficult to estimate, not only because smokers incur certain costs but may avoid others by dying early, and because smokers who die prematurely may forfeit productivity but, since the lethal effects of tobacco use are not immediate, society may be spared the cost of their pensions.

This brief account suggests that some measures enacted in the United States and the United Kingdom may be viewed as placing responsibility for health on the individual. At the same time, present-day health policy does not go nearly as far as it could, were it to embrace this doctrine without reservation. With a few exceptions, such as drinkers and smokers seeking liver transplants and assistance in reproduction, respectively, patients are treated according to their need regardless of their responsibility in creating the need. Though encouragement of healthier lifestyles has become a priority of the Department of Health and Human Services in the United States in recent years, we remain free to overeat, under-exercise, and smoke without paying penalties beyond the resulting illnesses themselves. And though taxes and other prepay mechanisms to cover the resulting health costs are not unknown, their use is inconsistent. Using existing policies as evidence, policy-makers can be understood to reject the assignment of responsibility for health at least as often as they rely on it.

6.2.1. *Personal responsibility and inequalities in health*

The correlation of health and longevity with social position—occupational and social status, educational level, and other indices of hierarchy—has been recognised for many decades, at least by social scientists. In recent years, this relation of health to socio-economic stratification has moved to the centre of public health concerns (Wilkinson 1996; Auerbach and Krimgold 2001). Up and down the socio-economic ladder, the better-off one is economically and socially, the better one's health and the longer one's life (Marmot et al. 1991, 1997; Evans et al. 1994; Wilkinson 1996). Death rates from 80 per cent of the eighty most common causes of death are higher for blue-collar workers than for white-collar workers (Wilkinson 1996); the differences in many cases are several-fold. Inequalities among social groups, also including racial groups, are as great in the United States and some other wealthy countries as the differences between wealthy countries and much poorer ones. 'As international evidence continues to accumulate documenting the relationship between socio-economic status and health,' Marmot et al. (1997) have written, 'a good case can be made that this is the major unsolved public health problem of the industrialized world'.

What do these findings suggest for health policy? On the assumption that those on the low end of the inequalities are biologically similar to those who are favoured, they seem to indicate that much opportunity for improved health exists for large segments of the population. If we know why the wealthy and healthy are doing so well, perhaps we can bring others up to their level.

This observation does not in itself entail that we *should* do so. That depends, in part, on the costs involved in efforts to narrow health inequalities, which might involve anything from paying for targeted health promotion to interference in labour markets to redistributing society's wealth and markers of status. But the implications for health policy (and social policy generally, given that the interventions required may lie outside of the domain of health care and public health) are not fully contained within a calculation of their costs and potential benefits. We also need a moral account, a compelling argument that health inequalities represent or constitute an injustice that places a claim on society's resources. Unless the inequalities associated with social position are unjust, interventions aimed at narrowing them would have to compete with other public health measures on the basis of ordinary standards used in setting priorities. If they are required to remedy an injustice, however, they might take higher priority, and might even be worth undertaking greater expenditure with lesser results.

What is the nature of this alleged injustice? For the most part, the public health literature has been concerned to document and to explain these group and individual variations. Perhaps the unfairness of adding illness and premature death to inferior social status seems obvious. These issues have only begun to attract attention from philosophers, but the few studies published to date (Marchand and Wikler 1998; Daniels et al. 2000) have located considerable complexity in the argumentation needed to establish this conclusion. For example, it is not clear that the injustice lies in the inequality per se or in society's failure to do more for those on the low end (regardless of the effect of such measures on inequality, for example, if the better off simultaneously benefit).

Also at issue is whether the differences in health status discovered in this research should be regarded as unjust only if they are the product of differences in social status which are themselves unjust. For example, one might argue that differences in health and longevity between racial or ethnic groups are unjust, and should be targeted by social policy, if they reflect racial or ethnic discrimination and stigma. Differences between racial groups not subjected to discrimination and stigma, or differences (however unlikely) in which stigmatised groups do better, would not count as injustices, on this view. Women's higher life expectancy might be such a case (Kekes 1997).

Similarly with class and other measures of social status: if the injustice of inequalities in health derives from the injustice (if any) of the social group differences which produce them, then we will regard differences in social position or class for health and longevity as unjust to the extent that we think that existing differences in control over work, income, occupational prestige, and other components of social position or class are themselves unjust. If high-status women have higher breast cancer rates because they postpone having children until they complete higher education, this class difference would not be unjust. And in a (mythical) society in which income varied only according to people's tastes for leisure versus labour (and its rewards)—a society in which income differences would be regarded as just by many people—any associated differences in health status might not be condemned as unjust, particularly if those who deliberated between leisure and labour were aware of these health consequences.

Alternatively, one might regard *any* group differences in health as unjust, perhaps unjust on their face, or else unjust in view of a comprehensive theory of justice that one accepts. For example, on the view that the norm of justice in the health 'sphere' of society is equality while in socio-economic competition there may be fair winners and losers, differences in socio-economic status might be deemed acceptable while the health inequalities they engender would be viewed as unjust (Walzer 1983).

On either view (though in varying circumstances), inequalities in health among social groups are likely to count as injustices, and hence to claim priority in the public health agenda. But the claim that inequalities in health represent injustices might be defeasible if the blame for the poorer health status of the less-favoured groups can be located in these individuals themselves. To those who claim that the inequalities between, say, racial groups, are an unjust product of unjust racism, those who stress personal responsibility may reply that racism would not have this consequence if members of the stigmatised group took better care of themselves. To those who find all social group differences in health objectionable, the response would be that people who differ in prudence should expect to differ in how healthy they remain. The locus of blame is key, for if blame is placed on the individual, social structure is exculpated, and the resulting suffering and premature death will not be counted as a social injustice. Narrowing health inequalities among social groups would thus not be of special urgency, either as a matter of prevention or of remedy.

The conclusion of the argument stressing personal responsibility need not be that public health should be unconcerned about the suffering of those on the low end of social group inequalities in health. Anyone who suffers illness and premature death deserves sympathy and, except for the most hard-hearted, some form of aid. But this is merely to say that their health needs will not receive priority among other health needs that might be targeted for public health action. It would require an additional step to maintain that locating blame for illness in the individual *reduces* the priority of giving them aid, relative to others who may suffer.

But this may be a step which some who stress personal responsibility would be logically impelled to take. The reasons supporting this extension of the argument point again to a locus of blame for illness. According to the lines of argument just presented, if social injustice (e.g. racism) is the source of an inequality in health, then, everything else being equal, those who suffer excess ill health due to their social position have a strong claim for remediation; and some will say also that inequalities in health which reflect even defensible differences in social status also deserve remediation. But more generally, most of us believe that health problems deserve social attention in their own right. In this most general case—the unremarkable and usual kinds of illness, injuries, and deaths—we may locate the 'blame' in nature, mediated by brute luck. The individual who becomes sick is simply in the wrong place at the wrong time, with the wrong kind of body with the wrong level of resistance to infection or injury. The individual becomes sick, or is injured, or dies, through no fault of her own, and our help is needed to combat the ills that nature has sent her way.

When the blame for a person's poor health can be placed on that person, it is no longer true that the blame rests in 'nature'; it is not a matter of brute luck, nor is this person sick through no fault of her own. From this perspective, the matter of personal responsibility for health does not merely lower the urgency of caring for an ill person (or preventing an illness that might befall a person) to that of ordinary medical distress, but lowers it still another rung on the ladder of moral importance. For some, it might negate the need for a social response altogether (though one would hope, in the name of decency, that an interpersonal response would still be forthcoming). In effect, this kind of thinking would remove whole tracts of the landscape of suffering from the health policy agenda.

The implications of this perspective for both domestic and international health policy are potentially vast. Roger Scruton (2000*a*, *b*), for example, has questioned the World Health Organization's effort to reduce smoking, one of the leading sources of disease and premature death worldwide, and a habit whose rapid spread in developing countries will kill many millions more in the next few decades unless effectively curbed. Scruton argues that smoking is 'in fact a voluntary activity and a source of pleasure, the risk of which entirely falls on the smoker'. Scruton does not extend the argument to AIDS, but it would seem to imply that governments should limit themselves to education on the risks of unsafe sex and needle sharing, rather than trying to curb these practices. And the same holds true for cardiovascular disease and the other main sources of reduced years of healthy life, insofar as they can be traced to choices, which are imprudent, so long as they are informed and voluntary. This way of thinking about public health might recommend measures under individual control, such as mosquito netting to guard against malaria, when they are alternatives to other disease reduction initiatives undertaken at public expense, such as eradication of mosquitoes, or even the treatment of malaria. Even more broadly, the same approach could distinguish patients who comply with medical advice from the noncompliant, and those who seek prompt attention when they experience warning signs of disease from those who decide to wait and see if the condition develops.

The tabulation of health statistics, too, would be changed were this viewpoint to inform health policy. WHO, whose tobacco policy Scruton (2000*a*, *b*) challenges, computes smoking-related morbidity and mortality in its estimate of the global burden of disease. For Scruton, it is a 'semantic trick' to so classify smoking, 'on the spurious round that the methods used to measure its effect belong to the science of epidemiology'. A nation's progress in health, either in terms of average healthy life expectancy or in the distribution of this quantity, would be tabulated only in terms of unavoidable illness, that is, illness for which nature or society is to blame. Deaths and illnesses attributable to personal choices, not being the responsibility of society, would not figure in these target-setting tabulations. Or, if we wished health statistics to count all suffering and premature death regardless of cause, that which is attributed to individual voluntary choice could be ignored in calculations of the value of interventions and in charting the progress of countries in advancing public health.

Similarly, the assignment of responsibility for health impinges on the content of human rights, specifically on the right to health, Article 12 of the Covenant on Economic, Social, and Cultural Rights, which governments worldwide have ratified. If social and economic inequalities are as powerful in determining health expectancies as current research indicates they are, then signatories to the Covenant would seem to be obligated to narrow these inequalities, or to find ways to reduce their impact on health and longevity. But if we assign responsibility for the excess mortality and morbidity associated with socio-economic inequality to individuals, on the premise that these misfortunes stem from differences in lifestyles, reflecting different personal priorities, tastes, and character traits, then we cannot demand remedial action by states bound by the Covenant.

The views expressed in these last few paragraphs are rarely expressed as bluntly as Scruton has done. Perhaps many of those who attach the greatest importance to personal responsibility for health would disown them. Still, they still might be entailed by the premises of their view. These extensions and further implications are worth noting to the extent that they help us to understand the view better (and also perhaps because they offer the possibility of a *reductio ad absurdum*). Though one might deny that these implications follow (and I would agree that some additional assumption would be required), I believe that they indicate the need to examine the basis for stressing personal responsibility for health. Since this view has not been stated with precision in writing on inequalities in health and social determinants of health, I will attempt to furnish an argument, which rests on current theories of justice. If I can show that this argument does not secure its conclusions, I hope to have shown that no weaker argument could do so.

6.3. LUCK, EGALITARIANISM, AND PERSONAL RESPONSIBILITY IN RECENT POLITICAL PHILOSOPHY

In the previous section, I sketched some potentially far-reaching health policy implications which might be drawn from the everyday intuition that people who take risks should bear the burden if harm results. These began with the claim that those who take risks should be made to pay for the costs of their care, and went on to the view that they should lose their place in the queue when care must be rationed. A different kind of implication is that inequalities in health and longevity, including those which mirror unjust social inequalities and discrimination, represent no injustice if the immediate source of the health inequality is the imprudence of the less favoured.

While the first of these has appeared in writing on public health over the past quarter century, the second view has barely been articulated, perhaps because public awareness of the research on the correlation of health and the social structure has been limited. But criticism has been voiced by conservative commentators of public health scientists for putting the blame on social injustice rather than individual irresponsibility. 'Behind all their talk of racism and sexism', according to one recent critic (Mac Donald 1998, 2000), [their] 'real prey is individual responsibility...the public health revisionists are generating a remarkable body of excuses for the most avoidable and dangerous behaviours...' An opinion piece in the *Wall Street Journal* editorial page attacked the claim that social injustice was the cause of excess morbidity among racial minorities, pointing instead to 'obesity, smoking, alcohol and drug use, reckless sexual behaviour' among other factors (Satel 1997). Similarly, that author, in her book-length critique of 'political correctness' in medicine, maintains that 'Social inequalities...do not literally produce the sedentary life-style, obesity, and risky behaviour that typically underlie many of the differences in health status between the less wealthy and the better-off' (Satel 2000: 30).

The exact dispute between these critics and their targets is not easy to pinpoint. They might disagree on how much of the difference in health status between social groups can be explained by differences in risk-taking behaviour. But the dispute might also centre on what to make of the contribution of behaviour to group differences, to the extent that it is an explanatory factor. The conservative critics see the answer lying not in remedies for social injustice, but in more prudent behaviour on the part of the poor—not only because this may be the more effective remedy, but because it places responsibility where (in their view) it belongs.

In so arguing, a left–right dispute entered the arena of public health that had been carried on in politics generally in the West for two decades. This controversy has engaged both popular politics and academic theorising. As Samuel Scheffler (1992, 1995) has noted, the conservative trend of the 1980s in politics in the

United States and United Kingdom traced in part to public dissatisfaction with the position taken by the left on the matter of personal responsibility. Scheffler links the stance toward personal responsibility taken by the political left (called liberals in the United States) with that of the academic political philosophy which also goes by that name. The welfare state is characterised by conservatives as offering a societal guarantee of at least minimal well-being regardless of an individual's prudence or effort, and faulted on that ground by politicians who led the right to victory in the Reagan and Thatcher years. For example, Newt Gingrich, a conservative in the US Congress, wrote that

By blaming everything on 'society', contemporary liberals are really trying to escape the personal responsibility that comes with being an American. If 'society' is responsible for everything, then no one is personally responsible for anything. (Gingrich 1995)

Not that this in itself demonstrates any rejection by the public of philosophical liberalism. The public remains largely unaware of this academic literature; philosophical liberalism was not the inspiration for most political liberals (though some of the architects of the War on Poverty of the 1960s later claimed to have been inspired by Rawls); and political liberals, as the programme of the moderate left, differ on points of doctrine with Rawlsian and other philosophical liberals. What the two sorts of liberalism have in common, and what puts them in opposition to the popular mood of the era, according to Scheffler, is precisely the lack of significance that they attach to personal responsibility, and to the related moral notion of desert. On this ground, Scheffler concludes that the dominant school of political philosophy of these decades is wholly out of sync with the thinking of much of the public.

Though Scheffler did not address personal responsibility for health, there is empirical evidence that much of the public accepts the notion that people should do what they can to stay healthy, and that those who fail to do should be given lower priority in deciding whom to treat. For example, Edwards et al. (2003) asked a sample of Welsh adults which factors should be taken into account in determining position on priority lists for treatment. Forty-one per cent chose self-inflicted bad health, agreeing that 'A patient who has contributed to his/her own ill health, through for example smoking or driving dangerously, should wait longer than a patient who has not contributed to his/her own ill health.' This was the eighth-highest factor in order of importance for determining position on priority lists. Forty-two per cent of a survey of 2000 adults by Bowling (1996) affirmed that people who contribute to their own illness (e.g. through smoking, obesity, or drinking) should have lower priority for health care. Dolan et al. (1999) encountered the same attitudes in the initial responses of about half the members of a series of focus groups in Yorkshire. Braakenheilm et al. (1990) report that half of a Swedish sample favoured priority for the prudent. Nord and Richardson (1995) found that 60 per cent of an Australian sample favoured priority to nonsmokers. But the interpretation of these findings is a complex matter, as I will discuss below.

Whether Scheffler is correct in his claim that theorists of justice in the Rawlsian tradition have attached little significance to personal responsibility is not entirely clear. It is true that in Rawls's *A Theory of Justice*, the role of personal responsibility is indeed circumscribed. Rawls argues that features of individuals or their circumstances that are morally arbitrary, or matters of luck, cannot serve as legitimate bases or justifying reasons for giving some individuals greater resources (such as income and wealth) than others. Thus, people who are born in favourable social circumstances, members of an advantaged social class, and those born with natural talents or aptitudes that are highly marketable, cannot be said to 'deserve' a greater share of income and wealth than others on these grounds (though society may choose to reward them for other reasons, for example, in the form of incentives). These are factors for which individuals are not responsible. Principles of justice, according to Rawls, should not reward individuals according to their good or bad fortune. What is fair, Rawls argues, is a system of equal rewards, or an equal distribution of income and wealth, unless rewarding the fortunate, for example, the better talented, proves to make everyone better off, especially the least fortunate. By this line of reasoning we arrive at Rawls's 'difference principle': inequalities in social goods are morally justified when even the worst-off benefit. Rawls suggests that the concept of 'desert' has a meaning and function only within the rules of justice of a society. These rules determine what individuals are entitled to, what are their legitimate expectations and claims on social resources, or what is deserved. Principles of justice, according to Rawls, should not be viewed as conforming to, or reflecting, some pre-institutional moral fact about what individuals deserve. As Christopher Woodward (1998) characterises Rawls's view, one looks to the theory to discover who deserves what, rather than the other way around.

But responsibility is not entirely absent from this view of justice. Rawls would hold individuals responsible for making do as best they can with their shares of social goods as determined by the principles of justice. For example, a person who has immoderate tastes or ambitions relative to others may find that her resource share goes less far in helping her realise aims in life, her 'good' or welfare. That she may fare less well than others in *this* regard is of no concern of justice, according to Rawls. Our preferences, as Rawls states, are our own concern or responsibility, and in this sense individual welfare is beyond the scope of social responsibility. What this implies about what justice requires in cases where individuals act imprudently as, for example, in 'squandering' their full resource shares, is open to argument. Clearly, Rawls rejects the view that expensive preferences should be collectively subsidised because the bearers of those tastes could thereby better realise their good or welfare. But the rejection of this view implies little about what the consequences should be, from the point of view of justice, of individuals acting recklessly or imprudently. Moreover, Rawls's theory assumes equal levels of need, abstracting away from actual interpersonal variations, and thus does not speak directly to the question of whether people should be expected to avoid creating health needs through prudent behaviour.

In much of recent post-Rawlsian writing on distributive justice, however, and in particular in a number of key contributions to liberal political philosophy that appeared in the wake of Sen's (1980) influential essay, 'Equality of What?', personal responsibility plays a key moral role. In his influential papers on equality, Ronald Dworkin (1981) tied distributive justice to the individual's willingness to take on certain risks. Dworkin distinguished between 'brute luck', the results of risks which are not deliberate gambles, and 'option luck', that which befalls a person as a result of gambles taken. In Dworkin's egalitarian schema, no one should be made to suffer on account of bad brute luck, while option luck, good or bad, may justly result in the increase or the reduction in a person's resources. But Dworkin imagines a scheme under which much of what would otherwise count as brute luck can be considered option luck. This is an insurance scheme, which each person is free to accept or to decline, at market prices. Those who decide to keep their resources rather than buying insurance against bad brute luck cannot later claim an entitlement to compensation should their brute luck turn bad.

This schema remains egalitarian, but only in respect to a restricted range of outcomes in which individual choice does not play a role. Subsequent writing in this vein reinforced the key premise that what egalitarian justice requires is not equal resources overall, but rather that no one should be worse off than others for no fault of his own; or, in another formulation, for reasons outside his control. This, of course, permits (and perhaps even requires) inequalities in what is one's fault, or for what is under one's control. In Gerald Cohen's words:

Egalitarianism does not enjoin redress of or compensation for disadvantage as such. It attends, rather, to involuntary disadvantage, which is the sort that does not reflect the subject's choice...the egalitarian asks if someone with a disadvantage could have avoided it or could not overcome it. If he could have avoided it, he has no claim to compensation. (Cohen 1989)

Cohen (1989), Richard Arneson (1989, 1997), and the other so-called luck egalitarians (Anderson 1999) thus propose a route for an egalitarian liberal theory of justice which promises to escape the alleged inattentiveness to the moral importance of individual choice, responsibility, and desert which Scheffler locates in Rawlsian philosophical liberalism. Here the emphasis on personal responsibility is as strong as in the right-of-centre political rhetoric of the past two decades: what results from free, informed choices, is a matter of personal fortune or misfortune. Where 'luck egalitarianism' parts company is over the distribution of well-being, or resources for well-being, for what is *not* the result of choice, that is, for what is brute luck. Luck egalitarians are strictly egalitarian here, whereas political conservatives are not: it is not part of the conservative view of the state that it should remedy cosmic injustice in this sense.

Luck egalitarians may differ from conservatives, also, in the degree to which they believe that that the plight of the poor and dispossessed in society (and that of the prosperous) is due to the consequences of choices they have freely made. It is a commonplace that more of one's station in life is attributed to the choices one has made, as we move rightward on the political spectrum. This is, as I will discuss shortly, a mixture of factual assumption and moral attitude. What is notable for the issue of personal responsibility for health, however, is that luck egalitarian philosophers have not been reluctant at all to assign responsibility to individuals in the domain of health. Indeed, choices involving health, such as smoking and drinking, have been the chief source of examples in this literature, as if the appropriateness of assigning personal responsibility in this domain were clearer than in others. Arneson, for example, would provide eyeglasses to a person born with myopia. But 'If a person became blind through deliberate and fully informed participation in a dangerous sport that often gives rise to injuries that result in blindness, it becomes questionable whether compensation is owed to him.' The clear implication of the use of these examples (none of the philosophical contributions addresses personal health policy issues as such) is that illness and premature death resulting from the choices one makes are one's private concern and place no claim on social assistance.

The luck egalitarians' lack of interest in health policy notwithstanding, this literature offers an elaborately reasoned rationale for an emphasis on personal responsibility in all the domains of health policy surveyed above. Those who lose in their gambles on health would deserve less consideration in rationing than those afflicted for reasons beyond their control; their worsened health state would not be counted as a social injustice; and, most generally, their sufferings might be understood as the price they paid for taking calculated risks. This is not to say that luck egalitarian writers are likely to see such policies as inherent in their approach; they tend to be left of centre, and their interest is for the most part on the egalitarian part of their message rather than on the inegalitarian implications I have alleged here. It is also open to luck egalitarians to recommend a pluralist view that combines or balances luck egalitarian provisions with a more traditional egalitarianism. John Roemer's approach to health resource allocation, for example, takes 'horizontal equity'—patients with similar needs receive similar treatment—as a starting point but uses luck egalitarian principles to choose among the many allocations that satisfy that requirement. (Roemer 2002; see also Roemer 1998) Nevertheless, these health policy conclusions tally with the medical examples that many luck egalitarians use, and it may be the case that what was intended as a largely egalitarian approach supports, in the end, a set of positions on health policy which are currently voiced only by the most conservative of commentators. As such, it represents the best-elaborated justification of these positions.

Nevertheless, I do not believe that these considerations make a plausible case for moving personal responsibility for health to the centre of health policy concerns, except in the sense of suggesting effective strategies of health promotion. In the final section, I offer objections to doing so, addressing both the intuitive argument drawn on by conservative commentators and also the philosophical considerations presented by the luck egalitarians.

6.4. A ROLE FOR PERSONAL RESPONSIBILITY FOR HEALTH?

The notion that people should bear responsibility for the consequences of their voluntary choices makes up part of the bedrock of our moral and political culture. It is, in John Roemer's words, 'the cost of freedom', the dues we pay when we assert our right to self-determination as free adult citizens. The same freedom that permits us to act on our personal tastes and preferences, pursuant to our individual goals, plans, and values, reduces the scope of excuses for these choices should they turn out badly. Just as we expect to be left alone to decide which risks to take, others expect to hold us accountable for the consequences. If the condition of evading or denying responsibility for the consequences of our choices were the denial of the freedom to choose, the price would often be too high.

In the field of health, personal responsibility can be life-giving. Because health and longevity depend so much on whether a person adopts healthy living habits, encouraging people to take good care of themselves is a key to a population free of avoidable infirmity and premature mortality. The first steps toward adoption of healthier living habits are understanding the causal links between behaviour and health, and accepting and acting upon the notion that to this large extent, we can control our state of health in the future.

Despite these considerations, I will argue that personal responsibility for health deserves but a peripheral role in health policy. This conclusion should be reached, in my view, whether or not we think that personal responsibility should be central to our thinking about distributive justice generally. I will begin with a brief account of arguments against emphasising personal responsibility in the theory of justice, for if we reject the broader view we have little reason to support it in the special case of health. On the chance that these arguments are not convincing, I proceed to offer reasons to reject any attempt to move from the general thesis to its application to health. I close with a word on how a very limited, but constructive, role for personal responsibility might be envisioned within health policy.

6.4.1. *Justice and responsibility*

A full assessment of the debate over the role of personal responsibility in the general theory of justice is not possible within the confines of the present chapter. But it is worth noting some of the grounds on which such objections might be made. As Elizabeth Anderson points out in her paper, 'What is the point of equality', some implications of luck egalitarianism are highly counterintuitive, and an important source of these problems is the view's preoccupation with individual choice. The fundamental idea, that bad (brute) luck deserves compensation but that the consequences of voluntary trades, gambles, risks, and tradeoffs do not, seems to yield appropriate concern on neither point. For example, such a regime would in effect punish many people who seem to have done no wrong, such as those who voluntarily refrain from work in order to care for dependents, or people who suffer when prudent risks go bad. These people will lose out in a luck egalitarian society because their deprivation stemmed from their free choices. On the other hand, luck egalitarianism might call for compensation to a person with better than average income who, through no fault of his own, had developed inalterable tastes for champagne and caviar. Anderson notes that while luck egalitarianism might seem at first sight to offer the best of capitalism and socialism by encouraging personal responsibility under the protection of a safety net against bad luck, it is also vulnerable to the charge that it combines some of the worst features of the two systems. In seeking to remove every difference in involuntary advantage, it is a utopian project to 'correct' for cosmic injustice, differences in prospects which are the fault of no person or society. At the same time, it assigns responsibility, and withholds assistance, regardless of need, whenever people make choices, standing in stern judgement of what, in actual human beings, is often a halting and uncertain effort to secure well-being. Its echo of the Elizabethan poor laws is a case in point; and the medical implications are another.

Given that most, if not all, of the philosophers contributing to the luck egalitarian literature hail from the left side of the political spectrum (in some cases, far from the centre), it is startling when the views they express on some issues exceed in their judgemental rigour positions which are prevalent even on the right. In this regard, the luck egalitarian position does not close the gap Scheffler alleged to exist between theorists of justice and contemporary popular political morality; it opens a new gap to the opposite side.

Again, the medical examples are the clearest example. The record shows that proposals to assign personal responsibility for health along the lines discussed in this essay have been relatively rare in any political milieu. Though proposals to this effect have appeared occasionally in the literature of medicine and bioethics, no significant figures in health policy or politics have taken up John Knowles's theme. Physicians, who in the United States lean toward the right, tend to be even more emphatic on the requirement that patients be cared for without regard to fault. The near-unanimity of liver transplant surgeons on the need to avoid 'moralizing' about the responsibility of alcoholics is particularly noteworthy, in light of the absolute need to establish priorities among patients whose lives hang in the balance.

It is true that some respondents in focus groups studied by health economists indicated that rationing should take into account the contribution of the individual to his or her own plight. But in nearly every case, those who voiced this sentiment were in the minority. Moreover, several investigators noted that support for assigning lower priority to individuals at fault waned during deliberation. (Nord and Richardson 1995; Dolan et al. 1999; Nord 1999) And the proposition has been rejected outright by some deliberative bodies seeking to establish basic principles for prioritisation (Nord 1999).

Even the minority view on personal responsibility for health which appears to tally with the luck egalitarian verdicts may, in the view of one group of researchers, stem from quite different premises. Ubel et al. (1999) sought to distinguish between three grounds for assigning lower priority to patients whose behaviour may have contributed to their susceptibility to illness or injury. These respondents declined to change their priorities when told that the capacity for treatment, that is, likelihood of recovery with a given amount of resources, was the same for both sets of patients. But they were unmoved also when told that, after all, the patients' behaviour had not in fact been a contributing factor in their ill health. The reason that these respondents favoured lower priority for treatment for the likes of alcoholics and addicts was that they did not think that the lives of people of this sort were as worthy of care. This position, of course, is antithetical to the egalitarian emphasis of the luck egalitarian viewpoint which, superficially, leads to similar conclusions on personal responsibility for health.

The lack of correspondence between the luck egalitarian view and conventional morality need not be understood as any kind of rebuttal of the former; ordinary thinking about these moral issues might be wrong. But in this case the charge against Rawls and other liberals, that their views are seriously out of step with mainstream opinion, does not recommend luck egalitarianism as an alternative.

In the view of luck egalitarianism, informed and voluntary choices establish a moral fact, that of individual responsibility, from which important consequences flow. The more plausible alternative is of course that the more fundamental consideration is that of need. And it is the need of patients, without regard to responsibility, that is counted as the only relevant consideration in conventional medical ethics, and apparently in the mind of most members of the public as well.

A theory of justice which does not give a central role to personal responsibility need not dismiss the moral significance of choice entirely. It can be given due emphasis on instrumental grounds. Where people, or whole societies, might be harmed by relieving people of responsibility for the consequences of their choices, this accountability can be imposed. But where the consequences of doing so would, on the whole, be adverse, there would remain no reason to do so. J. S. Mill (1965) as noted by Richard Arneson (himself a luck egalitarian), urged that assistance be given to the impoverished up to the point at which further aid becomes harmful (Arneson 1997). The point applies still more forcefully to health, since it is very unlikely that the threat of forfeiture of health care can serve as a deterrent to risk taking, and in particular that the harm that would be averted would be greater than that inflicted in denying care to the sick and injured.

6.4.2. *The context of personal responsibility for health*

These brief remarks do not tell against luck egalitarianism, or indeed against any theory of justice which has the consequence that individual responsibility for health should be assigned a central role in health policy decisions. This must be determined on the merits of these theories as general theories of justice. Though the medical examples are instructive, they appear in this literature only as illustrations; the tail does not wag the dog. This task cannot be undertaken here, but there are further considerations that tell against any attempt to put personal responsibility closer to the centre of the health policy stage, however well-founded the theory of justice which recommends doing so. These considerations are a mixture of practical and philosophical concerns.

Which actions are voluntary?

A moral viewpoint that puts great store on individual choice and responsibility must offer a criterion for determining which choices incur these obligations. The web of complications that stand in the way is, as we know from criminal law, extremely broad. But in criminal law we have at least a set of precedents and statutory specifications that guide us. In the case of personal responsibility for health, we have only the intuitions of one observer, set against that of another.

Moreover, actions only rarely have all the attributes—informed, voluntary, uncoerced, spontaneous, deliberated, etc.—that, in the ideal case, are preconditions for full personal responsibility. This is a particular problem in the case of lifestyles, which are matters of habit ingrained over many years and may have been learned from the individual's principal role models. The most dangerous elements of lifestyle, such as smoking or alcohol abuse, involve addiction, and the status of the smoker's decision to light up the next cigarette is anything but clear. One way around this problem is to assign personal responsibility on the basis of the initial decision to smoke, or the rational deliberation of the then-unaddicted individual to accept risk to health as the price of anticipated pleasure. This is the same strategy used by prosecutors of witchcraft in colonial Salem, Massachusetts, where both statute and common law viewed the acts of witchcraft as those of the inhabiting spirits and punished the witch for having permitted the devil to assume her shape, or by having communed with the devil by commissioning him to do acts of mischief. As with the magistrates in Salem, it is no easy matter to establish when and where this originating sin occurs, or to link the severity of the sentence to the degree of wrongful risk that we might imagine has been assumed.

At the most fundamental level, this requirement takes us directly to the ancient question of freedom of the will. Any policy debate which awaits resolution of these uncertainties is a long way from closure. John Roemer, a luck egalitarian theorist, has taken up the challenge and offers, in the abstract, a method. Once again, a health example—responsibility for the consequences of smoking—is chosen as a focus for discussion.

Roemer's elegant proposal (1993, 1995) imagines that among factors leading to the act of smoking we can sort those over which the individual has control from those over which this is lacking. The circumstances of one's birth; one's gender; and perhaps one's social class, for example, may not be matters of one's choosing. But all of these seem to influence a person's pattern of tobacco use. Roemer recognises that different societies will identify the locus of control differently: the factors counted in one culture as beyond individual control may be regarded otherwise elsewhere. Roemer suggests that each society list the factors it wishes to recognise as beyond control, which in turn will delimit a 'type'—for example, female schoolteachers, or male steelworkers. These 'types', subject to different factors beyond individual control, will display different ranges of behaviour; for example, the steelworkers might smoke more than the schoolteachers. But, in Roemer's view, their degree of responsibility is not proportionate. Instead, Roemer suggests that the median individual in each type (as measured, for example, in the number of cigarettes smoked per day) should be assigned null responsibility, with accounting in a positive or negative direction proceeding from this midpoint. Roemer does not propose any particular list of such factors, and indeed is not committed to the premise that this question admits of anything other than a conventional answer. Still, in Roemer's view, the proposal will ensure that, in every society, responsibility will be assigned in proportion to the degree of personal control, as understood by that society. In Roemer's words, this is 'A pragmatic theory of responsibility for the egalitarian planner'.

It is as a pragmatic theory for planning purposes, however, that the first questions arise. For the debate within societies, including Roemer's, over how much control individuals have over their behaviour, much of the controversy is precisely over which factors should be on this list. The prospect that different societies will construct their lists in different ways, however responsive to cultural differences, itself advertises the likelihood that all these lists will reflect not metaphysical bedrock—that is, whether the individual really does have control, or lacks it—but rather the consensus of opinion. A dissident who rejects this consensus will thus have no reason to change his or her views. Finally, it is not clear how finely these 'types' will be differentiated. Each individual's path to tobacco or obesity is distinct, channelled or inhibited by influences, opportunities, inclinations, and preferences unique to that person. Male steelworkers, even if they tend to smoke more than female schoolteachers, are an otherwise heterogeneous lot. If we classify like with exactly like, the groups will be too small and too homogeneous to admit of enough deviation from the median to generate Roemer's interesting result.

The question of what counts as 'a factor', that is, how precisely to account for a particular individual's behaviour, takes us directly back to the controversy, which the proposal was designed to resolve, over the possibility and scope of free choice given the apparent determinants in one's internal and external environments. Arneson, a luck egalitarian, moderates the policy impact of this approach in pointing out that responsibility and desert are proportional not only to the consequences of one's actions but also to the difficulty one faced in attempting to be prudent. Pill and Stott (1982, 1985) found that working class respondents trusted health information if obtained from someone they knew, but seldom otherwise; individuals vary, to some extent as a matter of chance, in the sources of information offered to them. These variations at the individual level are unlikely to be measurable at the societal level. And even when they are, we may not agree on their significance. Studies of the origins of class differences in health-related behaviour, for example, demonstrate that unhealthy habits of living are strongly predicted by poverty in childhood and throughout the lifespan (Lynch et al. 1997). Some people transcend these origins and life prudently; there is at least as much disagreement over the freedom of the others to do likewise as on any other issue in this complex debate.

Adverse effects of assigning responsibility

On a less metaphysical plane, an important consideration weighing against emphasis on personal responsibility for health is the potential harm that the enterprise might inflict upon the enterprise of health care, and on social policy on health affairs. One plausible ground for the resistance of physicians to basing treatment decisions on assessments of personal responsibility is the prospect that the very useful and virtuous first instinct of the doctor or nurse, that of sympathy and care for the suffering patient, might be attenuated—put on an unstable hold, as it were, until the verdict of fault comes in. All of us gain if and when doctors think of patients as patients (a point which tells also against financial screening of patients at the hospital door). The same point can be made for societies as a whole: it is not salutary for people to become used to withholding sympathy for sick fellow-citizens unless and until it is established that those who are sick could not have stayed healthy by acting more prudently.

Arbitrariness of fault-finding

The empirical findings of Ubel et al., mentioned above, point to a further reason for concern with the notion of assessing personal responsibility for health. Ubel's sample, it will be recalled, included people whose concern was less with the contribution to illness made by voluntary choice than with distaste for the kinds of people who were thought to make these choices. An examination of the small literature, beginning with Knowles, that has proposed a greater role for personal responsibility reveals that not all choices leading to illness are counted alike. Those that are targeted tend to be sins—sloth, gluttony, lust, to use their old-fashioned names—or to be behaviour, such as drug addiction, of the marginalised. We could, but do not, augment this list by adding other kinds of choices, also having a pronounced effect on health—of which we tend to approve. For example, the decision to have children, now that this involves a definite intention for many people, risks the health of the mother. A decision to postpone childbearing until advanced education has been completed markedly increases the risks for cervical and breast cancer. Daredevilry in sports and adventure risks life and limb, but the survivors are treated as heroes. If the moral principle underlying a move to give greater prominence to personal responsibility for health is that those who generate costs should pay for them, we should not expect that the only ones made to shoulder the costs are those who behave in ways that offend their neighbours. The point is not that a society must either demand compensation for all avoidable costs or else demand none. But the coincidence of two lists, that of lifestyles deemed burdensomely expensive and that of lifestyles deemed sinful, or of people deemed unworthy, suggests a different agenda from the stated one.

A sense of disproportion

Finally, a policy in which individuals are made to shoulder the burden caused by adverse consequences of choices they have made must make 'the punishment fit the crime': the burden reimposed on the risk-taker should be proportional to the burden imposed by the risk taking. But there is no metric to permit this. One problem is that similar behaviour in different people, and in different circumstances, represents quite different levels of risk (Japanese men, for example, are less likely to contract lung cancer from smoking than American men). Moreover, some habits which are unhealthy, even lethal for some are actually health-giving to others; alcohol is the outstanding example. And some habits, because they are taxed, may present a net economic gain to their societies. When cigarette taxes are high, for example, the added medical costs generated by the use of tobacco are more than offset by the payment of taxes and the elimination of pensions when smokers die. Those who have taken care of themselves, in that kind of regime, are the real threat to their neighbours' well-being.

Exaggeration of interpersonal differences

When critics of the emerging literature on the influence of social status on health attempt to explain away the evident health impact of social inequality, the thrust of their commentary is to shift responsibility away from social institutions and social structure and onto individuals. But to make this plausible, a series of exaggerations are required. First, almost all of the measured differences in health status between social groups is attributed to behaviour. Second, almost all of that behaviour is characterised as purely voluntary. But neither claim is supportable. Though it is certainly true that working class adults in the United Kingdom and United States smoke more and weigh more than their well-to-do fellow citizens, on average, these differences account for only part of the difference in health. One widely cited study which examined the leading risk behaviours put the figure at 15 per cent (Lantz et al. 1998). Though others give higher estimates (and there is not agreement on what these figures mean), no investigators explain virtually all health differences associated with social status to differing lifestyles. Moreover, where these behavioural differences do exist, the extent to which these can reasonably be viewed as free, informed, and voluntary choices is partial at best. Even assuming that some of the behavioural differences reflect different values, goals, or attitudes toward time, the remainder is occasion enough for concern over the fairness of the distribution of health.

In this light, proposals to attach importance in health policy to imprudent health-related behaviour involve a great deal of hand-waving. A sense of proportion is elusive. This should not be surprising. The administration of the criminal law, in which degree of responsibility must be determined as closely as possible, requires the elaborate and expense apparatus of the courts, attorneys, and lengthy trials. There is nothing comparable in the medical world, and there is no common law built of precedents, penalties attached to particular kinds of acts over many years, adopted in the interest of a smoothly functioning society. Nor is there likely to be, nor would it be desirable if there were to be.

6.4.3. *A positive role for personal responsibility for health*

Taken together, these considerations suggest that health policies that would give personal responsibility for health a central role face severe objections. The theory of justice which seems most supportive of this policy is questionable on its own terms, and in any case does not lend this support without a number of dubious accompanying assumptions. These reservations are joined by a number of objections of a more practical nature which suggest that a commitment to assessing personal responsibility for health might be wrong-headed, arbitrary, disingenuous, and even dangerous.

This account should not, however, end on that note. For a number of reasons, it is both practical and desirable that personal responsibility play a role (though not a central role) in public health and clinical medicine in the future.

One reason that personal responsibility for health should not be wholly ignored is the inherent desirability of free choice, and assumption of responsibility, for personal development and for the management of one's life course. Interpersonal variation in goals, preferences, and tastes—beyond the reckoning of the most omniscient managers—requires individual liberty so that circumstances can be tailored to the individual. Assumption of risk by the individual enables society to condone this freedom. This shouldering of the risk has numerous further benefits for the individual as well (though these can be overshadowed by seriously adverse consequences). As Thomas Scanlon has observed (1988), choosing freely tells others that one is the kind of being capable of doing so, and this is a prerequisite to participation as a person in a society of free and equal beings. Looked at from a different perspective, requiring that people take a measure of responsibility for some of the adverse consequences of their behaviour can and should be taken into account by the chooser at the time of decision, lest their deliberations be distorted in leaving out the consequences of their actions for others. If this deters some actions, as high taxes dissuade teenagers from smoking, this is often a further benefit.

Above all, the fostering of a sense of personal responsibility for health can be part of a programme of 'positive freedom' or 'empowerment', a realization that actions taken can have a marked and positive impact on one's health, with radiating good effects on other dimensions of life and on other people. There is a risk, in stressing what the individual can do to stay healthy, that an individual's actual power will be exaggerated, and consequently that people can come to blame themselves, wrongfully, when they fall ill (Crawford 1977, 1979; Wikler 1985). But there is nothing inherent in the prospect of health promotion that necessitates this double message, and there is no reason to hold back from development of techniques of education and motivation which enable those who would favour the tradeoffs required to avoid illness and injury to do so efficiently and confidently. Neither self-blame nor that of others need figure in personal responsibility for health thus conceived.

6.5. CONCLUSION

Nothing in the foregoing denies what many take to be obvious, viz., that some people burden themselves and others in avoidable and undesirable ways by taking unjustified risks with their health. These actions can be as free, informed, and voluntary as any other, though, under this description, they must also count as rash and foolish. Ordinary morality would license resentment by people burdened as a result of these actions, and I have not provided any philosophical argument to the contrary.

The intuitions supporting this moral judgement, however, are insufficient to justify a strong emphasis on personal responsibility for health in the domain of health policy. Neither philosophical nor practical considerations give sufficient support for a policy of excluding patients who are sick as a result of their own imprudence from health services. Moreover, health deficits should generally be counted alike regardless of their source in policies aimed at reducing inequalities in health traceable to social status, and in targeting the burden of disease in public health interventions.

The theme of personal responsibility for health, perhaps more fortuitously labelled personal *opportunity* for health, may yet come to play a constructive role in health promotion, an element in efforts to educate and inspire individuals to take an active, informed role in staying healthy. The ethics of public health have traditionally been oriented to the future, to positive outcomes of interventions that promise to relieve suffering. A theme of personal responsibility for health that focuses on what the individual may have done or not done to deserve assistance, however, begins its moral calculations with what has happened in the past. This account is difficult to square with the mission of public health as usually conceived, and if the conflict is not fully resolvable I suspect that the traditional values chart the best course for the future.

References

Anderson, Elizabeth S. (1999). 'What is the Point of Equality?', *Ethics*, 109(2): 287–337.

Arneson, Richard J. (1989). 'Equality of Opportunity for Welfare', *Philosophical Studies*, 56: 77–93.

——(1997). 'Egalitarianism and the Undeserving Poor', *Journal of Political Philosophy*, 5(4): 327–50.

Auerbach, James A. and Barbara K. Krimgold, (eds.) (2001). *Income, Socioeconomic Status, and Health: Exploring the Relationships*. NPA Report #299. Washington: National Policy Association.

Bowling, Ann, (1996). 'Health Care Rationing: the Public's Debate', *British Medical Journal*, 312(16 March): 670–4.

Braakenheilm, C. R. (1990) *Vaard paa lika vilkaar (Health Care on Equal Terms)* in J. Caltorp and C. R. Braakeheilm (eds.) Vaardens Pris (The Price of Care). Stockholm: Verbum forlag.

Cohen, Gerald A. (1989). 'On the Currency of Egalitarian Justice', *Ethics*, 99: 906–44.

Crawford, Robert. (1977). Individual Responsibility and Health Politics in the 1970s, in Susan Reverby and David Rosner (eds.), *Health Care in America: Essays in Social History*. Philadelphia: Temple University Press, pp. 247–68.

——(1979). 'You are dangerous to your health: The Ideology and Politics of Victim Blaming', *International Journal of Health Services*, 7: 663–80.

——Bruce Kennedy, and Ichiro Kawachi (2000). *Is Inequality Bad for our Health?* Boston: Beacon.

Department of Health and Social Services (UK) (1976). *Prevention and Health: Everybody's Business*. London: HMSO.

Dolan, P, R. Cookson, and B. Ferguson (1999). 'Effect of Discussion and Deliberation on the Public's Views of Priority Setting in Health Care: Focus Group Study', *British Medical Journal*, 318: 916–19.

Dworkin, Gerald (1981). 'Voluntary Health Risks and Public Policy', *Hastings Center Report*, 11: 26–31.

Dworkin, Ronald (1981). 'What is Equality? Part I: Equality of Welfare', *Philosophy and Public Affairs*, 10(3): 185–246.

——(1993). 'Justice in the Distribution of Health Care', *McGill Law Journal* 38: 883–98.

Edwards R. T., A. Boland, D. Cohen, C. Wilkinson, and J. Williams (2003). 'Clinical and Lay Preferences for the Explicit Prioritisation of Elective Waiting Lists: Survey Evidence from Wales', *Health Policy*, 63(3): 229–37.

Evans, Robert G., Morris L. Barer, and Theodore R. Marmor (1994). *Why are Some People Healthy and Others Not?* Hawthorne, NY: Aldine de Gruyter.

Gingrich, Newt (1995). *To Renew America*. New York: HarperCollins, p. 39.

Kekes, John (1997). 'A Question for Egalitarians,' *Ethics*, 107: 658–69.

Knechtle, Stuart et al. (1992). 'Liver Transplantation for Alcoholic Liver Disease', *Surgery*, 112: 694–703.

Knowles, John (1977). *Doing Better and Feeling Worse*. New York: W. W. Norton.

Lalonde, Mark (1974). *A New Perspective on the Health of Canadians. A Working Document*. Ottawa: Report of the Government of Canada.

Lantz P. M., J. S. House, J. M. Lepkowski, and D. R. Williams et al. (1998). 'Socioeconomic Factors, Health Behaviors, and Mortality: Results from a Nationally Representative Prospective Study of U.S. Adults', *Journal of the American Medical Association*, 279: 1703–8.

Leichter, H. M. (1991). *Free To Be Foolish. Politics and Health Promotion in the United States and Great Britain*. Princeton, NJ: Princeton University Press.

Lynch, J. W., G. A. Kaplan, and J. T. Salonen (1997). 'Why Do Poor People Behave Poorly? Variation in Adult Health Behaviors and Characteristics by Stages of the Socioeconomic Lifecourse', *Social Science and Medicine*, 44(6): 809–19.

Mac Donald, Heather (1998). 'Public Health Quackery', *City Journal*, Fall 8: 40–53.

——(2000). *The Burden of Bad Ideas: How Modern Intellectuals Misshape Our Society*. Chicago: Ivan R. Dee.

Marchand, Sarah and Daniel Wikler (1998). 'Class, Health, and Justice', *Milbank Quarterly*, Fall 1998.

Marmot, Michael G., G. Davey Smith, S. Stansfield, C. Patel, F. North, and J. Head (1991). 'Health Inequalities among British Civil Servants: The Whitehall II Study'. *Lancet*, 37: 1387–93.

Marmot, Michael, Carol D. Ryff, Larry L. Bumpass, Martin Shipley, and Nadine Marks (1997). Social Inequalities in Health: Next Questions And Converging Evidence, *Social Science and Medicine*, 44(6): 901–10.

Mill, John Stuart (1965). *Principles of Political Economy*. Toronto: University of Toronto Press, book V, chapter 11, section 13: 961. Originally published 1848.

Nord, Erik and Jeff Richardson, Andrew Street, Helga Kuhse, and Peter Singer (1995). 'Maximising Health Benefits Versus Egalitarianism: An Australian Survey of Health Issues', *Social Science and Medicine*, 41(10): 1429–37.

—— and —— (1999). *Cost-Value Analysis in Health Care*. Cambridge: Cambridge University Press.

Pill, Roisin and Nigel Ch. H. Stott (1982). 'Concepts of Illness Causation and Responsibility: Some Preliminary Data from a Sample of Working Class Mothers', *Social Science and Medicine*, 16: 43–52.

—— and —— (1985). 'Choice or Chance: Further Evidence on Ideas of Illness and Responsibility for Health', *Social Science and Medicine*, 20(10): 981–91.

Reiser, Stanley J. (1985). 'Responsibility for Personal Health: A Historical Persepective', *The Journal of Medicine and Philosophy*, 10: 7–17.

Roemer, John E. (1993). 'A Pragmatic Theory of Responsibility for the Egalitarian Planner'. *Philosophy and Public Affairs*, 22: 146–66. Reprinted in Roemer, John E. (1995). *Egalitarian Perspectives*. Cambridge: Cambridge University Press.

—— (1995). 'Equality and Responsibility', *Boston Review*, 20(2).

—— (1998). *Equality of Opportunity*. Cambridge MA.: Harvard University Press.

—— (2002). Equity in Health Care Delivery. Unpublished manuscript.

Satel, Sally (1997). The Politicization of Public Health. *The Wall Street Journal*, 12 December 1996.

—— (2000). *How Political Correctness is Corrupting Medicine*, New York, Basic Books.

Scanlon, Thomas (1988). 'The Significance of Choice', *The Tanner Lectures on Human Values, Vol. 8*. Cambridge: Cambridge University Press, pp. 149–216.

—— (1995). 'Comments on Roemer', *Boston Review* 20(2).

Scheffler, Samuel (1992). 'Responsibility, Reactive Attitudes, and Liberalism in Philosophy and Politics', *Philosophy and Public Affairs*, 21(4): 299–323.

—— (1995): 'Individual Responsibility in a Global Age', *Social Philosophy and Policy*, 12: 219–36.

Schenker, Steven, Henry S. Perkins, and Michael Sorrell (1990). 'Should Patients with End-Stage Alcoholic Liver Disease have a New Liver?', *Hepatology*, 314–19.

Scruton, Roger (2000*a*). 'The Risks of Being Risk-Free', *Wall Street Journal* (Europe), 7 January.

—— (2000*b*). *WHO, WHAT, and WHY: Trans-national Government, Legitimacy and the World Health Organization*. London: Institute of Economic Affairs.

Starzl, Thomas et al. (1988). 'Orthotopic Liver Transplantation for Alcholic Cirrhosis', *Journal of the American Medical Association*, 260(17), 4 November: 2542–4.

Surgeon General of the United States (1979). *Healthy People: Report on Health Promotion and Disease Prevention*. Washington, DC, Government Printing Office.

Sylvester, Rachel (1999). 'IVF Treatment to be Denied to Smokers', *The Independent* (London), 16 March 1999.

Tren, Richard, and Hugh High (2000). *Smoked Out: Anti-Tobacco Activism at the World Bank*. London: Institute of Economic Affairs.

Ubel, Peter A., Jonathan Baron, and David Asch (1999). 'Social Responsibilty, Personal Responsibility, and Prognosis in Public Judgments about Transplant Allocation', *Bioethics*, 13(1): 57–68.

Veatch, Robert (1980). 'Voluntary Risks to Health', *Journal of the American Medical Association*, 243 (January 4): 50–5.

Walzer, Michael (1983). *Spheres of Justice*. New York: Basic Books.

Wikler, Daniel (1978). 'Persuasion and Coercion for Health: Ethical Issues in Government Efforts to Change Life-Styles', *Milbank Memorial Fund Quarterly*, 56(3): 303–38.

—— (1985). 'Holistic Medicine: Concepts of Personal Responsibility for Health', in Stalker, Douglas, and Glymour Clark (eds.), *Examining Holistic Medicine*. Buffalo, NY: Prometheus Press.

—— (1987). 'Personal Responsibility for Illness', in T. Regan and D. Van DeVeer (eds.), *Health Care Ethics*. Philadelphia: Temple University Press.

—— and Dan E. Beauchamp (1995). 'Lifestyles and Public Health', in Warren Thomas Reich (ed.), *The Encyclopedia of Bioethics*. New York: Simon and Schuster Macmillan, pp. 1366–9.

Woodward, Christopher (1998). Egalitarianism, Responsibility, and Desert. *Imprints* 3(1): 25–48.

7

Relational Conceptions of Justice: Responsibilities for Health Outcomes

THOMAS W. POGGE

7.1. INTRODUCTION

My view on justice in regard to health is distinctive in two ways. First, I hold that the strength of our moral reasons to prevent or to mitigate particular medical conditions depends not only on what one might call *distributional* factors, such as how badly off the people affected by these conditions are in absolute and relative terms, how costly prevention or treatment would be, and how much patients would benefit from given treatment. Rather, it depends also on *relational* factors, that is, on how we are related to the medical conditions they suffer.

This point is widely accepted in regard to conduct: you have, for instance, stronger moral reason to make sure that people are not harmed by you than that they are not harmed through other causes (others' negligence or their own, say, or bad weather). And your moral reason to mitigate the injuries of an accident victim is stronger if you were materially involved in causing his or her accident. I assert an analogous point also in regard to any social institutions that agents are materially involved in upholding: in shaping an institutional order, we should be more concerned, morally, that it not substantially contribute to the incidence of medical conditions than that it prevent medical conditions caused by other factors. And we should design any institutional order so that it prioritises the mitigation of medical conditions whose incidence it substantially contributes to. In institutional contexts as well, moral assessment must then be sensitive not merely to the distribution of health outcomes as such, but also to how these outcomes are produced.

The latter consideration is needed to distinguish different degrees of responsibility for medical conditions and for their prevention and mitigation. What is morally significant here, in institutional as well as interactional contexts, is

This chapter was improved considerably by the thoughtful responses it received, especially from my commentator Sissela Bok, at the November 1998 Conference on The Foundations of Health Equity held at the Harvard University Center for Population and Development Studies. The final version greatly benefited from extensive and astute comments by Christian Barry, Mira Johri, and especially Fabienne Peter. It was composed with the help of a generous grant from the Research and Writing Initiative of the Programme on Global Security and Sustainability of the John D. and Catherine T. MacArthur Foundation.

something like the conventional distinction between positive and negative responsibility. However, the differentiations required are, even in interactional contexts, more complex than binary talk of positive and negative duties suggests; and they are, as we shall see, very much more complex in institutional contexts.

My second thesis builds upon the first. It is generally believed that one's moral reason to help prevent and mitigate others' medical conditions is stronger when these others are compatriots than when they are foreigners. Limiting this common view, my second thesis denies the moral significance of compatriotism with regard to the prevention and mitigation of medical conditions in whose incidence one is materially involved.

This thesis, too, is less controversial in regard to conduct: the strength of your moral reason to act so as to avoid injuring others' health and to help mitigate any of their medical conditions you helped cause is not affected by whether these others are compatriots or foreigners. Thus, for example, your moral reasons to drive carefully and to attend to victims of any accident you have caused do not weaken when you are traveling abroad. More controversial, by contrast, is the analogous point for institutional contexts, where—pursuant to the first thesis—we ought to ensure that any institutional order we help impose avoids causing medical conditions and prioritises the mitigation of any medical conditions it does cause. Here my second thesis holds that the stringency of this responsibility is not sensitive to whether the medical conditions at stake are suffered by foreigners or by compatriots.

To get a sense of how strong these theses are, we can link them by transitivity: Foreigners' medical conditions in whose incidence we are materially involved have the same moral weight for us as compatriots' medical conditions in whose incidence we are materially involved (second thesis).[1] Compatriots' medical conditions in whose incidence we are materially involved have greater moral weight for us than compatriots' medical conditions in whose incidence we are not materially involved (first thesis). Therefore, foreigners' medical conditions in whose incidence we are materially involved have greater moral weight for us than compatriots' medical conditions in whose incidence we are not materially involved (combined thesis).

In interactional contexts, this combined thesis is not likely to be very controversial. Suppose two children have been injured by speeding drivers and money is needed to pay for the expensive medical treatment necessary to

---

[1] This sentence must be read as including an implicit 'other things being equal' clause. In particular, I assume the same degree of material involvement. I also assume, here and in the next two sentences, similarity of medical conditions, of treatment options and cost, and of patients. Concerning this last respect, my second thesis does not, then, put every foreigner on a par with every compatriot. It does not deny that we have stronger moral reason to be concerned about injuries we have caused, or might cause, to a compatriot child than about like injuries to a foreign career criminal. I am merely asserting that the foreigner/compatriot distinction plays no role in explaining such a discrepancy, which should then, less misleadingly, be put as follows: We have stronger moral reason to be concerned about injuries we have caused, or might cause, to a child than about like injuries to a career criminal, regardless of what the citizenship of either may be.

restore their health and appearance completely. In one case, the child is a foreigner and you were the driver. In the other case, the child is a compatriot and someone else was the driver. My combined thesis entails that in a situation like this you have (other things being equal) stronger moral reason to buy the costly treatment for the foreign child.

In institutional contexts, by contrast, my combined thesis is likely to be quite controversial. It might be stated as follows: foreigners' medical conditions, if social institutions we are materially involved in upholding substantially contribute to their incidence, have greater moral weight for us than compatriots' medical conditions in whose causation we are not materially involved. This combined thesis is radical if social institutions we are materially involved in upholding do substantially contribute to the incidence of medical conditions abroad. Is this the case?

Many kinds of social institutions can substantially contribute to the incidence of medical conditions. Of these, economic institutions—the basic rules governing ownership, production, use, and exchange of natural resources, goods, and services—have the greatest impact on health. This impact is mediated, for the most part, through poverty. By avoidably producing severe poverty, economic institutions substantially contribute to the incidence of many medical conditions. Persons materially involved in upholding such economic institutions are then materially involved in the causation of such medical conditions.

In our world, poverty is highly relevant to human health. In fact, poverty is far and away the most important factor in explaining existing health deficits. Because they are poor, 815 million persons are undernourished, 1,100 million lack access to safe drinking water, 2,400 million lack access to basic sanitation,[2] more than 880 million lack access to health services, and approximately 1,000 million have no adequate shelter.[3] Because of poverty, 'two out of five children in the developing world are stunted, one in three is underweight and one in ten is wasted'.[4] Some 1,200 million persons, one-fifth of the world's population, are said to be living below the World Bank's international poverty line of US$32.74 purchasing power parity (PPP) 1993 per month, and 30 per cent below this threshold on average.[5] One-third of all human deaths are due to poverty-related causes.[6]

---

[2] UNDP (2002: 21, 29). Most of those suffering these deprivations are female (ibid.: 222–37).

[3] UNDP (1999: 22); UNDP (1998: 49). These figures relate to a world population of about 6,000 million.

[4] UN Food and Agriculture Organization, at www.fao.org/focus/e/sofi/child-e.htm.

[5] World Bank (2000: 23), and Chen and Ravallion (2001: 290, 293) (dividing the poverty gap index by the headcount index). Various flaws in the World Bank's poverty assessment exercise—including its use of general-consumption PPPs rather than PPPs based on a narrower set of commodities more closely related to the needs of the poor—make it likely that these figures for the year 1998 substantially understate the extent of global income poverty (Reddy and Pogge 2002). 'PPP' stands for 'purchasing power parity'.

[6] In 2000, there were 55.694 million human deaths. The main causes highly correlated with poverty were (with death tolls in thousands): diarrhoea (2,124) and malnutrition (445), perinatal (2,439) and maternal conditions (495), childhood diseases (1,385—mainly measles), tuberculosis

This massive poverty is not due to overall scarcity. At market exchange rates, the international poverty line corresponds today to about $10 per person per month in a typical developing country.[7] The 1,200 million persons living some 30 per cent below this line thus have an aggregate annual income of roughly $100 billion. By contrast, the aggregate gross national incomes of the 'high-income economies'—with 955 million people—amount to $25,506 billion (World Bank 2002: 235). However daunting the figure of 1,200 million poor people may sound, global inequality is now so enormous that even doubling or tripling the incomes of all these poor people solely at the expense of the high-income countries would barely be felt in the latter.[8]

It cannot be denied that the distribution of income and wealth is heavily influenced by economic institutions, which regulate economic cooperation and the distribution of a jointly generated social product. What can be said, and is said quite often, is that the economic institutions that substantially contribute to extreme poverty in the developing world are *local* economic institutions in whose imposition we, citizens of the developed countries, are not materially involved. Economists tirelessly celebrate the success stories of the Asian tigers or of Kerala, leading us to believe that those who remain hungry have only

(1,660), malaria (1,080), meningitis (156), hepatitis (128), tropical diseases (124), respiratory infections (3,941—mainly pneumonia), HIV/AIDS (2,943) and sexually transmitted diseases (217) (WHO 2001: 144–9). 'Worldwide 34,000 children under age five die daily from hunger and preventable diseases' (USDA 1999: iii). Attending here to the global health picture, I am focusing on the effects of absolute poverty (see generally Evans et al. 1994; Dreze and Sen 1995; WHO 2000: chapter 2; and Gwatkin 2000). It is worth remarking, however, that relative poverty (local socio-economic inequality) also plays an important role in the causation of medical conditions. For more details, see Black et al. (1990); Wilkinson (1996); as well as, in the present volume, Marmot and also Daniels et al.

[7] The exact amount varies from country to country. The World Bank counts such low incomes as sufficient to avoid poverty on the ground that the purchasing power of money is some three to seven times higher in developing countries than market exchange rates would suggest. Such comparisons of the purchasing power of different currencies reflect an average based on the prices of all commodities weighted by their share in international consumption expenditure. Such an average hides large differences across commodities: prices of services may be eighty times higher in a poor country than in the United States and prices of foodstuffs only three times higher. Averaging out differences of this magnitude makes sense for purposes of comparing countries' entire social products. The World Bank can thus plausibly equate India's per capita gross national income of $460 to 2,450 PPP, China's $890 to 4,260 PPP, Nigeria's $290 to 830 PPP, Pakistan's $420 to 1,920 PPP, Bangladesh's $370 to 1,680 PPP, Ethiopia's $100 to 710 PPP, Vietnam's $410 to 2,130 PPP, and so on (World Bank 2002: 234–5). For assessing very low incomes, however, these PPPs can be highly misleading, because such low incomes are and must be spent on basic necessities. Such necessities are generally cheaper in poor countries, but not as much cheaper as PPPs would suggest (Reddy and Pogge 2002).

[8] In fact, it is claimed that the 225 richest individuals could comfortably solve the problem out of their income from safe investments:

The additional cost of achieving and maintaining universal access to basic education for all, basic health care for all, reproductive health care for all women, adequate food for all and safe water and sanitation for all is … less than 4% of the combined wealth of the 225 richest people in the world. (UNDP 1998: 30).

their own institutions and hence themselves and their own compatriots to blame.[9] Even the philosopher John Rawls feels called upon to endorse the view that poverty has local explanations:

> The causes of the wealth of a people and the forms it takes lie in their political culture and in the religious, philosophical, and moral traditions that support the basic structure, as well as in the industriousness and cooperative talents of its members, all supported by their political virtues.... Crucial also is the country's population policy. (Rawls 1999*b*: 108)

It is quite true, of course, that local economic institutions, and local factors more generally, play an important role in the reproduction of extreme poverty in the developing world. But this fact does not show that social institutions we are materially involved in upholding play no substantial role. That the effects of flawed domestic institutions and policies are as bad as they are is often due to global institutions—to the institution of the territorial state, for instance, which allows affluent populations to prevent the poor from migrating to where their work could earn a decent living.[10] Global economic institutions reflect the highly uneven bargaining power of the participating countries[11] and thus tend to reinforce and to aggravate economic inequality.[12]

Global institutions also have a profound impact on developing countries' institutions and policies themselves. By assigning those who manage to gain effective power in a developing country the authority to borrow in the name of its people and to confer legal ownership rights in the country's resources,

---

[9] The Asian tigers—Hong Kong, Singapore, South Korea, and Taiwan—are the favourite examples of economists friendly to markets largely freed from taxes and regulations. Kerala, a state in India with a traditionally socialist government, is favoured by more left-leaning economists. The lesson suggested by these examples is that, with the right institutions and policies, any country can overcome severe poverty. [10] Cf. Carens (1987).

[11] For example: "Rich countries cut their tariffs by less in the Uruguay Round than poor ones did. Since then, they have found new ways to close their markets, notably by imposing anti-dumping duties on imports they deem 'unfairly cheap'. Rich countries are particularly protectionist in many of the sectors where developing countries are best able to compete, such as agriculture, textiles, and clothing. As a result, according to a new study by Thomas Hertel, of Purdue University, and Will Martin, of the World Bank, rich countries' average tariffs on manufacturing imports from poor countries are four times higher than those on imports from other rich countries. This imposes a big burden on poor countries. The United Nations Conference on Trade and Development (UNCTAD) estimates that they could export $700 billion more a year by 2005 if rich countries did more to open their markets. Poor countries are also hobbled by a lack of know-how. Many had little understanding of what they signed up to in the Uruguay Round. That ignorance is now costing them dear. Michael Finger of the World Bank and Philip Schuler of the University of Maryland estimate that implementing commitments to improve trade procedures and establish technical and intellectual property standards can cost more than a year's development budget for the poorest countries. Moreover, in those areas where poor countries could benefit from world trade rules, they are often unable to do so. ... Of the WTO's 134 members, 29 do not even have missions at its headquarters in Geneva. Many more can barely afford to bring cases to the WTO...." (*The Economist* 25 September, 1999: 89)

[12] 'The income gap between the fifth of the world's people living in the richest countries and the fifth in the poorest was 74 to 1 in 1997, up from 60 to 1 in 1990 and 30 to 1 in 1960.' (UNDP 1999: 3)

our global institutional order greatly encourages the undemocratic acquisition and exercise of political power in especially the resource-rich developing countries.[13]

National institutions and policies of developed countries, too, can strongly influence the developing countries' institutions and policies and their domestic effects. An obvious example is that, until quite recently, most developed countries (though not, after 1977, the United States) have allowed their firms to pay bribes to officials of developing countries, and even to deduct such bribes from their taxable revenues.[14] Such authorisation and moral support for bribery have greatly contributed to the now deeply entrenched culture of corruption in many developing countries.

If the institutions and policies of the developed countries and the global institutional order these countries uphold contribute substantially to the reproduction of poverty, then it is hard to deny that we citizens of developed countries are therefore materially involved in it as well. It is true, of course, that these institutions are, in the first instance, shaped by our politicians. But we live in reasonably democratic states where we can affect the selection of politicians and political programmes from among a wide range of alternatives, where we can participate in shaping political programmes and debates, and where politicians and political parties must cater to the popular will if they are to be elected and reelected. If we really wanted our country to shift its policies as well as national and global institutional arrangements toward avoiding extreme poverty abroad, politicians committed to this goal would emerge and be successful. But the vast majority of citizens of the developed countries want these policies and institutions to be shaped in the service of their own interests and therefore support politicians willing so to shape them. At least the citizens in this large majority can then be said to be materially involved in the reproduction of poverty and the associated health deficits.[15] And they, at least, have then stronger moral reason to discontinue their support, and to help the foreign victims of current institutions, than to help fund most services[16] provided

[13] Cf. Lam and Wantchekon (1999); Wantchekon (1999); and Pogge (2002: chapters 4 and 6).

[14] Only in 1999 did the developed states, under OECD auspices and under public pressure generated by a new NGO (Transparency International), adopt a *Convention on Combating Bribery of Foreign Officials in International Business Transactions* (www.oecd.org/home), which requires them to enact laws against the bribery of foreign officials. 'But big multinationals continue to sidestep them with ease' (*The Economist* 2 March, 2002: 63–5).

[15] It might be said that, in the larger rich countries, none of these citizens has real influence on the electoral success of politicians and political programmes they choose together. But this position is absurd. The outcome of the vote depends on the decisions of the citizens eligible to vote and on no one else. If such citizens did not count as materially involved and thus could bring about this outcome and any harms it foreseeably entails without being responsible therefor, then Nazis and criminals can invoke the same privilege: if enough of them act together, they can commit crimes in which none of them is materially involved. For further analysis of this mistake, cf. Parfit (1984: chapter 3).

[16] Social institutions which we are materially involved in upholding do substantially contribute to some medical conditions suffered by compatriots; and these medical conditions may then be on

under ordinary health programmes (such as Medicare) for the benefit of their compatriots—or so the view I have outlined would suggest.[17]

This summary of my larger view on health equity was meant to be introductory, not conclusive. Seeing what is at stake, I would expect even the most commonsensical of my remarks about the explanation of global poverty to be vigorously disputed; and I certainly do not believe that this brief outline can lay such controversies to rest. At most I would hope that it may inspire some readers to think further about these issues and may also provide some context for the more focused and intricate discussion to follow. This discussion is devoted specifically to the explication and defence of my first thesis.

7.2. TWO CONCEPTS OF JUSTICE

I begin with a look at the concept of justice, whose structure is basically the same, I think, as that of the concepts of equity and fairness. The concept of justice is a predicate, and so we might ask first what kinds of entities are capable of being just or unjust. To have a name for such entities, let me rephrase the question: what kinds of entities are possible *judicanda* under the headings of justice, fairness, equity?[18] In ordinary usage, the concept of justice is primarily applied to four kinds of *judicanda*: to *subjects* such as persons and groups, to the *conduct* of such subjects (acts and omissions: decisions, policies, wars, accusations, and so on), to *social rules* (e.g. social institutions, laws, conventions, practices, economic arrangements, educational and health-care systems),[19] and to *other states of affairs* insofar as they are not already

a par with foreigners' medical conditions in whose incidence we are materially involved. To gain economic advantages for a majority of citizens, for example, we often legally authorise activities that impose considerable risks on persons who can neither consent to, nor benefit from, these activities. We have especially strong moral reason to prevent and to mitigate the resulting harms (e.g. harms to children from legally authorised pollution or motorised traffic).

[17] Superficially similar conclusions are sometimes defended on cost/benefit grounds, by reference to how thousands of children in the developing countries can cheaply be saved from their life-threatening diseases at the cost of terminal care for a single person in a developed country. Representative examples of such lines of argument are Singer (1972); Rachels (1979); Kagan (1989); and Unger (1996). My view, by contrast, turns on the different ways in which we are related to the medical conditions of others and it may therefore tell us to favour foreigners even if costs and benefits are equal. Two notable pioneers of this line of thought are O'Neill (1975) and Nagel (1977). Both emphasise our active involvement in the reproduction of poverty. See also Pogge (1989: 32–6, 276–80, 2002, 2004).

[18] The word *'judicandum'* is Latin and means 'that which is to be judged'. I am using it in exactly this sense, to single out the things to which an evaluative predicate applies. I have hope for the reader's indulgence, because there is no good English word for this purpose. G. A. Cohen (1997) has used the word 'site' to refer to types of such things. He distinguishes four sites in particular: basic structures (schemes of social institutions), ethi (plural of 'ethos'), conventions, and personal conduct.

[19] When we speak of just states, societies, or organisations, we typically think of them under the third rubric, referring to their internal mode of organisation, their 'basic structure' or institutional scheme. But we can also think of them under the first rubric, as organised collective subjects, and can then judge them on the basis of their policies and attitudes toward outsiders.

included under any of the first three rubrics (e.g. facts or combinations of facts, even the world at large, particularly including distributions). Occasionally, the concept of justice is also applied to the feelings and emotions of persons (as in 'unjust anger') and to natural phenomena (such as an avalanche, hurricane, lightening, or epidemic).

The concept of justice can function as a one-place predicate and grammatically does so function in most cases. But it can also function as a two-place predicate— A is just or unjust toward B—and this use is actually more fundamental.[20] For the concept of justice, like those of fairness and equity, essentially involves the idea of one or more parties at the receiving end. It is incoherent to hold that a certain *judicandum* is unjust, but unjust toward no one.[21] Justice thus always is justice *toward* certain *recipients* (as I will call them). And we can then say of subjects, conduct, or social rules that they are just toward some and unjust toward others, or we can assess their overall justice by balancing their treatment of their various recipients.

The idea of recipients, of those who have justice claims on a particular *judicandum*, immediately suggests the question what these recipients have and do not have, and what they ought to have or not to have—the question what their claims on the *judicandum* are. Let me use the expression 'goods and ills' for such items.[22] Taking this question into account, we see that the concept of justice can also function as a *three*-place predicate—A is just toward B in regard to the distribution of C (to/among B)—and that this use is actually more fundamental still. For the concept of justice, like those of fairness and equity, essentially involves the idea of something being done or happening to certain recipients. It is incoherent to hold that a certain *judicandum* is unjust to someone, B, without being able to point to any goods or ills that B either has-but-should-not-have or lacks-but-should-have.

The concept of justice as explicated thus far—fundamentally a three-place predicate, with frequent but derivative one-place and two-place predicate employments—dominates current discussions of justice. According to this concept, justice is a feature of certain entities (*judicanda*), which is dependent on what distribution of relevant goods and ills they produce among certain

---

[20] It is more fundamental in the sense in which the two-place predicate use of the word 'mother' is more fundamental than its one-place predicate use: one cannot understand what it is to be a mother without understanding what it is to be the mother of someone. Contrast the word 'sad,' whose one-place predicate use can be understood without understanding its two-place predicate use in 'A is sad about B.'

[21] I am not denying, of course, that there can be an unjust law that is never enacted and thus never does anyone an injustice. My point is rather that someone who calls this proposed law unjust, perhaps to prevent its enactment, is committed to showing that there are some recipients toward whom the law, if enacted, would be unjust. Similarly, I am not denying that a man can be unjust even though he has never been unjust toward anyone. He may merely be disposed to injustice. But this *means* that he is disposed to be unjust *towards others*.

[22] As the word 'conduct' is meant to include the null-case of omissions, so the expression 'goods and ills' is meant to include the null-case of someone receiving nothing (being denied a good or being spared an ill).

recipients. The comparative assessment of alternative health-care systems, for instance, is based on the distribution of health outcomes each of these systems is expected to produce. One might call this the concept of *passive* justice, because it focuses moral attention on those by whom justice and injustice are experienced or suffered.

There is an important alternative to the concept of passive justice, an alternative concept that is fundamentally a *four*-place predicate. This concept adds an essential place for (what I call) the *agents* of justice, for those who have or share moral responsibility for the justice or injustice of the *judicandum*. Pursuant to this alternative concept, it is incoherent to hold that a *judicandum* is unjust without being able to point to any agent or agents, D, who is/are responsible for its injustice or for making it (more) just. In order to stress the contrast, I call this the concept of *active* justice, because it diverts some attention from those who suffer justice and injustice to those who produce them.[23] In what follows, I try to show that we should self-consciously employ the concept of active justice—'the active concept,' as I shall also, more economically, call it.

To show this, I will display the changes this shift would induce in our thinking about justice. I am not claiming that these changes, especially the more profound ones, are either forced by the new concept or made impossible by the old one. Which concept we employ matters mainly psychologically; but it still matters a lot. The concepts we use condition what we pay attention to, and this in turn greatly influences our theorising.[24]

Substantively, the shift in concepts matters in various ways, which can best be clarified by considering, first, its effects on how we might be inclined to structure conceptions or theories of justice, or subfields such as justice in regard to health. Using the active concept, such a theory would seek plausible answers to a plurality of interdependent questions in *four* dimensions, roughly as follows:

A Who or what is capable of being just, or who or what is to be made (more) just? This is the most fundamental question of *judicanda*.

---

[23] Meant to be provocative, the active/passive terminology may seem to be tendentious, even somewhat misleading, in that the new concept focuses attention on both: agents and recipients of justice. The rationale offered in the text—that the new concept is 'more active' than the old one because some of the attention that the concept of passive justice focuses on recipients is diverted from them to the agents of justice—may seem lame. I have thought of using relational/distributional instead of active/passive, but this seems even less satisfactory.

[24] Given this importance of concepts, one might mark the shift to the active concept of justice by replacing the word '*judicandum*' with '*justificandum*' (that which is to be made just) derived from the Latin *facere* (to make) and *justum* (just). I realise that using it in this sense could be confusing in that justification—which in old English still signified the administration of justice—is today understood as a verbal activity characteristic of lawyerly types. I find it tempting to restore the word to its old meaning nonetheless. Doing so would protest the perennial tendency to substitute the appearance for the reality—in this case, sliding from justification, making things just, to justification, making things appear just. Moreover, no other word could capture quite so precisely the shift from the passive to the active concept.

D1   Who can have (or share) moral responsibility for achieving and maintaining the justice of *judicanda*? This question concerns the possible *agents* of justice or equity.[25]

D2   Which agents have moral responsibility for achieving or maintaining the justice of a particular *judicandum*? This question concerns the *scope of responsibility* with regard to particular *judicanda*.[26]

D3   What moral responsibilities do particular agents have for achieving and maintaining the justice of a particular *judicandum*? This question concerns the *allocation of responsibility* with regard to particular *judicanda*.[27]

B1   Who can have a claim to justice, can experience justice or injustice? This question concerns the possible *recipients* of justice or equity.[28]

B2   Which recipients have justice claims on a particular *judicandum*? This question concerns the *domain of recipients* with regard to particular *judicanda*.[29]

---

[25] One may think that this question is of interest mainly in the case of social rules, not in that of subjects and their conduct. But this is not so. The question is of great importance in the assessment of disorganised and organised collective subjects (mobs, corporations) and of their conduct (Thompson 1980). And even in the case of individual subjects, the question is by no means trivial: we may have responsibilities in regard to the developing character and conduct of others (e.g. our children). And we may even have responsibilities in regard to the character and conduct of our own future self—for example, a responsibility to shape ourselves into persons who *notice* morally significant features of our environment and then *act deliberately* in response to them (Bok 1996).

[26] This scope might, in the limit, include only a single agent—as when, for instance, a judge alone is responsible for the justice of her verdict. Even in this limiting case, the next question (**D3**) still arises: What is the judge required to do, and what is she not required to do, toward achieving a just verdict?   [27] It is interestingly addressed, for instance, in Murphy (2000).

[28] As is perhaps obvious, a recipient of justice can, even in the same context, be an agent of justice as well. Agents and recipients may overlap or even coincide—as when the members of a group share a collective responsibility for the justice of the rules they jointly impose upon each.

[29] This domain may include only a single recipient, as when one innocent man is convicted through an unjust verdict. In this limiting case, the question of metric (**C2**) may still arise (we may want to know, for example, how great an injustice this was, in comparison to other unjust verdicts that, say, involved excessive punishment or acquittal of a guilty person). But in this limiting case the question of aggregation across recipients (**C3**) evidently does not come into play.

It is worth distinguishing these single-recipient cases from ones whose domain includes a plurality of recipients whose situations are assessed in a non-comparative way. With regard to criminal-verdict producing procedures, for example, we may well believe that the verdict (conviction or acquittal) each defendant ought to receive is entirely independent of what verdicts are received by other defendants and also that how much the conviction of an innocent defendant or the acquittal of a guilty defendant detracts from the justice of such a procedure is entirely unaffected by what happens to other (innocent or guilty) defendants. (The conviction of an innocent person is not rendered morally more acceptable by the fact that other similarly innocent persons are also convicted.) Despite such non-comparative assessment, aggregation across recipients is still necessary. In judging the justice of criminal-verdict producing procedures, one must decide how to weight the two kinds of errors they are liable to produce—for example, one must decide on an 'exchange rate' between miscarriages of justice that result in an innocent person being convicted of murder and miscarriages of justice that result in the acquittal of a person guilty of murder.

In the case of most *judicanda*, justice is partly or wholly comparative, such that whether recipients within its domain have more or less than justice requires depends, in part or entirely, on

C1 What claims of justice do particular recipients have upon a particular *judicandum*? This question concerns the *allocation of claims* with regard to particular *judicanda*.

C2 By what yardstick are we to assess the claims that particular recipients have upon a particular *judicandum*—whether they are being treated as (or better or worse than) justice demands? This question concerns the *metric* of justice or equity (including intra-recipient aggregation) with regard to particular *judicanda*.[30]

C3 How are we to calculate an overall shortfall from justice when the domain includes several recipients being treated either better or worse than justice demands? This question concerns the *aggregation across recipients* of deviations from justice or equity.

This new way of structuring conceptions of justice makes it easier to appreciate further respects in which the shift from the passive to the active concept is likely to matter. One consequence is minor: employing the passive concept, one may view it as unjust when avalanches, lightening, hurricanes, epidemics, or lions strike down some but not others (or sometimes as just, perhaps, when evil persons get hurt). If we employ the active concept, such entities—assuming their dispositions and behaviour are not the responsibility of anyone—are not capable of being just or unjust,[31] and therefore drop out of the class of potential *judicanda*, as do states of affairs insofar as they are not under human control.

how much other recipients within its domain actually have. With procedures for meting out punishments or medical treatments, justice is partly comparative—non-comparative insofar as they are governed by the requirements that punishments should go only to guilty persons duly convicted and medical treatment only to persons in need thereof, and comparative insofar as whether particular punishments are of appropriate severity depends in part on how others are punished for similar crimes and whether treatment options made available to particular patients are of appropriate quality depends in part on what treatment options are available to others.

[30] This is a broader version of the 'equality of what' question pioneered by Amartya Sen (1982, 1992). G. A. Cohen (1989) speaks of the 'currency' of (egalitarian) justice. The question has generated an extensive literature, including the first three chapters of Dworkin (2000); Rawls (1982); Arneson (1989); Elster and Roemer (1991); Nussbaum and Sen (1993); Roemer (1996). See also Galston (1980) and Griffin (1986). In most theories, the metric of justice for assessing basic structures is closely related to some notion of human flourishing or quality of life. It is important to bear in mind, however, that the moral quality of distributions of relevant goods and ills may be sensitive to the distribution of items other than these goods and ills. Thus a given distribution of goods and ills may be considered the morally better the closer a correlation there is between recipients' quality of life (goods minus ills) and their quality of character (virtue). And the metric of justice may then include factors other than those whose distribution the relevant *judicandum* can affect.

[31] The devastating *effects* of a hurricane, or the fact that a disease outbreak turned into an epidemic, may still be traceable to an injustice in factors under human control, such as a flawed economic or health-care system under which safe buildings or vaccines are unaffordable to the poor. This illustrates once more the important point that the effects of one causal factor (e.g. a hurricane) can importantly depend on other causal factors (cf. text accompanied by note 10 above).

7.3. TREATING RECIPIENTS JUSTLY VERSUS PROMOTING A JUST DISTRIBUTION

A more important consequence is that the active concept focuses attention on who bears responsibility for a particular *judicandum* and also allows new complexities in the moral relations between *judicanda* and recipients. To begin with the former point: while the passive concept encourages neglect of questions of responsibility or at best the vague suggestion that all agents have moral reason to promote the justice of all *judicanda*, the active concept invites differentiations and allows for various kinds of agent-relativity. Thus, some agents may have responsibilities with respect to the justice of a particular *judicandum* and others may not; unlike you, I may have no moral reason to seek to prevent or to remedy a minor injustice in your spouse's conduct toward your children. There may also be gradations, as when moral responsibility with regard to the justice of some *judicandum* varies from agent to agent within its scope; being privileged or influential may strengthen moral responsibilities while being poor, disabled, or burdened with many other responsibilities may weaken them. Furthermore, as this last thought suggests, there may be a competition among *judicanda*—one may have responsibilities with regard to achieving and maintaining the justice of several *judicanda* and may then have to decide how much of an effort one ought to make with regard to each. These issues concerning responsibilities and their prioritisation are crucial for giving justice a determinate role in the real world. And they tend to be overlooked from the start, or grossly oversimplified, when the topic is approached in terms of the concept of passive justice.[32]

Let us proceed now to relations between *judicanda* and recipients. Here, the choice of concept can make a major difference to how *judicanda* are assessed. Employing the concept of passive justice, one will focus on a *judicandum*'s relative impact on its recipients—specifically on the difference it makes, relative to its feasible alternatives, to what these recipients are able to have or to be. Roughly speaking, a *judicandum* is considered just in proportion to its relative impact on the quality of the distribution of relevant goods and ills among its recipients: to be just is to promote a good distribution. The concept of passive justice thus leads easily to *purely recipient-oriented* conceptions of justice. The active concept, by contrast, suggests a conception of justice as *relational*, as involving a relation between particular agents and recipients mediated through a *judicandum*: to be just is to give equitable treatment. By drawing attention to what we owe to each other,[33] to each agent's specific responsibilities for particular *judicanda* and thus toward their particular recipients, the active concept leads us away from the idea that a concern for the justice of a *judicandum* is

---

[32] Witness Rawls's generic natural duty to promote just institutions (1999a: 99, 216, 293–4), which leaves all such more specific questions of responsibility out of account.

[33] An allusion to Scanlon (1999).

simply a concern for its relative impact on the quality of the distribution of relevant goods and ills among its recipients. Rather than tie justice to an out-come, to a state that does or does not obtain—what would justice be like, what ought recipients to be able to have or to be?—the active concept presents justice as something that is or is not done: by particular agents, through a *judi-candum*, to particular recipients.

The significance of this shift can be illustrated in terms of two fundament-ally different ways of understanding contemporary egalitarian liberalism. One variant sees the core of egalitarian liberalism in the idea that no citizen ought to be worse off on account of unchosen inequalities. This idea, duly specified, defines an ideal society in which no person is worse off than others except only as a consequence of free and informed choices this person had made. In such a society, social institutions, and perhaps all other humanly con-trollable factors as well, are then to be aimed at promoting such a solely choice-sensitive overall distribution of quality of life.[34] The other variant sees the core of egalitarian liberalism in the idea that a liberal society, or state, ought to treat all its citizens equally in terms of helps and hindrances. Such *equal* treatment need not be *equality-promoting* treatment. Pre-existing inequalities in, for example, genetic potentials and liabilities—however unchosen by their bearers—are not society's responsibility and not to be corrected or compens-ated at the expense of those favoured by these inequalities.

The health equity theme provokes the most forceful clash of these two vari-ants of egalitarian liberalism. One side seems committed to the indefinite expansion of the health-care system by devoting it to neutralising (through medical research, treatment, alleviation, and compensation) all handicaps, dis-abilities, and other medical conditions from which persons may suffer through no fault of their own. The other side seems committed to the callous (if not cruel) view that we, as a society, need do no more for persons whose health is poor through no fault of ours than for persons in good health.[35]

Most contemporary theorists of justice take the purely recipient-oriented approach, though they do not explicitly consider and reject the relational alter-native. Much of the current debate is focused on the question how we are to

---

[34] The main champion of the argument that all such factors—social institutions and practices, conventions, ethi, and personal conduct—should be pressed in the service of promoting a just distribution so understood is G. A. Cohen (1989, 1992, 1997, 2000). For a detailed critique of this view, see Pogge (2000).

[35] Advocates of the first view could also be accused of callousness in that the huge demands they make in behalf of persons whose health is poor through no fault of their own will, in the real world, shrink the domain of recipients, typically in line with national borders. The billions of dollars required for providing our compatriots with all the 'services needed to maintain, restore, or compensate for normal species-typical functioning' (Daniels 1985: 79) would suffice to protect countless millions who now die from poverty-related causes, such as malnutrition, measles, diarrhoea, malaria, tuberculosis, pneumonia, and other cheaply curable but all-too-often fatal diseases. On my view, as sketched above, citizens in affluent countries have stronger moral reason to prevent and mitigate the latter medical conditions suffered by foreigners than most of the former medical conditions suffered by compatriots.

judge the justice of overall distributions or states of affairs in a comparative way.[36] This focus may well be a residue of the long dominant consequentialist idea that we should assess subjects, conduct, and social rules solely by their effects on how well the world goes. Much current theorising about justice involves the closely related thought that the justice of subjects, conduct, and/or social rules should be assessed by their effects on the quality of the overall distribution of goods and ills among the recipients of the relevant *judicandum*. In both cases, our interest in outcomes is indirect. How well the world goes is of little practical import in and of itself, but becomes quite important if we judge the moral quality of subjects, conduct, and/or social rules by their impact on how well the world goes. Similarly, the moral quality of overall distributions is of little import in and of itself, but becomes quite important if we judge the justice of subjects, conduct, and/or social rules by their impact on the moral quality of overall distributions of goods and ills (or quality of life).

But *should* we judge the justice of subjects, conduct, and/or social rules solely by their impact on the quality of such overall distributions? *Should* such distributions be our primary *judicanda*? With respect to subjects and their conduct, most would reject the purely recipient-oriented mode of assessment. Among the timeworn staples of ethics classes are gruesome organ redistribution stories designed to elicit the response that it is *not* true that subjects and conduct that aim at or produce the best overall distributions are always just. Abstractly considered, a situation in which everyone has at least one eye and one kidney is surely morally better than (an otherwise similar) one in which some, through no fault of their own, have no functioning eye or kidney while many others have two. Redistributive subjects and conduct aiming at such an abstractly better distribution are nonetheless, however, considered gravely unjust.

With respect to subjects and their conduct, cases of this sort may be used to draw the conclusion that we ought to distinguish between *treating recipients justly* and *promoting a good distribution among recipients* and, more generally, between how subjects *treat* and how they *affect* their recipients. The moral significance of this distinction can be illustrated, for instance, with matched doing/allowing scenarios such as the following: In Scenario 1, John has two functioning kidneys and Susan has none. A doctor is able to give one of John's kidneys to Susan. In Scenario 2, John has one functioning kidney and Susan has none. A functioning kidney becomes available from a donor, and the doctor can give this kidney to John or to Susan. (Other things are presumed to be equal in these two scenarios and, in particular, John and Susan both urgently want all the kidneys they can get.) Now, in terms of their distributional effects, the two doctor's decisions are on a par: In each scenario, the doctor decides whether the final distribution of kidneys between John and Susan will be 2:0 or 1:1; and a decision in favour of Susan is then in both scenarios

---

[36] Cf. the literature listed in note 30 above.

equally promoting of a good distribution. In terms of how the doctor would be treating John and Susan, however, the scenarios differ dramatically. A decision in favour of Susan treats John unjustly in Scenario 1 but not in Scenario 2; and a decision in favour of John treats Susan unjustly in Scenario 2 but not in Scenario 1. Or so our intuitive judgements would suggest.

With respect to social rules, a similar distinction would seem to be called for, and for similar reasons. Just social rules for the allocation of donated kidneys favour those who, through no fault of their own, have no functioning kidney over those who have one; and such rules thereby promote a better distribution of kidneys over recipients. Just social rules do not, however, mandate the forced redistribution of kidneys from those who have two to those who have none, even though doing so would likewise promote a better distribution of kidneys over recipients. Similarly, social rules producing a better distribution of kidneys are not for this reason more just if they do so by engendering severe poverty that compels some people to sell one of their kidneys in order to obtain basic necessities for themselves and their families. So the fact that medical conditions are intrinsically identical does not show that they are morally on a par. The moral weight of renal failures that an institutional scheme avoidably gives rise to may depend, for example, on how patients came to be dependent on a single kidney. Was the other one forcibly taken from them through a legally authorised medical procedure (forced redistribution)? Were they obliged to sell it to obtain food? Or did it atrophy on account of a genetic defect? How important the avoidance, prevention, and mitigation of renal failures is for the justice of an institutional scheme depends greatly on which of these scenarios it would exemplify.[37] Once again, treating recipients justly does not boil down to promoting the best distribution among them—what matters is how social rules *treat*, not how they *affect*, the set of recipients.

This simple thought has been remarkably neglected in contemporary work on social justice. It is not surprising, of course, that it plays no role in consequentialist theorizing. Consequentialists, after all, hold that social rules (as well as subjects and their conduct) should be judged by their effects on the overall outcome, irrespective of how they produce these effects. Consequentialists hold, that is, that the justice of social rules is determined exclusively by the quality of the overall distribution (of goods and ills, or quality of life) produced by these rules. What is remarkable, however, is that supposedly deontological approaches, such as that developed by Rawls and his followers, likewise make the justice of social rules depend exclusively on the overall distribution these rules produce.

---

[37] This point has profound implications for the topic of health-care rationing, discussed by Brock and Kamm in the present volume. We should, for instance, design the institutional scheme of our society to give priority to the mitigation of medical conditions whose incidence it substantially contributes to. The discussion and defence of this implication would be worth another essay.

To make clear what is at stake here, consider the ambiguous claim that the justice of a social order depends on how it affects the overall distribution of goods and ills among its recipients. Rawls agrees with one understanding of this claim: the moral assessment of a social order should be based on what overall distribution of goods and ills it, in comparison to its feasible alternatives, would produce among its recipients—*and on nothing else*, he would add. This much is built into the centrepiece of his theory, his proposal that we should judge any social order from the standpoint of prospective participants each of whom cares only about the quality of life he or she can expect under each of the feasible alternatives.[38] Through his addition to the first understanding of the claim, Rawls rejects the other possible understanding of it: he leaves aside as morally irrelevant *in what way(s)* a social order affects the distribution of goods and ills. By judging social orders in this purely recipient-oriented way, Rawls ensures from the start that they are judged exclusively by their 'output' in terms of what overall distribution of quality of life they produce among their participants—without regard to how they may bring it about that particular social goods or ills end up with particular persons.

7.4. A PROBLEM FOR PURELY RECIPIENT-ORIENTED CONCEPTIONS OF SOCIAL JUSTICE

To clarify further the recipient-oriented bias I believe to be common among consequentialist and supposedly deontological discussions of the justice of social rules, let me venture a little farther into Rawls's theory and, in particular, its way of handling natural inequalities among recipients.

Rawls's project is to propose and defend a public *criterion of social justice*, that is, a public criterion for judging feasible institutional structures in moral terms. His central thesis is that we should morally endorse that criterion of social justice which parties in the *original position* would endorse prudentially. He imagines these parties to deliberate in behalf of prospective participants— but behind a *veil of ignorance*, so that they know nothing specific about the particular persons they are supposed to represent. The parties are made to assume, however, that every prospective participant has three fundamental

---

[38] 'The persons in the original position try to acknowledge principles which advance their systems of ends as far as possible. They do this by attempting to win for themselves the highest index of primary social goods, since this enables them to promote their conception of the good most effectively whatever it turns out to be. The parties...strive for as high an absolute score as possible'. (Rawls 1999a: 125)

By 'social order' I mean here—appropriate to Rawls's theory—a public criterion of justice together with the important and pervasive social institutions ('basic structure') it would favour under particular historical, cultural, and technological conditions. As conditions change, a criterion of justice may require institutional reforms in the basic structure. Such reforms, so long as they are guided by the same criterion of justice, do not count as modifying the social order (as the term is here understood).

interests, which Rawls sees as closely connected to their role as citizens in a democratic society and hence as not being partisan to any particular religious, philosophical, or ethical world-view or way of life. Rawls calls these the *three higher-order interests*, suggesting both that they are interests in the content and fulfilment of other interests (like second-order desires are desires about desires) and also that they are deep, stable, and normally decisive.

The first two higher-order interests are interests in developing and exercising *two moral powers*,[39] namely

a capacity for a sense of justice and a capacity for a conception of the good. A sense of justice is the capacity to understand, to apply, and to act from the public conception of justice which characterizes the fair terms of cooperation. Given the nature of the political conception as specifying a public basis of justification, a sense of justice also expresses a willingness, if not the desire, to act in relation to others on terms that they also can publicly endorse. . . . The capacity for a conception of the good is the capacity to form, to revise, and rationally to pursue a conception of one's rational advantage or good.[40]

The third higher-order interest is 'to protect and advance some determinate (but unspecified) conceptions of the good over a complete life',[41] that is, the interest to be successful in the pursuit of one's major projects and ambitions, whatever these may be.

Rawls then argues that the parties, deliberating in behalf of prospective citizens with these three interests, would be especially concerned to avoid very bad outcomes, that is, institutional schemes under which the fundamental interests of some would remain unfulfilled. They would thus prudently seek agreement on a criterion of justice that rules out such institutional schemes as unjust.

This structuring of the decision problem clearly brings out that Rawls shares the consequentialists' presumption that the justice of alternative ways of organising a society is to be judged exclusively by the overall distribution of goods and ills that each such social order would produce. To be sure, he departs from typical consequentialists (utilitarians) in regard to the metric of individual advantage—substituting higher-order interest fulfilment for pleasure-minus-pain or desire satisfaction. And he departs from typical consequentialists also in regard to aggregation across recipients—substituting a heightened concern to avoid very bad outcomes for their simpler concern with maximising the average.[42] But he shares with consequentialism the purely recipient-oriented mode of theorising about justice.

How is this shared presumption problematic? Let me illustrate by bringing Rawls's contractualist machinery to bear on the question—highly relevant to our health equity theme—whether and how social institutions should be

---

[39] Rawls (1996: 74, 2001: 192).   [40] Ibid. (1996: 19, cf. 2001: 18–19).
[41] Ibid. (1996: 74, cf. 2001: 192).
[42] These are the two features Rawls himself adduces as the ones that render his theory distinctive and deontological (Rawls 1999*a*: 26–27, 220).

responsive to natural inequalities. It is evident that the extent to which a person's higher-order interests (especially the third) are fulfilled depends not merely on her share of social goods but also on her natural endowments. Someone genetically predisposed toward good health, cheerfulness, intelligence, and good looks is better able to advance her conception of the good than someone who is genetically predisposed toward sickliness, melancholy, low intelligence, and ugliness. How, if at all, would the parties in the original position take account of this fact? Let us grant that genetic manipulations are currently unfeasible and leave them aside. Even so, the parties can still raise the floor of higher-order interest fulfilment by selecting a public criterion and social order under which the naturally disfavoured are favoured in the distribution of social goods and ills. By effecting a negative correlation between the social and natural distributions, social institutions can raise the floor by ensuring that no one is both naturally and socially disfavoured.

Let me illustrate this point in a simple numerical model. Suppose that the value of persons' natural endowments and social position each vary from 0 (very poor) to 10 (very ample) and that a person's expected higher-order interest fulfilment (EHOIF) is the sum of the two values minus 1/20 of their product:

EHOIF = $N + S - NS/20$

Given this formula, EHOIF among persons could vary between 0 ($N = 0$; $S = 0$) and 15 ($N = 10$; $S = 10$).

However, if social institutions can be designed to produce a negative correlation between persons' N-values and S-values, it may be possible to raise both the average and the floor of EHOIF. Suppose, for instance, that it is possible to shape social institutions so that—through special subsidies, tax credits, and tax deductions, preferences in admission and hiring, and so on—they produce higher S-values for those whose N-values are low, in such a way that, for each person,

$$S \geq \frac{(150 - 20\,N)}{(20 - N)^{43}}$$

If this could be accomplished, then *all* citizens' expected higher-order interest fulfillment would fall within the top half of the range (EHOIF ≥ 7.5). And the same concentration of social resources on the naturally disfavoured would also raise *average* EHOIF as well because, the lower a person's N-value is, the more a given increase in his or her S-value (from 4 to 5, say) will add to his or her EHOIF.[44] Being exclusively concerned with prospective citizens' EHOIF

[43] This requires, for example, that those with $N = 0$ must have at least $S = 7.5$ (150/20), those with $N = 1$ must have at least $S = 6.842$ (130/19), those with $N = 2$ must have at least $S = 6.111$ (110/18), those with $N = 3$ must have at least $S = 5.294$ (90/17), those with $N = 4$ must have at least $S = 4.375$ (70/16), those with $N = 5$ must have at least $S = 3.333$ (50/15), those with $N = 6$ must have at least $S = 2.143$ (30/14), and those with $N = 7$ must have at least $S = 0.769$ (10/13).

[44] To be sure, this is an implication of my stipulated formula. This stipulation does, however, strike me as generally plausible: social goods, such as money and the social bases of self-respect, really do tend to have greater marginal importance for the naturally disfavoured.

and especially with avoiding the lower levels of EHOIF, the parties would therefore have reason to aim for a criterion of social justice that calls for such a negative correlation of S and N.

Rawls claims, nonetheless, that his parties would agree on a criterion of social justice that does not prefer basic structures that favour the naturally disfavoured along the lines just sketched. Instead, Rawls's criterion of justice assesses each social order exclusively on the basis of the distribution of *social* primary goods it produces: 'a hypothetical initial arrangement in which all the social primary goods are equally distributed ... provides a benchmark for judging improvements' (Rawls 1999*a*: 54–55). Information about the distribution of natural primary goods, such as 'health and vigor, intelligence and imagination' (ibid.: 54), is left aside entirely. Thus, while Rawls's contractualist machinery, in line with the concept of passive justice, reflects a purely recipient-oriented conception of justice, the public criterion he 'derives' therefrom does not.

In fact, this public criterion seems to be vaguely inspired by a relational conception of justice associated with the active concept—as when Rawls comments on its disregard for natural primary goods: 'The natural distribution is neither just nor unjust' (ibid.: 87). This comment may express the idea that citizens creating and upholding a social order bear responsibility for any very low social positions it may produce, but not for any very poor natural endowments, which can be viewed as so-to-speak preexisting.

How might we react to Rawls's apparent inconsistency? First, we might defend him by arguing that natural characteristics are not correlated with the ability of persons to fulfil their higher-order interests. This line strikes me as wholly unpromising. Genetically based mental deficits—such as lower intelligence or ability to concentrate—typically reduce a person's capacity to understand, to apply, and to act from a public conception of justice as well as her capacity to form, to revise, and rationally to pursue a conception of the good. Even more clearly, such deficits, and melancholy and ugliness as well, tend to reduce substantially persons' success in advancing whatever particular conception of the good they may have chosen to pursue.

Second, one might reject Rawls's exclusive emphasis on the distribution of *social* goods and ills as simply a mistake to be corrected. In this vein Amartya Sen has argued that, since natural differences among persons evidently affect the quality of life they can expect, these natural differences should be taken into account—for example, by replacing Rawls's social-primary-goods metric with a capabilities metric.[45] To this critique, Rawls has responded that, for purposes of a first approximation, he had been meaning to leave severe natural handicaps and disabilities aside and that the remaining natural disadvantages— Sen mentions differential caloric and textile needs, conditioned by differences in metabolic rate and body size, respectively—generally do not render persons unable to be fully cooperating citizens (Rawls 1996: 182–6). It is hard to see

---

[45] Sen (1980, 1992) criticises Rawls's theory from outside, but, as we have seen, his critique can also be supported by appeal to Rawls's own original position.

the relevance of this second point, but perhaps Rawls is suggesting that, apart from severe handicaps and disabilities, natural differences are relatively minor so that their accommodation within a public criterion of social justice is not worth the cost in terms of increased complexity and divisiveness. But this response strikes me as implausible: many quite ordinary natural handicaps—such as ugliness or a disposition toward melancholy and depression—are anything but minor (in their tendency to reduce EHOIF). And even if severe natural handicaps of mind and body can be ignored in a first approximation, they cannot be left aside in the final version of the theory which is to serve as a public standard by reference to which citizens are to shape and reform their common social institutions.

7.5. THE SEMICONSEQUENTIALIST ALTERNATIVE

Third, one might resolve the tension in Rawls's work in favour of his proposed criterion of social justice and thus at the expense of his purely recipient-oriented machinery for deriving this criterion. One might say that the purpose of a social order is not to promote a good overall distribution of goods and ills or quality of life, but to *do justice to*, or to *treat justly* all those whose shared life is regulated by this order. Just treatment of participants requires a just allocation of the benefits and burdens of social cooperation, not promotion of the best attainable distribution of all (social and natural) goods and ills that may bear on persons' higher-order interest fulfilment or quality of life. Natural inequalities precede, so to speak, social institutions, as persons already have their natural endowments and handicaps when they enter society. And just social institutions should not then make the naturally favoured subsidise the naturally disfavoured any more than a just administrator or civil judge should seek to allocate benefits and burdens under her control so as to even out natural inequalities. Pushed all the way, this sort of reasoning would lead to the conclusion that there is nothing unjust about a society that has a just economic system, satisfying Rawls's second principle perhaps, but then leaves the allocation of medical care (as well as of the means of mitigating melancholy, homeliness, low native intelligence, and their effects) entirely to the market.

This kind of self-consciously semiconsequentialist conception of social justice—which does not make the distribution of quality of life the primary *judicandum* and according to which social rules, rather than promote a good overall distribution among their participants, ought to treat them justly along the lines I have sketched—is missing from current discussions of social justice.[46]

[46] The adjective 'semiconsequentialist' is introduced in Pogge (1989: 47 *et passim*). A semiconsequentialist conception of social justice is there defined as one that asserts (1) that any (social) benefits and burdens a social order brings about are always more important than any (natural) goods and ills it merely lets happen (so that the latter can figure at most as a tie-breaker in assessing the justice of social orders); and (2) that any (social) benefits and burdens a social order brings about are of equal importance for assessing the justice of this order (benefits and

The semiconsequentialist approach articulates an important intermediate attitude toward natural handicaps and disabilities. It rejects, on the one hand, the quest for the social order that would generate the best overall distribution of quality of life by using social benefits to *compensate* for natural handicaps and disabilities. It also rejects, on the other hand, conceptions of social justice like those advocated by Nozick and Gauthier, who celebrate or at least condone social institutions under which natural handicaps and disabilities would, via lesser bargaining power, be *compounded* by severe social burdens and disadvantages. A semiconsequentialist approach aims for the best overall distribution of *social* benefits and burdens only, regardless of the preexisting distribution of natural endowments. Neither compensating nor compounding natural inequalities, Rawls's two principles constitute a semiconsequentialist criterion of social justice in this sense. But rather than self-consciously justify its semiconsequentialist character, Rawls marshals in its defence a contractualist machinery that, as we have seen, inescapably favours a social order that would use social benefits to compensate for natural handicaps and disabilities.

The idea of a semiconsequentialist conception of justice is important for exposing the prevailing bias toward purely recipient-oriented conceptions of social justice, important in making room for the thought that a social order that treats its participants justly need not be the one that promotes the best attainable overall distribution among its participants. While importantly correct on this point, the idea is nonetheless too crude in two respects. First, the distinction between natural and social components of human quality of life cannot be drawn clearly enough, and is not significant enough, to bear the great moral weight here placed upon it. Natural and social factors interpenetrate in their effects, so that given social benefits and burdens may have vastly differential impacts on persons who differ in natural endowments (as when the absence of proper sidewalks with curbs is catastrophic for the blind and only a nuisance for the sighted). And natural factors are by no means independent of social factors which, for instance, influence mating patterns and thereby the instantiated genotypes of the next generation—not to speak of mutations and birth defects due to pollution and other socially produced environmental factors. It is then incorrect, or at least overly simplistic, to view serious handicaps and disabilities as burdens that persons bring along with them when they enter society.

Second, semiconsequentialism is still too close to purely recipient-oriented conceptions of social justice by accepting the notion that at least the benefits and burdens a social order allocates to persons should be assessed by the impact they tend to have upon persons' overall quality of life. This again is too simple. For, quite apart from their impact on quality of life, it makes a considerable moral difference whether such benefits and burdens are, for example, *mandated*

burdens a social order establishes thus never have more weight than equivalent benefits and burdens it foreseeably engenders). There is a detailed discussion in Chapter 4 of the implications of a semiconsequentialist conception of social justice for the design of a just health-care system.

by a social order (e.g. prescribed by law) or merely come about pursuant to such an order through the decisions interacting persons make under its rules.[47]

If these two complications are to be taken into account, then the most plausible general structure for a conception of social justice would involve weighting the impact that social institutions have on relevant quality of life according to how they have this impact. Let me illustrate this structure by distinguishing, in a preliminary way, six basic ways in which a social order may have an impact on the medical conditions persons suffer under it. In my illustration, I will use six different scenarios in which some particular medical condition suffered by certain innocent persons can be traced to the fact that they, due to the arrangement of social institutions, avoidably lack some vital nutrients V (the vitamins contained in fresh fruit, perhaps, which are essential to good health). The six scenarios are arranged in order of their moral weight, according to my intuitive, pre-reflective judgement.[48]

In Scenario 1, the nutritional deficit is *officially mandated*, paradigmatically by the law: legal restrictions bar certain persons from buying foodstuffs containing V. In Scenario 2, the nutritional deficit results from *legally authorised* conduct of private subjects: sellers of foodstuffs containing V lawfully refuse to sell to certain persons. In Scenario 3, social institutions *foreseeably and avoidably engender* (but do not specifically require or authorise) the nutritional deficit through the conduct they stimulate: certain persons, suffering severe poverty within an ill-conceived economic order, cannot afford to buy foodstuffs containing V. In Scenario 4, the nutritional deficit arises from private conduct that is *legally prohibited but barely deterred*: sellers of foodstuffs containing V illegally refuse to sell to certain persons, but enforcement is lax and penalties are mild. In Scenario 5, the nutritional deficit arises from social institutions *avoidably leaving unmitigated the effects of a natural defect*: certain persons are unable to metabolise V due to a treatable genetic defect, but they avoidably lack access to the treatment that would correct their handicap. In scenario 6, finally, the nutritional deficit arises from social institutions *avoidably leaving*

---

[47] This problem is discussed at length in Pogge (1995: esp. section V). The main thought there is that, if we view all social benefits and burdens as on a par, then justice would permit, even require, that we authorise our officials deliberately to produce social burdens where doing so reduces social burdens overall. Such authorisations would be especially problematic in the domain of the criminal law: Should there be rough interrogations of suspects, lower standards of evidence, strict-liability criminal statues, the death penalty for drunk drivers? Yes, would be the answer, if and to the extent that such measures reduce risks and dangers for the representative citizen overall—the criminal-justice system is to be designed so as to minimise the sum of two burdens: the expected burden from harms inflicted by criminals plus the expected burden from harms inflicted by the authorities. But widely shared fundamental moral convictions revolt against this answer.

[48] Other things must be presumed to be equal here. Medical conditions become less weighty, morally, as we go through the list. But less weighty medical conditions may nevertheless outweigh weightier ones if the former are more severe or more numerous or more cheaply avoidable than the latter. In this way, an advantage in reducing Scenario 4 type deficits may outweigh a much smaller disadvantage in engendering Scenario 3 type deficits, for example.

unmitigated the effects of a self-caused defect: certain persons are unable to metabolise V due to a treatable self-caused disease—brought on, perhaps, by their maintaining a long-term smoking habit in full knowledge of the medical dangers associated therewith—and avoidably lack access to the treatment that would correct their ailment.

This differentiation of six ways in which social institutions may be related to the goods and ills that persons encounter is preliminary in that it fails to isolate the morally significant factors that account for the descending moral weight of the relevant medical conditions. Lacking the space to do this here, let me merely venture the hypothesis that what matters is not merely the *causal* role of social institutions, how they figure in a complete causal explanation of the deficit in question, but also (what one might call) the implicit *attitude* of social institutions to the deficit in question.[49] To illustrate: a high incidence of medical conditions caused by domestic violence may show a society's legal order to be unjust if such violence could be substantially reduced by appropriately training police, prosecutors, and judges and by instructing them to enforce existing criminal statutes vigorously and to impose serious punishments (Scenario 4). But the same abuse of the same women would indicate a much greater injustice, if it were not illegal at all—if spouses were legally free to beat each other or, worse, if men were legally authorised to beat the women in their households (Scenario 2).

My preliminary classification is meant to suggest a scalar understanding of negative and positive responsibility: the lower a rank institutionally avoidable medical conditions occupy on the proposed ordering, the more positive, and hence the less weighty, is the responsibility of those who cooperate in the coercive imposition of a social order giving rise to these conditions.[50]

This preliminary classification is surely still too simple. In some cases one will have to take account of other, perhaps underlying causes; and one may also need to recognise interdependencies among causal influences and fluid transitions between the classes.[51] Bypassing these complications here, let me emphasise once more the decisive point missed by the usual theories of social justice: To be morally plausible, a criterion of social justice must take account of—and its application thus requires information about—the particular relation between social institutions and human quality of life, which may determine

---

[49] This implicit attitude of social institutions is independent of the attitudes or intentions of the persons shaping and upholding these institutions: only the former makes a difference to how just the institutions are—the latter only make a difference to how blameworthy persons are for their role in imposing them.

[50] To illustrate: whether it is unjust for social institutions not to entitle indigent persons to treatment for a certain lung disease—and, if so, how unjust this is—may be greatly affected by whether this disease is contracted through legally authorised pollution by others (Scenario 2) or self-caused through smoking in full awareness of its risks (Scenario 6).

[51] The case of smoking, for instance, may exemplify a fluid transition between Scenarios 2 and 6 insofar as private agents (sellers of tobacco products) are legally permitted to try to render persons addicted to nicotine.

whether some institutionally avoidable deficit is an injustice at all and, if so, how great an injustice it is. Such a criterion must take into account, that is, not merely the comparative impact a social order has on the distribution of quality of life, but also *the manner in which* it exerts this influence. If this is right, then it is no more true of social rules than of subjects and conduct that they are just if and insofar as they promote a good overall distribution. Appraising overall distributions of goods and ills (or of quality of life) may be an engaging academic and theological pastime, but it fails to give plausible moral guidance where guidance is needed: for the assessment and reform of social rules as well as of subjects and their conduct.

7.6. CONCLUSION

Bearing in mind that the material introduced in the preceding five paragraphs requires much more reflection and deliberation, let me close with the following suggestions. Social institutions can be said to contribute substantially to medical conditions if and only if they contribute to their genesis through Scenarios 1–3. Supposing that at least the more privileged adult citizens of affluent and reasonably democratic countries are materially involved in upholding not only the economic order of their own society but also the global economic order, we can say two things about such citizens: pursuant to my second thesis, they have equally strong moral reason to prevent and mitigate compatriots' medical conditions due to avoidable poverty engendered by domestic economic institutions and to prevent and mitigate foreigners' medical conditions due to avoidable poverty engendered by global economic institutions. And pursuant to my combined thesis, they have stronger moral reason to prevent and mitigate foreigners' medical conditions due to avoidable poverty engendered by global economic institutions than to prevent and mitigate compatriots' medical conditions that are not due to mandated, authorised, or engendered deficits.

In the United States, some 40 million mostly poor citizens avoidably lack adequate medical insurance. Due to their lack of coverage, many of these people, at any given time, suffer medical conditions that could be cured or mitigated by treatment not in fact accessible to them. This situation is often criticised as manifesting an injustice in the country's social order. Now imagine that the poverty of the 40 million were so severe that it not only renders them unable to gain access to the medical care they need (Scenarios 5 and 6), but also exposes them to various medical conditions owing specifically to poverty-related causes (Scenario 3). This additional feature, which plays a substantial role for some fraction of the 40 million, considerably aggravates the injustice. And this additional feature is central to the plight of the world's poorest populations. These people generally lack access to adequate care for the medical conditions they suffer, of course. But the main effect of an extra $50 or $100 of annual income for them would not be more medical care, but much less need for such care. If they were not so severely impoverished, they would not suffer in the first place most of the medical conditions that, as things are, they also cannot obtain adequate treatment for.

I have tried to lend some initial plausibility to the view that such poverty-induced medical conditions among the global poor are, for us, morally on a par with poverty-induced medical conditions among the domestic poor and also of greater moral weight than not socially induced medical conditions among poor compatriots unable to afford adequate treatment. In the first two cases, but not in the third, we are materially involved in upholding social institutions that avoidably contribute substantially to the incidence of medical conditions and of the countless premature deaths resulting from them.

References

Arneson, Richard (1989). 'Equality and Equality of Opportunity for Welfare', *Philosophical Studies*, 56: 77–93.

Black, Douglas Sir, J. N. Morris, Cyril Smith, and Peter Townsend (1990). 'The Black Report', in Townsend, Peter, and Nick Davidson (eds.), *Inequalities in Health*. London: Penguin.

Bok, Hilary (1996). 'Acting Without Choosing', *NOÛS*, 30: 174–96.

Carens, Joseph (1987). 'Aliens and Citizens: The Case for Open Borders', *Review of Politics*, 49: 251–73.

Chen, S. and M. Ravallion (2001). 'How Did the World's Poorest Fare in the 1990s?', *Review of Income and Wealth*, 47: 283–300.

Cohen, G. A. (1989). 'On the Currency of Egalitarian Justice', *Ethics*, 99: 906–44.

——(1992). 'Incentives, Inequality, and Community', in Grethe Peterson (ed.), *The Tanner Lectures on Human Values XIII*. Salt Lake City: University of Utah Press.

——(1997). 'Where the Action Is: On the Site of Distributive Justice', *Philosophy and Public Affairs*, 26: 3–30.

——(2000). *If You're an Egalitarian, How Come You're so Rich?* Cambridge, MA: Harvard University Press.

Daniels, Norman (1985). *Just Health Care*. Cambridge: Cambridge University Press.

Dreze, Jean and Amartya Sen (1995). *India: Economic Development and Social Opportunity*. Delhi: Oxford University Press.

Dworkin, Ronald (2000). *Sovereign Virtue*. Cambridge, MA: Harvard University Press.

Elster, Jon and Roemer, John (eds.) (1991). *Interpersonal Comparisons of Well-Being*. Cambridge: Cambridge University Press.

Evans, Robert G., Morris L. Barer, and Theodore R. Marmor (1994) (eds.) *Why Are Some People Healthy and Others Not? The Determinants of Health of Populations*. New York: Aldine de Gruyter.

Galston, William (1980). *Justice and the Human Good*. Chicago: University of Chicago Press.

Gauthier, David (1986). *Morals by Agreement*. Oxford: Clarendon Press.

Griffin, James (1986). *Well-Being*. Oxford: Clarendon Press.

Gwatkin, D. R. (2000). 'Health Inequalities and the Health of the Poor: What Do We Know? What Can We Do?', *Bulletin of the World Health Organization*, 78: 3–15. Also at www.who.int/bulletin/tableofcontents/2000/vol.78no.1.html.

Kagan, Shelly (1989). *The Limits of Morality*. Oxford: Oxford University Press.

Lam, Ricky and Leonard Wantchekon (1999). 'Dictatorships as a Political Dutch Disease', Working Paper, Yale University.

Murphy, Liam (2000). *Moral Demands in Non-Ideal Theory*. Oxford: Oxford University Press.

Nagel, Thomas (1977). 'Poverty and Food: Why Charity Is Not Enough', in Peter Brown and Henry Shue (eds.), *Food Policy: The Responsibility of the United States in Life and Death Choices*. New York: The Free Press.

Nozick, Robert (1974). *Anarchy, State, and Utopia*. New York: Basic Books.

Nussbaum, Martha and Amartya Sen (eds.) (1993). *The Quality of Life*. Oxford: Oxford University Press.

O'Neill [Nell], Onora (1975). 'Lifeboat Earth', *Philosophy and Public Affairs*, 4: 273–92.

Parfit, Derek (1984). *Reasons and Persons*. Oxford: Oxford University Press.

Pogge, Thomas W. (1989). *Realizing Rawls*. Ithaca: Cornell University Press.

——(1995). 'Three Problems with Contractarian-Consequentialist Ways of Assessing Social Institutions', *Social Philosophy and Policy*, 12: 241–66.

——(2000). 'On the Site of Distributive Justice: Reflections on Cohen and Murphy', *Philosophy and Public Affairs*, 29: 137–69.

——(2002). *World Poverty and Human Rights*. Cambridge: Polity Press.

——(2004). ' "Assisting" the Global Poor', in Deen K. Chatterjee (ed.), *The Ethics of Assistance: Morality and the Distant Needy*. Cambridge: Cambridge University Press.

Rachels, James (1979). 'Killing and Starving to Death', *Philosophy*, 54: 159–71.

Rawls, John (1982). 'Social Unity and Primary Goods', in Amartya Sen and Bernard Williams (eds.), *Utilitarianism and Beyond*. Cambridge (UK): Cambridge University Press.

Rawls, John (1996) [1993]. *Political Liberalism*. New York: Columbia University Press

——(1999*a*) [1971]. *A Theory of Justice*. Cambridge, MA: Harvard University Press

——(1999*b*). *The Law of Peoples*. Cambridge, MA: Harvard University Press.

——(2001). *Justice as Fairness: A Brief Restatement*. Cambridge, MA: Harvard University Press.

Reddy, Sanjay and Thomas W. Pogge (2002). 'How *Not* to Count the Poor', unpublished paper available at www.socialanalysis.org.

Roemer, John (1996). *Theories of Distributive Justice*. Cambridge, MA: Harvard University Press.

Scanlon, Thomas M. (1999). *What We Owe To Each Other*. Cambridge, MA: Harvard University Press.

Sen, Amartya (1981). *Poverty and Famines*. Oxford: Oxford University Press.

——(1982). 'Equality of What?', *Choice, Welfare and Measurement*. Cambridge: Cambridge University Press.

——(1992). *Inequality Reexamined*. Cambridge, MA: Harvard University Press.

Singer, Peter (1972). 'Famine, Affluence and Morality', *Philosophy and Public Affairs*, 1: 229–43.

Thompson, Dennis (1980): 'Moral Responsibility of Public Officials: The Problem of Many Hands', *American Political Science Review*, 74: 905–16.

UNDP (1998). *Human Development Report 1998*. New York: Oxford University Press.

——(1999). *Human Development Report 1999*. New York: Oxford University Press.

UNDP (2002). *Human Development Report 2002*. New York: Oxford University Press. Also at www.undp.org/hdr2002.

Unger, Peter (1996). *Living High and Letting Die: Our Illusion of Innocence*. Oxford: Oxford University Press.

USDA (1999). *US Action Plan on Food Security*. www.fas.usda.gov/icd/summit/pressdoc.html.

Wantchekon, Leonard (1999). 'Why do Resource Dependent Countries Have Authoritarian Governments?', Working Paper, Yale University, www.yale.edu/leitner/pdf/1999–11.pdf.

WHO (2000). *The World Health Report 2000. Health Systems: Improving Performance*. Geneva: WHO Publications. Also at www.who.int/whr/2000.

—— (2001). *The World Health Report 2001*. Geneva: WHO Publications. Also at www.who.int/whr/2001.

Wilkinson, Richard (1996). *Unhealthy Societies: The Afflictions of Inequality*. London and New York: Routledge.

World Bank (2000). *World Development Report 2000/2001*. New York: Oxford University Press. Also at www.worldbank.org/poverty/wdrpoverty/report/index.htm.

—— (2002). *World Development Report 2003*. New York: Oxford University.

References

8

Just Health Care
in a Pluri-National Country

PHILIPPE VAN PARIJS

Justice in health care is an important issue for a number of reasons. Some of these are obvious, others less so. I shall here illustrate one of the less obvious ones by showing how the choice of a conception of justice in health care can crucially affect the conquest of a city and the survival of a country. This is not science fiction of a sort philosophers relish in concocting. This is about the fate of my own country in the last few years, today, and in the difficult years to come. Nor is it a parochial issue whose relevance is confined to a handful of anomalous corners of the world. Let us bear in mind that the world's estimated 6,000 living languages only have 211 sovereign countries to house them. Moreover, as economic globalisation tightens its grip on small and medium-sized nation-states, redistributive institutions organised entirely at the national level will become increasingly difficult to sustain, and one will have to think about how best to conceive of social justice or solidarity, *inter alia* in matters of health care, at a level that exceeds the nation-state.

8.1. HEALTH CARE CONFLICT IN A BI-NATIONAL FEDERAL STATE

Belgium was born in 1830 as a strongly unitary state on the French model, with French as the sole official language. In 1994, after a long and strenuous sequence of constitutional reforms, it became a complex federal state based on two distinct partitions of the population into three regions and into three communities, each with its own parliament and government. The regions took control over most 'territorial' powers such as public infrastructure, environmental and economic policy, while the communities were put in charge of such 'non-territorial' matters as education, culture, and (some aspects of) social policy. The three regions are Flanders, nearly 6 million inhabitants, mostly Dutch-speaking, very prosperous; Wallonia, nearly 3.5 million inhabitants, mostly French-speaking, in worse economic shape; and Brussels, the national capital, 1 million inhabitants, mostly French-speaking, the second richest region of the European Union in terms of GDP per capita but nonetheless with a per capita income below the country-wide average, owing to over half its jobs being filled by commuters. None of the three communities coincides with any of the three regions. The Flemish community consists of all residents of Flanders, and Brussels' small Dutch-speaking minority; the German community consists of the (60,000) residents of a handful of communes in the Eastern part of Wallonia; and the French community consists of all other residents of Wallonia and of Brussels' large French-speaking majority.

Despite this comprehensive devolution, the whole of Belgium's comparatively generous welfare state, including its high-quality health care system, has always been, and so far remains at the federal level, the bulk of it being funded by proportional social security contributions levied at the same rates throughout the country. But there are reasons to believe that this situation is unstable. At about the same time as the country became federal, statistical data revealed that the Walloon population had a per capita consumption of publicly funded health care significantly higher than the Flemish population. This could be attributed in part to its demographic structure (more elderly people), and to its economic situation (more unemployment). But it was also due in part to medical habits that turned out to be more expensive in Wallonia than in Flanders. For example, more diagnostic tests were routinely performed on the basis of similar symptoms, and more specialist services were routinely used for the same pathology.[1] Unsurprisingly, once these figures were known and appropriately advertised by Flemish journalists and politicians, a feeling of injustice quickly developed among Flemings: Why should they subsidise the Walloons' more expensive 'tastes'?

When two statistically identifiable segments of a population are covered by the same publicly organised health insurance system, the existence of large differences of per capita levels of health care consumption is not necessarily a problem: the differences may simply reflect inequalities in objective health risks beyond people's individual and collective control. But there is bound to be a problem if, for given health risks, the two segments—whether defined along linguistic, professional, provincial, or any other lines—consume unequally. In the case of linguistically distinct groups, this inequality might be due to some deep-seated cultural differences between members of the two groups. More plausibly, in the present context, it may be due to the influence of institutional differences, now under the control of regional or community authorities, such as an academic training of Walloon doctors that favours a wide spectrum of diagnostic tests, or a higher ratio of specialists to general practitioners in the Walloon population. Whatever the cause of the divergence (with given objective risks), the viability of a common insurance system requires— both for efficiency and for equity reasons—that it should be neutralised. The response to the challenge presented by the disturbing statistical data is

---

[1] See Schokkaert and Van de Voorde (1998) for a well-documented and dispassionate analysis.

therefore straightforward, it would seem: one must tighten the monitoring of the application of the common norms, so as to ensure a more uniform interpretation (by health care organisations, doctors, and patients) of what entitlements are generated in given objective circumstances, by virtue of the centrally funded health insurance package.

The challenge, however, is deeper than what this straightforward response can handle. First of all, objective medical needs themselves may be significantly influenced by the use regions and communities are making of the powers that have already been devolved to them in areas other than health care. Careless town-planning may foster psychiatric disorders; ill-guided economic and social policy may partly account for high unemployment and the associated health hazards; sloppy environmental and traffic regulations may increase casualties; and the way schools are managed is likely to affect teenagers' smoking, drinking, and drug-taking habits. For the overall design to be fair and efficient, it is therefore not sufficient to make the health care system work in a uniform way, for given objective needs. Differences in objective needs themselves are, at least in part, the responsibility of regions or communities.

Second, quite apart from being insufficient, it is not obvious at all that the uniform application of common norms is desirable. For the three regions of the country, or more plausibly still, its two main linguistic communities, could easily develop significantly distinct conceptions of the overall share of public resources to be devoted to health care and of the specific make up of the package of services that these resources should be used to provide free of charge, or at a subsidised rate. How much, if anything, should be covered by way of dentistry, cosmetic surgery, acupuncture, fertility treatment, abortion, hospital comfort, or physiotherapy? Where does the border lie between the admissible and the murderous easing of an elderly person's death? On all these issues, there is bound to be some disagreement within any linguistic community, but distinct cultural traditions and public debates could easily generate median answers that differ markedly from one community to another.

8.2. THE DUALISM OF SOLIDARITIES

These two difficulties are inherent in the 'unitarist' response outlined above, but can be dealt with at one swoop by a coherent, principled approach which tends to be associated, in the Belgian debate, with the most radical Flemish organisations, but which can boast strong credentials, as we shall see, from the most respectable of philosophical sources. This approach, which I shall label 'dualistic' rests on a sharp dichotomy between solidarity between the members of one people, and solidarity between peoples. I shall argue against it below, but I first want to spell it out in what I believe to be its most attractive version.

According to this dualistic conception, inter-individual solidarity *within one people* can be conveniently understood along the lines of insurance behind a veil of ignorance. In the particular case of health care, the relevant thought experiment can be phrased as follows. We accept to abstract from our particular situation among all those in which the members of our people could find themselves, and we wonder what we would insure against, and for how much, on the background of a shared conception of what counts as being ill, and what treatment ill health requires. Put differently, it can be viewed as counter-factual reciprocity: I do this for you, not because you will give me something equivalent in exchange (whether certainly or probabilistically), but because I believe I *could have been* in your position, and you in mine (since we are members of the same people), and I trust that (as a member of the same people, sharing the same conception of what counts as being ill, etc.) you would then have done for me what I now do for you. As defined by this solidarity, justice within one people is of course far more demanding, morally speaking, than actuarial fairness. But it does not reach beyond the borders of one's people, characterised in a mutually reinforcing way by identification ('I could have been her'), and by a common culture ('in matters of health care at any rate, we care about roughly the same things to roughly the same extent'). This does not mean that there is no room for solidarity *between peoples*. But instead of being opaquely camouflaged as inter-individual solidarity, it should be circumscribed to specific risks societies as such are exposed to, such as famines, floods, epidemics, and highly adverse economic conditions.

Such a sharply dualistic approach was strikingly articulated by the federation of Flemish cultural associations which vigorously launched the public debate on the partition of Belgium's welfare state in the early 1990s.[2] What it implies for the organisation of the health care system is clear. Rather than trying to enforce uniformity more strictly, one should rather allow each people, each linguistic community, to make its own choices, bearing of course the full financial consequences of these choices. The just organisation of health care would then require each people to determine its own guaranteed health care package, and to fund it with its own money. Both problems left unsolved by the 'unitary' approach are then easily solved. The fact that objective medical needs are affected by the use each community makes of its decentralised powers no longer offers opportunities for free riding and irresponsibility. Nor does the fact that one community may have more expensive 'tastes' with given objective needs. Moreover, this approach grants each community full freedom to develop its own vision of a just and adequate health care system. If one of the two communities is doing so badly that it qualifies as needy, solidarity across communities is called for. But this residual solidarity would henceforth cease to be exercised specifically via the health care system, and be amalgamated into a transparent general solidarity grant to the destitute community.

---

[2] See OVV (1991), and Pieters (1994) and Bertels et al. (1998) for a detailed blueprint and argument.

8.3. BREAK-UP AND RECONQUEST

If consistently and thoroughly implemented, this conception of justice in health care has dramatic consequences for the fate of Belgium, and particularly of its capital city, Brussels. To understand this, a few figures should be helpful.[3] Whereas the relative sizes of the Flemish and francophone communities are about 60 and 40 per cent, respectively, their contributions to the funding of the country-wide health care system (about 1,300 euros per capita annually in 1997) are about 64 and 36 per cent and their share in total health care expenditure about 57 and 43 per cent. A corollary is that over 10 per cent of the francophones' consumption is funded by net transfers from the Flemings because of lower per capita contributions, and nearly another 6 per cent because of higher per capita spending. The entire gap between revenues per capita, and much of the somewhat smaller gap between expenditures per capita can be explained by Wallonia's weaker economic and demographic situation.

Under the 'unitary' approach of norm uniformisation, net transfers stemming from unequal incomes or from objective differences in medical needs would be left untouched, and the loss to the francophones would therefore be limited to a small fraction (attributable to their 'expensive tastes') of the 6 per cent of excess per capita consumption. Under the 'dualistic' approach, on the other hand, each community would be organising its own health care system, and the loss to the francophones would be given by the total of all current net transfers, and hence amount to nearly 16 per cent of their consumption.

Moreover, under this 'dualistic' approach, there is no good reason to stop here. What can be said about the organisation of a people's health care system can easily be generalised to its educational system, its child benefit, pension, and public assistance schemes. In all these areas, it should be up to each people to work out and implement, with its own resources, its vision of solidarity, with the total direct loss in net transfers easily reaching 5 per cent of Wallonia's GDP.[4] Now that Belgium has long lost its colonies, has little need for an army, and has given up its currency, it is hard to see how it could survive the shock of the dismantling of its common welfare state. Or at least, the break up of the country would seem unavoidable, assuming dualists got their way, if some solution could be found for Brussels, where the two communities are tightly intertwined: the divorce will not go through, and the

---

[3] All estimates of proportions are based on d'Alcantara (1995: 490–1), which relates to the 1990 situation, with a 20%/80% assumption about the shares of the two communities in the populations, revenues and expenditures of Brussels and with the small German community amalgamated, along with the rest of Wallonia, into the French community. Absolute magnitudes are based on the 1997 figures provided on the web site http://belgium.fgov.be ('*La sécurité sociale: Données statistiques et financières*'). See also Van Gompel (1998) and Docquier (ed.) (2000) for updates on net transfers.

[4] I am here abstracting from any indirect cost, such as the loss of Walloon jobs resulting from the emigration of purchasing power across the linguistic border or the economic consequences of a dramatic fall in the funding of the education system.

bickering will linger on unless some mutually agreeable arrangement is found for the couple's child.

But precisely, the very same dualistic conception provides the theoretical underpinnings for a reconquest of Brussels by Flanders, which would elegantly (though not painlessly) settle the matter. Brussels used to be a Flemish-speaking city, and is completely surrounded by Flemish territory, but basically as result of having been the capital of a francophone state, less than 20 per cent of its current population have Flemish as their mother tongue. Moreover, it is hard to see how the 'Frenchization' of the city could fail to continue, as cheaper, safer, greener, and more Flemish suburbs are bound to exert a strong attraction on a large fraction of Brussels's shrinking Flemish minority. Yet, it can be reversed. Here is the recipe.

First implement the dualist conception of solidarity outlined above, so that each of Belgium's two main linguistic communities organises and funds at least its own health care, child benefit, and education systems. Next, rather than making membership of a community an ascriptive matter of mother tongue, let Brussels households choose, as they can now, which community they belong to, and hence which package of health insurance, schools, and child benefits they will have access to, jointly with the obligation to contribute to their funding. Making the choice of these three items a joint choice is quite natural, as education is already, for obvious reasons, devolved to the linguistic communities (though still centrally funded), and the right to child benefits (currently up to age twenty-five and centrally funded) is subjected to school or university attendance. Given the huge difference between per capita incomes in Flanders and Wallonia, the Flemish benefit-contribution package is bound to be worth far more than what the francophones can offer: the gap should reach about 2,500 euros annually for a family of four.[5]

At this sort of level, powerful financial incentives are in place for Brussels families to move over from the French to the Flemish community—especially when bearing in mind that the majority of these families, if weighted by the number of children, is of recent immigrant origin. Given the key importance of the language of schooling, and taking a number of snowball effects into account— decline and demoralisation of the French schools, return of Flemings to Brussels, etc.—the 're-Flemishization' of Brussels will then follow in the space of one or two generations, at least if enough material resources and paedagogical acumen are channelled into Dutch-language schools to help them cope with the massive

[5] With the communities fully in charge of the funding of education, health care, and child benefits, the Flemish community could offer 250 euros per capita more than now to its members with unchanged contributions (or tax them 250 euros less with unchanged benefits and services), while the French community will have to reduce the value of its services by 400 euros per capita (or collect 400 euros more in contributions with unchanged benefits and services). Hence an annual differential of 650 euros per person, depending on which community one chooses to belong to. Estimates on d'Alcantara (1995), supplemented by the *Exposé général du budget 1998* (Bruxelles: Services du premier ministere 1997) and *Les séries statistiques* (Bruxelles: ONAFTS 1997).

influx of non-native pupils. The region of Flanders could then simply absorb the city-region of Brussels, which it (oddly but, it would then turn out, quite aptly) chose as its official capital when Belgium became a federal state. And the decisive condition would then be satisfied for Belgium itself to wither away.

8.4. THE LAW OF PEOPLES

This completes my illustrative demonstration of how a conception of justice, and particularly a conception of justice in the area of health care, can unexpectedly prove to matter greatly to the reconquest of a city, and the fate of a country. While much in the example is idiosyncratic, the challenge it illustrates cannot easily be dismissed as having only local or anecdotal interest. As pointed out above, pluri-national polities are the rule rather than the exception, and increasingly so. Moreover, the dualistic conception which did much of the work in the above demonstration cannot be reduced to an ad hoc construct advertised by a handful of organisations in a tiny portion of the world in order to rationalise their self-interested demands. For the twentieth century's most influential political philosopher is defending a dualistic conception of social justice which bears far more than a superficial resemblance to it. John Rawls's *Law of Peoples* (1999) rests on a dichotomy between two 'original positions'—one with representatives of the members of one people, and one with representatives of the various peoples—which closely parallels the two solidarities outlined above. And it generates distributive outcomes—the difference principle (or some other liberal-egalitarian distributive principle) within each people versus the far less demanding duty of assistance between peoples in case one of them became 'burdened' by adverse circumstances—which closely parallel those following from the dualism of solidarities—an elaborate system of institutionalised inter-individual transfers within each people versus an explicit, transparent grant to the government of a needy people.

A closer examination—which I shall not undertake here (see Rawls and Van Parijs 2003)—would no doubt come up with some significant differences, but these would emerge on a firmly common background, constitutive of what I am here calling a dualistic approach: a sharp distinction needs to be made, when discussing social justice in general, and justice in health care in particular, between those persons whom it makes sense to imagine sitting in the same original position, putting themselves in the others' shoes, reaching an agreement, behind a self-imposed veil of ignorance, on what to insure for, and what not, and those who belong to different peoples, and are therefore only indirectly linked through the far weaker duty of solidarity which connects their respective peoples. Thus, quite apart from its intuitive plausibility, the dualistic view articulated by the federation of Flemish cultural organisations turns out to be endorsed by John Rawls himself.

And yet, it should be resisted. This is not because there is something outrageous about the death of a country—a mere artefact which there is no need to revere as a fetish—or about the linguistic reconquest of a city—no more objectionable than its prior conquest, in the course of the last couple of centuries, through the social and economic pressure to learn a more prestigious language. My firm conviction that the dualistic view should be resisted has two different sources. First, as a citizen of a pluri-national state whose survival is at risk, and at the same time of a multinational political entity—the European Union—which is undeniably more than a confederation of states, yet has no professed intention or objective prospect of becoming one country or one people—I cannot help finding the notion of 'people' far too contingent, too fragile, too much a matter of degree, to allow a conception of justice to be structured by a dichotomy which gives it a central role. Second, although I fully recognise the difficulty, and in most cases the undesirability, of developing a public health insurance system across the borders of populations with different languages, and hence, in all likelihood, diverging public debates, I also feel that it would be a serious regression if the relatively generous inter-individual transfer system that currently exists across linguistic borders in pluri-national welfare states such as those of Belgium or Canada were to be dismantled, and that it would be a bad, thing, as far as justice is concerned, if no similar system could be institutionalised in countries in which it does not yet exist.

Yet, the intuitions which inspire this resistance can be naturally accommodated within an approach that would remain, in a general sense, 'Rawlsian', that is, not only liberal-egalitarian, but also concerned to respect the prerogative of different 'peoples' to design their solidarity systems, and in particular their health care systems, in accordance with their views as to what an illness is, for example, and what treatment it requires. There is no doubt more than one way of trying to articulate a 'Rawlsian' resistance in this sense. I shall present one, which directly follows from the particular liberal-egalitarian conception of social justice I tried to defend in *Real Freedom for All*, thus seizing this opportunity to spell out the latter's central implications for the just allocation of health care, and to test its plausibility in this area.

8.5. MAXIMIN GIFTS, AND UNDOMINATED DIVERSITY

The conception of social justice as 'real freedom for all' essentially consists in the combination of two simple ideas, each of which I find very appealing, though unacceptable if not supplemented by the other.[6] The first of these ideas is the maximin distribution of gifts. Whether deliberately or unwittingly, whether structurally or randomly, countless gifts are made to us in the course of our lives, mainly today through the jobs and other market opportunities which our talents and other forms of luck give us very unequal access to. There is no reason to expect the spontaneous distribution of these gifts to be fair. Fairness does not

[6] For the sake of brevity, I am here leaving out a third simple idea—universal self ownership—which operates as a prior constraint on the other two (see Van Parijs 1995: chapter 1).

mean that we should all receive identical, or equally valuable gifts. But it does require—this is the first simple idea—that the value of the gifts received by the person who receives least should be sustainably maximised. This criterion naturally leads in a market society to giving each an unconditional cash endowment at the highest per capita level that can be sustained through predictable taxation. This endowment could conceivably be given in the form of a one-off payment that could be turned into a regular payment by those who so wish—higher for men than for women, though, because of the latter's higher life expectancy. I favour instead a regular instalment over people's lifetime, equal for all at a given age.[7] One way of motivating this preference consists in assuming that spreading the income guarantee over their whole lifetimes in this fashion is what people would do if asked to make up their minds *ex ante*, with full knowledge of the consequences of every option but without knowing which statistical category (man or woman, etc.) they belong to.[8] Another rationale, metaphysically more demanding perhaps, rests on the claim that later selves need to be protected against earlier ones: a just society cannot countenance destitute elderly people who owe their destitution to their squandering youth.

This first simple idea—the maximin distribution of gifts—fits my considered moral judgement quite well, or rather would do so if one could disregard handicaps or, more broadly, significant differences in capacities that are not, or not fully, reflected in unequal market rewards. This is where the second simple idea kicks in. It is called for to handle cases in which the assumption of equal talents is far off the mark. If we have unequal capacities, if some of us are handicapped as a result of genetic defects, accidents at birth, unfavourable family environments, etc. justice cannot be achieved by giving all an equal cash grant, be it at the highest sustainable level. It requires a more targeted compensation to the less well endowed. According to what criterion? I propose *undominated diversity*.[9] Let us define a person's comprehensive endowment as the set of all the external resources he or she is given, and of all the (internal) capacities he or she is endowed with. Undominated diversity is satisfied if for any two members A and B of the community considered, there is at least one member of the community who prefers A's comprehensive endowment over B's, and at least one who prefers B's over A's. In other words, undominated diversity

---

[7] I am here stating dogmatically a sequence of claims for which I argue in Van Parijs (1995). Chapter 2, in particular, defends the idea of a regular payment or basic income—James Tobin's 'demogrant', James Meade's 'social dividend'—against the related idea of a basic endowment, which can be traced back to Thomas Paine (1796) and has been recently revived by Ackerman and Alstott (1999). See Van Parijs et al. (2001) for a recent discussion.

[8] Daniels (1996: 262) argues along the same line on the basis of his 'prudential lifespan account' (to which I return below): 'the prudent course of action would be to allocate their (the planners') fair share in such a way that their standard of living would remain roughly equal over the life-span'.

[9] The criterion is vindicated at length, and defended against its rivals, in chapter 3 of Van Parijs (1995). It constitutes a generalisation and reinterpretation of a notion put forward by Bruce Ackerman (1980) in connection with liberal genetic engineering.

amounts to the absence of a unanimous preference among endowments within the community. If instead the existing diversity is 'dominated', say because of a unanimous preference for A's comprehensive endowment over B's, one must channel external resources from A to B up to the point when there is at least one person who prefers B's comprehensive endowment to A's.

To convey the underlying intuition, I shall briefly sketch four perspectives from which this criterion can be motivated. First, some may find appealing the idea that for redistribution from A to B to be justified, all one needs is that a majority should prefer A's comprehensive endowment to B's. But this can mean requiring a transfer from A to B despite the fact that both A and B find A's endowment worse than B's. For those who want to rule out this possibility while sticking to a majoritarian approach, undominated diversity is a natural criterion to adopt.

Others may instead be attracted by the notion of envy-freeness: a distribution of endowments is just if no one envies anyone else's endowment. But this criterion is generally unsatisfiable if people possess at the same time different talents and different tastes. For those who are bothered by this limit, while wishing to stick as much as possible to the envy-freeness approach, undominated diversity is again a natural option. For undominated diversity is nothing but *potential* envy-freeness: saying that undominated diversity obtains is equivalent to saying that, for each member of any pair (A, B) of people in the community, there exists at least one preference schedule actually held in the community such that, were A to adopt it, he or she would not envy B's endowment, and there also exists at least one such schedule such that, were B to adopt it, he or she would not envy A's endowment.[10]

Others still may be tempted by a conception of justice as equality of welfare, or at least as equality of potential welfare or of opportunity for welfare. But whether for epistemic reasons or for deeper ethical reasons, they may become persuaded that welfare levels are incommensurable across individuals. They then have to reduce their ambition from a complete ordering to a very partial ordering corresponding to the intersection of all individual orderings. This is exactly undominated diversity.

Last but not least, among those who believe for other reasons—typically, the treatment of expensive tastes and adaptive preferences—that equality of welfare or of potential welfare is not even a prima facie characterisation of social justice, there is a temptation to focus exclusively on the distribution of goods or external resources. But such an exclusive focus would overlook unjust inequalities in people's capacity to turn goods into valuable functionings. The pursuit of justice rather consists, at least in part, in the equalisation of people's basic capabilities. But what counts as a basic capability, and what tradeoffs, if any, can be allowed for between different levels of different basic capabilities?

---

[10] See Fleurbaey (1994, 1995) and the appendix to Van Parijs (1995: chapter 3) for more formal discussions of various ways of weakening envy-freeness.

One possible answer rests on a perfectionistic conception of the nature of human beings and their needs. But there is also a liberal, nonperfectionistic answer: undominated diversity.[11]

To work out the most plausible version of the criterion of undominated diversity, some tightening of the formulation is required, at least in the form of a restriction of relevant preferences to well informed or 'reasonable' ones, and some loosening is required too, for example, to exclude redistribution that would turn out to be counterproductive because of adverse incentive effects (the analogue to preferring leximin over strict equality for a one-dimensional variable). Thus trimmed and tuned, the criterion easily justifies the targeted redistribution of resources for the benefit of specific categories of 'disabled' people. This redistribution may take the form of handicap-tested cash transfers, but also of collective investments in special schools, adapted technology, handicap-friendly public infrastructure, or even of the spreading of a general ethos of tactful help: being blind can be quite a different experience depending on whether one lives in a society in which everyone looks away or drives past when a blind person is struggling to cross a street, and in one in which she can always count on a helping arm.

In its most defensible specification, undominated diversity remains a very weak criterion of equality. My firm intuitions about social justice are far too egalitarian to find it attractive as a full characterisation of what justice requires. But I find it exceedingly appealing if it is consistently combined with the first simple idea, more specifically if it is made a constraint on the sustainable maximisation of the external endowment that must be unconditionally granted to all in order to maximin what we are given.

8.6. HEALTH INSURANCE AS A COMPONENT OF THE BASIC ENDOWMENT

What relevance does all this have for just health care? I mentioned that the maximinning of gifts naturally leads to an unconditional cash basic income. But the presumption in favour of an all-cash endowment can easily be overridden in favour of at least a modest in-kind component. Trivially, one of the most vital gifts we receive every second or two is the air we breathe, and nobody would find it a particularly clever idea to fit an oxygen meter onto our noses, and make us pay a fee for each gallon we inhale (even though some market freak might well have suggested that this would be the efficient thing to do). A less facile but no less persuasive case can be made for a health-insurance package as a further in-kind component. The argument for constraining part of the endowment in this way can be based on the existence of various external benefits of making health insurance obligatory for all. This may have to do, for example, with adverse selection problems that hamper voluntary schemes,

[11] See, for example, Sen (1985); Van Parijs (1990); and Sen (1990) on the connection.

with public good aspects in the control of epidemics, and with administrative advantages in the treatment of emergencies. The case can also rest, in a mildly paternalistic vein, on the plausible assumption that anyone fully aware of the probability of health problems, their costs and other consequences, would devote some of her basic income to a basic health insurance package. The guiding question should be: supposing I did not know anything about my own specific risks of needing any particular form of health care, while knowing everything about the probabilities of the various risks, their consequences, and the cost of the various available cures, what types of treatment would I want to be covered, and to what extent, by an insurance scheme to which everyone would be obliged to subscribe, all this bearing in mind that its cost will be deducted from the basic income given to all.[12] Under reasonable assumptions about risk aversion, the overall level of the highest sustainable basic income, and the degree to which people in a given society have a shared conception of what health is, and what illness requires, a substantial basic health insurance package can be expected to be justified in this way.

What form should the health insurance package, thus justified, take? It could in principle take the form of an undiminished cash benefit with an obligation to insure or, at the other extreme, of the direct free provision of care to all by public sector employees. Or it could take a number of intermediate forms such as a standard insurance package that directly pays private care providers or reimburses the patients for at least part of the expenses. Should it be means-tested or universal? Just as a cash basic income could be given in the form of a negative income tax, free or subsidised access to health care could either be granted to all irrespective of incomes, or phased out as household income increases. From Tawney ('A policy for the poor is a poor policy') to Atkinson (1998), the pitfalls of means-testing have often been emphasised (stigma, poverty trap, rate of take up, dynamics of political support). The resulting strong presumption in favour of universality can conceivably be overridden, however, either because of an inefficient tax system that fails to claw back the benefits granted to the better endowed or because of the political weight of the persistent illusion that a policy concentrating on the poor is bound to be more cost-effective.

This forms the background on which undominated diversity can now operate. But to see how it does, it is essential to clarify the relevant time scale. Handicaps demanding targeted transfers can be present at birth, but also appear in the course of a person's life. To assess whether any of them is dominated, people's endowments are to be compared over their entire lives, not at the particular stages of life they happen to be. This is why undominated diversity does not mandate massive transfers to the very old. But since one cannot wait for someone's life to be completed to decide whether any targeted transfer

---

[12] Just as the spreading of the basic endowment over the lifespan, this allocation of part of it to a specific health care package is justified by a 'prudential lifespan account' of a sort similar to Norman Daniels's (1988, 1996).

should be made to or from her, one will constantly have to operate on the basis of presumptive anticipations. Becoming crippled or blind or indeed dying at age five will not be assessed in the same way, by the standards of undominated diversity, as being similarly affected at age ninety. Through this path, undominated diversity justifies an age-sensitive allocation of health care resources which discards the irresponsible or hypocritical 'Life is sacred' or 'Health has no price', without implying any instrumentalistic commitment to the maximisation of aggregate welfare, let alone of economic performance.

Whether existing from birth or arising from some later accident, disabilities of all sorts can be expected to be alleviated by the health care package justified as part of everyone's basic endowment. The extent of dominated diversity will therefore be substantially reduced, not only relative to a situation in which there is no redistribution whatever, but also relative to one in which the whole of the highest sustainable basic income takes the form of a uniform cash grant. But it is unlikely to have vanished altogether. Even with the correction resulting from care which has seemed cost-effective enough to be made part of the basic package, it is still likely that what can be presumed about the make up of some people's lifetime endowments will make these worse, in everyone's eyes, than some other people's, and some targeted distribution, over and above the basic income, will therefore be mandated.[13] As mentioned before, this targeted redistribution need not take a cash form, and may quite plausibly take the form of medical care focused on a specific condition.

Of course, working out the concrete implications of the thought experiment that defines undominated diversity, just as working out those of the thought experiment that specifies the basic health insurance package, needs to rely on countless empirical conjectures, and will never supply more than approximate guidance. But the conjunction of both provides, I believe, a coherent and plausible framework which can guide the identification of relevant arguments and sensible policies. Rather than trying to argue why this framework may prove more satisfactory than those proposed, in a broadly similar spirit, by Norman Daniels (1985, 1988); Erik Rakowski (1991); Ronald Dworkin (1993, 1994); and others, I now return, on the background it provides, to the issue of just health care in a culturally divided society.

8.7. JUST HEALTH CARE IN CULTURALLY DIVIDED SOCIETIES

Let us first consider the general question of how cultural diversity in matters of health care affects the operation of the framework just sketched. Suppose,

[13] The more generous and medically effective the basic health insurance package, the smaller the need for targeted transfers. And the less targeted redistribution is needed, the more generous the basic endowment can be, and hence also its health insurance component. As economic prosperity, medical efficiency and/or cultural diversity increase, one may therefore expect the demands of justice to require less and less targeted transfers. (On the other hand, better genetic diagnosis, for example, may make it possible, or easier to detect cases of undominated diversity which would otherwise have gone uncompensated.)

for example, that one segment of the society concerned regards biological parenthood as an essential part of a successful life, whereas the other does not. It is clear that both of the thought experiments introduced above will yield different results, depending on whether they are performed at the level of the society as a whole or within each of its two segments separately. Some fertility treatments will be part of the basic package in one of these groups, whereas it will not be (or only at a lower level) in the society as a whole. Furthermore, persistent infertility will turn out to be a handicap, to be compensated by appropriate means, in the former context, but not in the latter, where undominated diversity will therefore be easier to satisfy. This example illustrates the following general point: the more culturally diverse the society concerned, the more meagre the health care package that will be justified, either as part of everyone's endowment, or as part of a targeted transfer to those members of the society who can be identified as handicapped.[14] At the limit, extremely high levels of cultural diversity would shrink the health care package into insignificance, and secure undominated diversity even in the absence of any transfer. Hence, keeping culturally different parts of a society together blocks the just institutionalisation of more generous health care systems, while splitting a society along cultural lines would enable each part to justly develop its own distinct and more generous system.

Yet, this shrinking of the health care package does not translate into a corresponding shrinking of the overall level of redistribution, as whatever is no longer redistributed in a targeted form is now to be redistributed to all, while whatever was redistributed in kind must now be redistributed in cash.[15] The crucial point is that while the thought experiments which specify the just pattern of in-kind provision and the demands of undominated diversity require some degree of cultural homogeneity to have any bite, the one which underlies the justification of a basic income does not. To justify strong redistributive demands, it does not require that we should be homogeneous in terms of what we care about in life, but only that we should view ourselves as rival recipients of gifts, which we are unequally positioned to capture for reasons we recognise

---

[14] Here is another example, which shows at the same time how broadly undominated diversity can be interpreted. In various countries, some financial aid is given to people who have a close relative (parent, partner, child) requiring intensive care and feel morally obliged to sacrifice some or all of their professional activities in order to look after that relative—sometimes at the cost of great material hardship. In a society in which we all feel this moral obligation, undominated diversity can justify this if we extend the understanding of a person's endowment to cover features of his or her situation, such as the fact that he or she has a badly handicapped child. But it is enough for some people to sincerely not care, to feel no such obligation, for undominated diversity to lose its bite. The more culturally diverse the society, the more likely this is to happen and the poorer this scheme's prospect of being justified.

[15] The former shift does entail a small fall in net redistribution, as contributors are now also among the beneficiaries. The latter shift does not. Admittedly, giving part of the basic income in the form of health care may boost its highest sustainable level (e.g. because of its effect on the spreading of epidemics), but the components of the package that could plausibly produce such an effect would not cease to be justified as a result of increased cultural diversity.

are arbitrary. The chasing of the same jobs, outlets, inputs or investments, exposure to the same externalities, the imposition of political borders which protect the living standards of some, and prevent others from improving their fates, all this contributes to making such a picture of ourselves compelling, and hence also the need to secure a fair distribution of the value of this wide variety of gifts. How much of what she values each person will be guaranteed access to depends on the price structure, and hence on the overall pattern of preferences, including society's cultural constellation. But whatever diversity obtains, there is no reason to expect the real value of the highest sustainable basic income to shrink as a result of greater diversity.[16]

Against this background, it is certainly conceivable to give culturally more homogeneous segments of a society the option of working out their own distinct health care system. One convenient way of doing so, assuming that the level of coverage (as distinct from the pattern of care that is being covered) is about the same in the various segments, consists in giving the government of each of these segments a centrally funded capitation grant with which it can directly finance or indirectly reimburse the services the relevant thought experiments justify providing. Applied to the Belgian situation described at the start, this conception would be sympathetic to a community's desire to have its distinct health care system, if it feels prevented from designing it as it wishes, owing to the cultural diversity generated by linguistic distinctness, and the associated separation of public debates. But there is no reason why a poorer community should have to fund the whole of its health care system 'with its own money', except to the extent that it wishes to devote to health care a larger per capita share of total resources than the other communities. This fact may considerably reduce the attraction of a separate system for those whose main objective is not to make room for autonomy but to curtail net transfers. Yet, it may still present enough advantages to offset any economies of scale that derive from the existence of a joint system, and all the transitional and permanent administrative complications of a separation.

Even if it spreads to other sectors of the welfare state, a separation of this sort would have an impact on the fate of Belgium and its capital very different from the one sketched above in connection with the 'dualistic' conception. First, a strong federal state would of course still be essential to secure a fair distribution of resources, by collecting taxes (or social security contributions) throughout the country according to people's ability to pay throughout the country, and allocating the revenues to each community according to the size of its population, possibly weighted, for example, by the relative levels of medical expenditure for the various age groups, so as to capture at least this aspect of the 'objective' health risks. Second, the mechanism for a linguistic reconquest of Brussels would be switched off. For even if every Brussels

[16] I am here abstracting from the possible effect of cultural diversity on general economic performance as discussed for example by Alesina and La Ferrara (2003).

household were still made to choose between the health-care-and-child-bene-fit-and-education systems of the two communities, the small difference in the financial advantage of joining one rather than the other would lack the mus-cle needed to precipitate a massive conversion to the Flemish community.[17]

Even more important are two further differences with the 'dualistic' scenario. First, now that the project of turning Belgium into a single (francophone) nation has long been shelved, and that a full recognition of the two languages has gradually led the two linguistic communities and their public debates to drift apart, the dualist approach justifies a dismantling of Belgium's trans-regional transfer system. By contrast, according to the alternative approach just sketched, this system does not need to be dismantled but only reconfigured in a lump-sum direction, so as to prevent the autonomy granted to each community from giving rise to unfair compensation and inefficient incentives. Something closely analogous to what would emerge from such a reconfiguration—rather than an extension of national solidarity onto a higher scale through the construction of a European welfare state—is also exactly what is needed in such larger multi-national polities as the European Union.

Second, while recognising that more homogeneous polities can and must go for a more refined solidarity, this alternative approach does not ascribe to the notion of a 'people' the momentous importance it is given by the dualist approach. As soon as significant potential mobility and other interdependen-cies exist, the demand for a fair distribution of external resources extends across the borders of states and cultural communities. It calls for the preser-vation and development of institutions for collecting, across these borders, a significant share of resources which would otherwise be appropriated by some because of the luck of being born within particular borders, of speaking a par-ticular language, of possessing particular marketable talents, or of having acquired the right skill at the right time, etc. And it calls for an allocation of these centrally collected resources either directly to individuals or to the more decentralised authorities in charge of education and health systems. At these more local levels, cultural homogeneity should durably remain greater, espe-cially if political authorities have the power and will to enforce the adoption of the local language by anyone wishing to permanently settle within the bor-ders of its territory.[18] And because of this greater homogeneity, justice will

---

[17] Allocating people who share the same territory to tightly separate health care and education systems may be undesirable for other reasons. However mild, this is a form of permanent 'apartheid' (unlike the temporary one involved in the reconquest scenario) which hampers the people's ability to work out and realise a coherent social project with an unavoidable territorial dimension. For this and other reasons, the sort of federalism that is needed to durably accommodate the autonomy of distinct peoples within one country is of the territorial type, rather than of the 'personal' type imagined in Karl Renner's (1918) pioneering attempt to reconcile national diversity and democracy, and very partially implemented in Belgium's federalism of Communities.

[18] Possibly at a heavy and increasing cost to themselves (see Van Parijs 2000).

allow at this level—indeed mandate—more generous in-kind provision and more targeted distribution.

   This is what I meant by a 'Rawlsian' approach—not only liberal-egalitarian but also 'peoples-friendly'—which neither makes a sharp dichotomy between solidarity within one people and solidarity across peoples, nor fosters the dismantling of existing transfer systems across the borders of peoples. The adoption of this alternative account requires one not to think about health care systems, and the other aspects of our welfare states, exclusively in terms of 'solidarity', fundamentally understood as compensation for a (counterfactual) risk, and conceivably formulated in terms of some original-position-type thought experiment. The alternative account does retain something of this notion, mainly under the thin guise of undominated diversity. But the fact that the latter must operate on the background of a fair distribution of external resources profoundly changes the overall picture—and secures a sound normative basis for the defence, reform, and development of generous redistribution schemes in an increasingly globalised world.

References

Ackerman, Bruce A. and Anne Alstott (1999). *The Stakeholder Society*. New Haven: Yale University Press.

——(1980). *Social Justice in the Liberal State*. New Haven and London: Yale University Press.

Alesina, Alberto and Eliana La Ferrara (2003). *Ethic Diversity and Economic Performance*; Harvard University: Department of Economics.

Atkinson, Anthony B. (1998). *Poverty in Europe*. Oxford: Blackwell.

Bertels, Jan, Dany Pieters, Paul Schoukens, and Steven Vansteenkiste (1997). *De Vlaamse Sociale Zekerheid in 101 vragen en antwoorden*. Leuven: Acco.

d'Alcantara, Gonzalez (1995). 'Interregionale verschillen', in Marc Despontin, and Marc Jegers (eds.), *De sociale zekerheid verzekerd?* Brussels: VUB Press, pp. 485–507.

Daniels, Norman (1985). *Just Health Care*. Cambridge: Cambridge University Press.

——(1988). *Am I My Parents' Keeper? An Essay on Justice Between the Young and the Old*. Oxford: Oxford University Press.

——(1996). 'The Prudential Lifespan Account of Justice Across Generations', in N. Daniels (ed.), *Justice and Justification*. Cambridge: Cambridge University Press, pp. 257–83.

Docquier, Frédéric (ed.) (1999). *La Solidarité entre régions. Bilan et perspectives*. Bruxelles: De Boeck Université.

Dworkin, Ronald (1993). 'Justice in the Distribution of Health Care', *McGill Law Journal*, 38: 883–98.

——(1994). 'Will Clinton's Plan Be Fair?', *New York Review of Books*, 13 January 1994: 20–25.

Fleurbaey, Marc (1994). 'L'Absence d'envie dans une problématique post-welfariste', *Recherches économiques de Louvain*, 60(1): 9–42.

180 III: Responsibility for Health and Health Care

180 III: Responsibility for Health and Health Care

Fleurbaey, Marc (1995). 'Three Solutions for the Compensation Problem', *Journal of Economic Theory*, 65: 505–21.

OVV (1991). 'Standpunt: Sociale zekerheid, een niet-federale bevoegdheid', Brussels: Overlegcentrum voor Vlaamse Verenigingen, October 1991: 6. (French translation: 'La sécurité sociale: une compétence non fédérale', *La Revue nouvelle* 11, 1993: 65–8.)

Paine, Thomas (1796). 'Agrarian Justice', in P. F. Foner (ed.), *The Life and Major Writings of Thomas Paine*. Secaucus, NJ: Citadel Press, 1974, pp. 605–23.

Pieters, Danny (1994). *Federalisme voor onze sociale zekerheid*. Leuven: Acco.

Rakowski, Eric (1991). *Equal Justice*. Oxford: Oxford University Press.

Rawls, John (1999). *The Law of Peoples*. Cambridge, MA: Harvard University Press.

—— and Philippe Van Parijs (2003). 'Three letters on *The Law of Peoples* and the European Union', *Autone de Rawls*, special issue of *Revue de philosophie économique*, 8: 7–20.

Renner, Karl (1918). *Das Selbstbestimmungsrecht der Nationen, in besonderer Anwendung auf Oesterreich*. Leipzig and Wien: Franz Deuticke.

Schokkaert, Erik and Carine Van de Voorde (1998). 'Interregionale financieringsstromen, defederalisering en solidariteit in de Belgische ziekteverzekering', *Acta Hospitalia*, 4: 63–81.

Sen, Amartya (1985). *Commodities and Capabilities*. Amsterdam: North-Holland.

—— (1990). 'Welfare, Freedom and Social Choice: A Reply', *Alternatives to Welfarism. Essays in Honour of Amartya Sen*, special issue of *Recherches Economiques de Louvain*, 56: 451–86.

Van Gompel, Johan (1998). 'Interregionale financiële stromen in België herbekeken', *KuLeuven*, December 1998.

Van Parijs, Philippe (1990). 'Equal Endowments as Undominated Diversity', *Alternatives to Welfarism. Essays in Honour of Amartya Sen*, special issue of *Recherches Economiques de Louvain* 56: 327–56.

—— (1995). *Real Freedom for All. What (if anything) Can Justify Capitalism?* Oxford: Oxford University Press.

—— (2000). 'The Ground Floor of the World. On the Socio-Economic Consequences of Linguistic Globalization', *International Political Science Review*, 21(2), 2000: 217–33.

—— et al. (2001). *What's Wrong with a Free Lunch?* Boston: Beacon Press.

ETHICAL AND MEASUREMENT PROBLEMS IN HEALTH EVALUATION

PART IV

ETHICAL AND
MEASUREMENT PROBLEMS
IN HEALTH EVALUATION

9

Disability-Adjusted Life Years: A Critical Review

SUDHIR ANAND AND KARA HANSON

9.1. INTRODUCTION

The disability-adjusted life year (DALY) has emerged in the international health policy lexicon as a new measure of the 'burden of disease'. The conceptual framework for DALYs is described and justified in the paper 'Quantifying the burden of disease: the technical basis for disability-adjusted life years' (Murray 1994). Developed as an input into the World Bank's *World Development Report: Investing in Health* (1993), DALYs are being used as a tool for policy-making in a wide range of countries (Bobadilla and Cowley 1995). According to some, the DALY concept has 'the potential to revolutionize the way in which we measure the impact of disease, how we choose interventions, and how we track the success or failure of our intervention' (Foege 1994: 1705).

DALYs combine 'time lived with a disability and the time lost due to premature mortality' (Murray 1994: 441). Years lost from premature mortality are estimated with respect to a standard expectation of life at each age. Years lived with disability are translated into an equivalent time loss by using a set of weights which reflect reduction in functional capacity, with higher weights corresponding to a greater reduction. In both cases, time spent in the state is adjusted using a set of 'value choices' (Murray 1994: 430) which weight time lived at different ages and at different time periods differently (through age-weighting and discounting, respectively). Because DALYs are defined in terms of time lost, they are a 'bad' which should be prevented, averted, and minimised.[1]

Anand's research was supported by the John D. and Catherine T. MacArthur Foundation, and by the Department of Economics, University of Oxford. We are extremely grateful to Ramesh Govindaraj, who was involved in the early stages of this project and provided valuable substantive and editorial comments. For helpful comments or discussion, we are also very grateful to Lincoln Chen, Roger Crisp, William Hsiao, Jonathan Levin, Michael Lockwood, Sanjay Reddy, Michael Reich, Dan Robinson, Amartya Sen, and Devinder Sivia.

[1] The terminology of DALYs can be misleading: more of a 'life-year' (even 'adjusted') is generally regarded as a 'good', which should be maximised and not minimised. The World Bank, and Murray himself, are victim to this terminological confusion (e.g. see World Bank 1993: 213; and Murray 1994: 441).

Disability-adjusted life years are claimed by Murray to be superior to measures that ignore time lived with disabilities and consider mortality alone in assessing disease burden, such as potential years of life lost (PYLL). Further, DALYs are considered to be an 'advance' over other composite indicators, such as quality-adjusted life years (QALYs), because the value choices incorporated in the DALY are made explicit: 'The black box of the decision-maker's relative values is then opened for public scrutiny and influence' (Murray 1994: 430). The present chapter constitutes a response to Murray's invitation to debate the specific values which have been adopted in the construction of the DALY.

The proponents of DALYs use the metric for at least two separate exercises: (1) the 'positive' exercise of measuring the burden of disease; and (2) the 'normative' exercise of resource allocation. The burden of disease is simply measured as the sum of DALYs attributable to premature mortality or morbidity. For resource allocation, Murray suggests that DALYs be used 'in conjunction with the literature on cost-effectiveness of health interventions' so as to facilitate 'using estimates of the burden of disease in determining health resource allocations' (Murray 1994: 442). In using DALYs for this purpose, the object is to minimize aggregate DALYs subject to a given budget.

Murray (1994: 429) states:

'The intended use of an indicator of the burden of disease is critical to its design. At least four objectives are important.

—to aid in setting health service (both curative and preventive) priorities;
—to aid in setting health research priorities;
—to aid in identifying disadvantaged groups and targeting of health interventions;
—to provide a comparable measure of output for intervention, programme and sector evaluation and planning.

Not everyone appreciates the ethical dimension of health status indicators. ... Nevertheless, the first two objectives listed for measuring the burden of disease could influence the allocation of resources *among individuals*, clearly establishing an ethical dimension to the construction of an indicator of the burden of disease' (emphasis added).

The attractions of applying a universal formula, not only to measure the burden of ill-health, but also to decide how much money should be spent in controlling which disease, and how much money should be spent in doing research on different diseases, are clear enough. However, we argue in this chapter that the conceptual and technical basis for DALYs is flawed, and that the assumptions and value judgements underlying it are open to serious question. Our concerns relate to the use of DALYs for both quantifying the global burden of disease and allocating resources on the basis of DALYs prevented. We shall argue that the appropriate information sets for the two exercises are quite different.

The 'burden' of disease as defined by Murray is a measure of ill-health which reflects functional limitation and premature mortality, and is adjusted for age, sex, and time of illness. This notion would seem to be closer to the aggregate quantity of ill-health than to the 'burden' as commonly understood. Although this may appear to be a semantic quibble, it has substantive implications. If the goal were measurement of the actual 'burden' of illness, more information would be needed about the circumstances of individuals who experience ill-health—for example, the support provided through public services, private incomes, family and friends—and not just their age and sex. Moreover, if the object of public sector resource allocation were to minimise *this* 'burden' of ill-ness, such considerations would clearly be relevant. Even if the object were simply to measure the quantity of illness—an exercise that has some inde-pendent value—we argue in this chapter that age-weighting and discounting are inappropriate procedures.

This highlights a more general problem with the DALY information set. By 'information set' we mean the set of variables that is used to quantify an indi-vidual's contribution to the burden of disease,[2] or that may be used for resource allocation, depending on the exercise at hand. In the DALY frame-work the information set used for both these separate exercises is the same, and consists of age, sex, disability status, and time period. A principle is enun-ciated of 'treating like health outcomes as like' along these dimensions (Murray 1994: 431). However, it is not at all obvious that one would wish to treat those who are *unlike* along some of these dimensions *differently*. We will argue that, in measuring an individual's contribution to the burden of disease, age and time period are irrelevant distinctions to make.

For the exercise of resource allocation, in contrast to that of measuring the quantity of ill-health, a further issue concerns the treatment of those who are *different* along dimensions *not* included in the DALY information set. Here, the DALY framework fails to make relevant distinctions between those who are unlike along dimensions that are surely important for resource allocation, such as income and socio-economic status.

Finally, the *use* of variables that are included in the information set can dif-fer depending on whether the purpose is measuring the burden of disease or allocating resources. In the DALY framework, a person with a preexisting dis-ability—such as a physical handicap—contributes less to the disease burden (for an illness independent of her disability) than an able-bodied person. On a cost-effectiveness basis she will receive lower priority, yet her claim on public resources should be greater precisely on account of her preexisting disability. In general, we show that if the existing DALY information set is used in con-junction with the criterion of aggregate DALY-minimisation, the implications for resource allocation will be inequitable.

Our chapter is structured as follows: Section 9.2 considers the implications of using DALYs as a measure of disease burden, and assesses each of Murray's 'value choices' in the order in which he presents them; Section 9.3 turns to the

---

[2] Henceforth we use the term 'burden of disease' in Murray's narrow sense of quantity of ill-health.

problems of resource allocation in the health sector based on the DALY framework; Section 9.4 is in conclusion.

9.2. MEASURING THE BURDEN OF DISEASE: IMPLICATIONS OF THE DALY FRAMEWORK

9.2.1. *What is the burden?*

The DALY approach measures the burden of illness through reduction in 'human function' (Murray 1994: 438). The 'multiple dimensions of human function' are mapped onto a unidimensional scale between 0 (perfect health) and 1 (death) along which six discrete disability classes are distinguished. Human function is represented by ability to perform certain activities of daily living, such as learning, working, feeding, and clothing oneself. The space in which ill-health is assessed is limitation in these activities rather than, for example, that of pain or suffering which would be the relevant categories in a utility-based framework.[3] Another space for assessment might be reduction in well-being, a notion that is broader than utility and is captured by general 'capability to function'—including physical functioning.[4] Of course, there will be utility or well-being consequences associated with reduction in human function, but these are not the basis for the DALY metric.

An often-cited advantage of DALYs, and similar composite indicators such as QALYs, is that they allow fatal and non-fatal health outcomes to be combined into a single indicator. A necessary condition for a finite scale which has perfect health (or quality of life) at one end and death at the other is that the values of all health states—including death—be bounded. In the DALY scale death differs from disability merely by reducing human function to nought. While having an indicator that combines states of imperfect health with death is clearly convenient, there is an obvious information loss in reducing death to simply another health state. Some will argue that the two events are incommensurable, and that a lexical priority attaches to life over death. At any rate, this suggests that information about mortality and morbidity should be presented separately—even if tradeoffs were conceded between the two events.

Disability-adjusted life years attempt to measure the burden of disease in a somewhat narrow sense. As discussed in Section 9.1, they represent the quantity of ill-health experienced by individuals through functional limitation and premature death. The burden that is measured does not reflect individuals' differential ability to cope with their functional limitation. Moreover, burdens which fall on family, friends, and society at large (e.g. the economic cost of illness)

---

[3] A framework based on limitation in physical (or mental) activities would also tend to emphasise the importance of conditions such as locomotor disability and chronic degenerative disease relative to those which do not result in (or extend beyond) reduction in human function (e.g. depression or psycho-social stress).
[4] The terminology of 'functioning' was initially proposed by Sen (1985), and is broader than that associated with health alone.

are not included. Only in the use of unequal age-weights does there appear to be an attempt to capture the indirect health burden of illness. We return to the rationale for and ethical implications of unequal age-weighting in Section 9.2.3.

Disability-adjusted life years use standardised maximum life expectancies (80 years for men and 82.5 years for women) which are considerably higher than the levels of life expectancy currently achieved in developing countries. Using these standardised life expectancies either in measuring the global burden of disease or in cost-effectiveness analysis implicitly assumes that health interventions alone are capable of achieving an increase in life expectancy to these higher levels. It is clear that many non-health circumstances will also need to change for life expectancy to rise to the level used in the DALY calculations. These interventions would have to address the socio-economic determinants of health. They would include raising incomes, increasing female education, improving water supply and sanitation conditions, improving workplace safety, and reducing accidents and violence. Hence the burden that is measured by DALYs is the *burden of disease and underdevelopment*, and not that of disease alone.

9.2.2. *Standard expectation of life and gender gap*

To calculate the DALYs from morbidity and premature mortality, a standard expectation of life at birth of 82.5 years is chosen for women and of 80 years for men. This gap is considerably smaller than the observed gender gap in life expectancy in low mortality populations, for example, Japan which has a gender gap of some six years. However, the gender gap of 2.5 years is argued to correspond purely to the 'biological difference in survival potential between males and females' (Murray 1994: 434), factoring out the effects on life expectancy of males' greater exposure to social and other risk factors. It is, nonetheless, an arbitrary choice.[5]

The assumed gender gap in life expectancy may have important implications for the estimation of the disease burden of women relative to that of men. World Bank (1993: 28) estimates that '[F]emales have about a 10 per cent lower disease burden per 1,000 population than males for the world as a whole'. The smaller the gender gap, *ceteris paribus*, the smaller will be the female contribution to the burden of disease relative to the male contribution. If the true biological gap happens to be greater than 2.5 years, then the calculations in Murray et al. (1994) and World Bank (1993) will understate the burden of disease of females relative to that of males.

[5] The literature on the 'biological-genetic' difference between the sexes acknowledges there to be significant disagreement regarding the relative contributions of biological factors and environmental or social ones (Waldron 1983; Holden 1987; Collins 1992). Murray's (1994: 434) attempt to isolate the contribution of biological factors in longevity is based on the observation of narrowing gender gaps among higher income quintiles in urban Canada, and a gender difference in the highest income quintile of 4–5 years. This gap is then projected 'forward', without explanation, to the assumed gap of 2.5 years.

Table 9.1. *The value of time lost from an infant death*

	Years lost	Age-weighted years lost[a]	DALYs, that is, age-weighted and discounted (at 3% per annum) years lost[a]
Female	82.5	85.42	32.45
Male	80	84.14	32.34
Gap	2.5	1.28	0.11
Gap relative to male (%)	3	1.5	0.3

[a]The age-weighting function used in Murray (1994) is $f(x) = 0.16243xe^{-0.04x}$.

While DALYs take account of higher female life expectancy in calculating years lost to premature mortality, the valuation of these years can be sharply reduced by age-weighting and discounting. As an illustration, Table 9.1 shows the estimate of time lost, and of its value, from the death of a female and a male infant, respectively. The female advantage in life expectancy of 3 per cent is reduced by age-weighting to 1.5 per cent, and is further reduced by discounting to 0.3 per cent in the calculation of DALYs.

9.2.3. *Age-weighting and the value of time lived at different ages*

Age-weighting assigns a different value to time lived at different ages. Thus in the construction of a DALY, a year lived at age two counts for only 20 per cent of a year lived at age 25 where the age-weighting function is at a maximum, while that lived at age 70 counts for 46 per cent of the maximum. In a human capital framework, age-weighting might be justified in terms of the differential productivity of an individual at different stages of his life cycle. This approach allows one to impute a money value to life and to disability according to the respective (discounted) income streams foregone. Although it provides a consistent justification for age-weighting (and for discounting), valuing people's lives in terms of a money metric—through their instrumental worth in production—is hard to defend ethically. Murray (1994) himself explicitly rejects the human capital approach, arguing that it 'inadequately reflects human welfare' (Murray 1994: 435).[6] What, then, is the basis for assigning different relative values to years of life lost at different ages?

---

[6] He also seems to suggest an 'apparent inconsistency in the application of the human capital concept'—'even though it would only be logically consistent' to '...weight time by other human attributes that correlate with productivity such as income, education, geographical location or even, in some economies, ethnicity' (Murray 1994: 435). There is no inconsistency here, apparent or real, and if the human capital approach is adopted time should indeed be weighted according to productivity.

Murray (1994) views 'unequal age weights as an attempt to capture different social roles at different ages', arguing that '[H]igher weights for a year of time at a particular age does not mean that the time lived at that age is *per se* more important to the individual, but that because of social roles the social value of that time may be greater' (p. 435). He claims that 'social roles vary with age' because the 'young, and often the elderly, depend on the rest of society for physical, emotional and financial support' (Murray 1994: 434). How 'different roles and changing levels of dependency with age' (Murray 1994: 434) are supposed to affect the burden of illness to the individual is far from clear to us. We take it that unequal age weights do not constitute a differential *intrinsic* valuation of years lived at different ages. Rather, there appears to be an *instrumental* justification for valuing the time of people in middle age-groups more highly than that of the young or elderly. Presumably ill-health among the middle age-groups also has an indirect effect on the health of the young and elderly because the latter depend on the former for care.[7]

However, if age-weighting is supposed to reflect an instrumental valuation of people's time, even if solely in terms of its health impact, then a host of other instrumentalities that have health impacts will need to be incorporated. From the viewpoint of preventing ill-health the 'social value' of time will clearly differ for different occupation groups in the population. For example, doctors' and nurses' time could be argued to be more valuable than that of other professions. More indirectly, the time of people who have a greater capacity to contribute, through taxation, to the size of the health budget should be valued more highly. However, a person's occupation or tax bracket are not part of the information set used to calculate DALYs, and nor are other (e.g. social and economic) factors which directly and indirectly influence individuals' health.

Murray (1994) apparently believes that '[U]nequal age weights [also] has broad intuitive appeal', and goes on to state that 'informal polling of tuberculosis programme managers by the author in an annual training course has revealed that everyone polled believes that the time lived in the middle age-groups should be weighted as more important than the extremes' (1994: 435). But what precise question were his group of programme managers asked? Did it concern an intrinsic valuation of time lived at different ages or an instrumental valuation? How do we know that it is not reflecting their view of income levels and productivity through the life cycle? Were they made aware of the implications of age-weighting for resource allocation? It is not obvious

---

[7] Note that for the purpose of measuring the burden of disease, higher weights placed on the middle age-groups according to this instrumental justification will lead to double-counting. Any consequential health effects should already have been recorded when the burden of disease is measured. On the other hand, for the purpose of resource allocation, avoiding ill-health for a mother will also avoid the consequential ill-health of her child. In this case, allocating resources to the mother will generate health benefits in excess of those that accrue to her alone. Hence for the purpose of resource allocation, age-weighting might be justified by Murray in a way that it cannot be for measuring the burden of disease.

to us that the author has properly solicited from his programme managers their value judgements concerning age-weighting *per se*.

It is also not at all clear that the programme managers were provided with (adequate) information about *other* adjustments made in the DALY formula to life years lived. It is possible, for instance, that they had in mind different functional capacities at different ages, in other words, a higher level of functioning in the middle age-groups compared to either end. But reduction in 'human function' will be captured separately and independently through Murray's disability weights (see Section 9.2.4). Even if function and age were correlated (and followed the shape of the age-weighting function), applying age weights on top of disability weights would amount to penalising reduced functional capacity twice over.

Murray (1994: 436) posits an age-weighting function of the form $Cxe^{-\beta x}$ where x is age, $\beta = 0.04$, and the normalisation constant $C = 0.16243$. Without discounting (q.v. Section 9.2.5), the sum of age-weighted time lived beyond age a, $V(a)$, is given as

$$V(a) = \int_{a}^{a+L(a)} Cxe^{-\beta x}\,dx,$$

where $L(a)$ is interpreted differently in the case of morbidity and premature mortality. In the former, $L(a)$ is the duration of an illness occurring at age a; in the latter, $L(a)$ is the expectation of life at age a (i.e. the expected years lost from premature mortality).[8] By differentiation with respect to a, it can be shown that

$$V'(a) = Ce^{-\beta a}\{[a + L(a)]\,e^{-\beta L(a)}\,[1 + L'(a)] - a\}.$$

In the case of an illness of constant duration, $L(a)$ will be constant and $L'(a) = 0$.[9] In this case, $V'(a) > 0$ whenever $a < L/(e^{\beta L}-1)$. In other words, the value of time lost from an illness of constant duration will be increasing in

---

[8] Note that the expression $V(a)$ corresponds to the age-weighted value of the expected time lost at age a, which assumes that everyone at age a will live exactly $L(a)$ more years. However, the expected loss is the expected value of age-weighted time lost—which will differ from the above.
[9] In discussing the loss from premature mortality rather than from illness of constant duration, the *World Development Report* (1993: 213) asserts that '[I]n the absence of discounting, [therefore,] the greatest loss of DALYs [sic] from premature death occurs from infant deaths.' This is not correct because the mean age at death, $a + L(a)$, where $L(a)$ is the expectation of life at age a, is not constant. According to the Model Life Table West Level 26 that is used, mean age at death $a + L(a)$ increases with a, while life expectancy $L(a)$ decreases with a (see Murray 1994: Table 1, 435). In other words, we have $-1 < L'(a) < 0$. Applying the formula for $V'(a)$ in the text to value the time lost from death at age $a = 0$ we have

$$V'(0) = CL(0)e^{-\beta L(0)}\,[1 + L'(0)]$$
$$> 0 \text{ because } 1 + L'(a) > 0 \text{ for the entire age range.}$$

This shows that the greatest number of DALYs from premature death arises *not* from infant deaths (at age $a = 0$) but from death at a higher age. Indeed, undiscounted but age-weighted DALYs will continue to *increase* until age a^* given as the solution of

$$[a^* + L(a^*)]e^{-\beta L(a^*)}\,[1 + L'(a^*)] = a^*.$$

the early years of a person's life (from age 0) to some maximum. This leads to the inevitable conclusion within the cost-effectiveness framework that, given a choice between treating two persons with the same illness and the same cost of treatment, more DALYs will be prevented if the older person of age $L/(e^{\beta L}-1)$ is treated rather than an infant. With the given value of $\beta = 0.04$ and an illness lasting one year, that is, $L = 1$, maximum DALYs are prevented at age 24.5. These implications of age-weighting are thoroughly unacceptable, and we can see no reason for valuing time lived at different ages differently. A principle of universalism of life claims (Anand and Sen 2000) would argue strongly for a common intrinsic valuation of human life, regardless of the age at (or time period in) which it is lived.

9.2.4. *Disability weights*

In the DALY framework, the effects of illness are captured through six disability classes which assign increasing weights associated with the extent of loss of physical functioning. Murray (1994: 439) states that 'weights for the six classes have been chosen by a group of independent experts'.[10] As in the case of age weights, the meaning attached to the different weighting of health states depends in an important way on the precise question that was asked of these 'experts'. Their responses would also depend on understanding the use to which such estimates would be put.

In Murray's formulation, DALYs suffered by individual i are a function of both his life expectancy L_i (at age a) and his disability weight D_i. Between the values of $D_i = 0$ which represents perfect health and $D_i = 1$ which represents death, six discrete disability categories are defined (Murray 1994: 438). The weights D_i may be referred to as 'uncompensated' disability weights.

A more appropriate measure of burden must take account of the way in which individual and social resources can compensate for the level of disability experienced. The individual's actual loss of functioning will depend on both his uncompensated disability state and the factors which affect his capacity to cope with that disability (given his circumstances). 'Compensated' disability weights would depend *inter alia* on the individual's income (e.g. whether he can employ somebody to prepare his meals and provide other assistance with his activities of daily living), and on the provision of local services to facilitate his daily activities. The latter might include designated parking, transport services for the disabled, etc. Compensated disability weights would come closer to reflecting the true burden of disability as experienced by the individual. The DALY approach does not distinguish between the quantity of ill-health and the 'burden' associated with it.

---

[10] No information is provided which would allow an assessment of the statistical or scientific basis for selecting the weights and, thus, of their validity. This same criticism applies to the choice of the age-weighting function, the estimate of disability duration associated with each disease, and other parameters.

A final question about the construction of disability weights relates to the manipulations necessary to restrict the maximum disability weight for an individual to 1. In particular, although DALYs are aggregated across individuals, problems caused by co-morbidity (an individual experiencing multiple illnesses) are not adequately dealt with in the framework, and can lead to an overestimation of the total disease burden.[11]

As they stand Murray's disability categories do not distinguish functionings associated with illness and those associated with age (but no illness). For example, the most severe disability class (Class 6) involves disability states in which an individual 'needs assistance with activities of daily living such as eating, personal hygiene or toilet use' (Murray 1994: Table 2, 438). Infants are not capable of feeding themselves: does this imply they are disabled? Do they by virtue of the functional limitations of their stage of development contribute to the burden of disease?[12] If disability weights are to be usable and consistent, they should be defined so as to avoid confounding age with disability.

9.2.5. *Time preference and the discounting of future life*

In the DALY formula, future years of life lived are valued less than present years. With the recommended 3 per cent discount rate,[13] this implies that one life saved today will be worth more than five lives saved in 55 years. Discounting future lives in this way would justify many forms of environmental degradation today which benefit the present generation at the expense of future generations. For example, the benefit today of economic activities which emit greenhouse gases at present rates could well outweigh the harm done to future generations from global warming if future lives are valued at only *one-fifth* of present lives.

We can see no justification for an estimation of the time lost to illness or death which depends on when the illness or the calculation occurs. Suppose a person experiences an illness today and another person, identical in all respects, experiences an illness of exactly the same description next year. Discounting amounts to concluding that the quantity of the (same) illness is lower in the latter case. This does not accord with intuition or even with common use of language.

As in the case of age-weighting, a logically consistent defence of discounting could be provided if the human capital approach to valuing life were adopted.

---

[11] Because of the disease- and not individual-specific estimation of the disease burden, an individual can turn out to have a cumulative disability weight greater than 1. While states worse than death might be possible in some evaluation spaces (pain, suffering, etc.), in the DALY space of physical functioning this is impossible.

[12] See Section 9.2.3 above on the confounding of age and disability.

[13] In choosing a discount rate of 3 per cent, Murray (1994: 440) argues that: 'This is consistent with the long-term yield on investments. There is also a precedent in the World Bank Disease Control Priorities Study that used a 3 per cent rate'. Below we argue that the yield on investments has little to do with discounting health outcomes.

Life would then be reducible to a monetary value, and discounting it justified because of the opportunity cost of money. But Murray (1994) eschews this framework yet invokes economic cost-benefit arguments to defend 'social time preference' (1994: 440).

Because life cannot be reduced to money, the usual arguments for discounting money do not apply to discounting DALYs. Yet Murray (1994) fails to distinguish between discounting DALYs (or utility) and discounting money (or consumption). Hence the usual cost-benefit reasons presented by him for discounting future consumption (money)—for example, by appeal to the marginal utility of consumption falling with expected future growth of consumption—are irrelevant to discounting utility or DALYs. Moreover, it is difficult to see how pure time preference in the discounting of future utility or future DALYs can be justified.[14]

The only defensible argument for treating future periods differently rests on the possibility that the world might end. A construction which could accommodate uncertainty is the minimization of expected (in the statistical sense) undiscounted DALYs.[15] Under this objective function lives in each period are weighted by the probability that the world will exist in that period.[16] Note that a 3 per cent discount rate implies a 50 per cent chance that the world will end in 23.4 years. Even a 1 per cent discount rate implies there is a 50 per cent chance that the world will end in 69.7 years. How many people would be willing to take an odds-on chance that the world will end within their, or their

[14] See Anand and Sen (2000: Section 5(b)) for a critique of pure time preference, that is, the discounting of future utility or well-being itself. Even if individuals themselves should happen to have a positive rate of pure time preference, there is no reason for a government to use pure time discounting in social decision-making. Social decision-making need not necessarily be 'welfarist' (Sen 1979); indeed the DALY approach itself is not obviously consistent with individuals' health behaviour—individuals do not minimise DALYs. In the case of pure time discounting, for example, Harrod (1948: 37–40) argued that 'On the assumption ... that a government is capable of planning what is best for its subjects, it will pay no attention to pure time preference, a polite expression for rapacity and the conquest of reason by passion'.

In rejecting pure time discounting, Pigou (1932: 29–30) noted that 'there is wide agreement that the State should protect the interests of the future *in some degree* against the effects of our irrational discounting and of our preference for ourselves over our descendents. The whole movement for 'conservation' in the United States is based on this conviction. It is the clear duty of Government, which is the trustee for unborn generations as well as for its present citizens, to watch over, and, if need be, by legislative enactment, to defend, the exhaustible natural resources of the country from rash and reckless spoliation.'

A similar argument against pure time discounting applies in the context of health-sector planning: since future generations are not here to represent their preferences, the government should act as trustee in protecting their interests—in particular, the value of the life years they will live.

[15] Of course, strong assumptions would be needed to justify this extension of the DALY-minimisation criterion to conditions of uncertainty. Moreover, if the probability of the world ending can be represented by a Poisson process, the minimisation of expected undiscounted DALYs will be functionally equivalent to as-if-discounting of future lives. But note that this is not the same as *valuing* future lives less than present lives.

[16] Incidentally, if planet Earth were to be struck by a comet, such as Shoemaker-Levy 9, the burden of illness would immediately vanish: there would be *no* people with any illness.

children's, lifetime? We reckon that the discount rate implied by the probability of the world ending within the planning horizon for DALY calculations is infinitesimally small. For any practical purpose, the assumption of a zero discount rate is likely to command more assent than even a very small one.

It appears to us that Murray's positive arguments in support of discounting are based largely on attempts to avoid some awkward implications of the use of undiscounted DALYs for cost-effectiveness analysis. The first of these states that 'if health benefits are not discounted, then we may conclude that 100% of resources should be invested in any disease eradication plans with finite costs as this will eliminate infinite streams of [undiscounted] DALYs which will out-weigh all other health investments that do not result in eradication' (Murray 1994: 440). Quite apart from whether it is necessary to invest 100 per cent of resources to eradicate diseases, we fail to see how this statement provides an argument for discounting DALYs. In the burden of disease framework it would seem a desirable outcome to eradicate a disease, for precisely the author's goal of minimising aggregate ill-health.

Murray also invokes the so-called 'time paradox', arguing that if health benefits are not discounted then 'one will always choose to put off investing in a health project until the future' because '...the budget could be invested and yield a positive return' (1994: 440). Whether or not any 'time paradox' arises,[17] if Murray's concern is that, without discounting, present health outcomes will be sacrificed in favour of future health outcomes—leading to an undesirable inequality between generations—then this concern for equity should be incor-porated directly in a temporally neutral way. One way of making the criterion sensitive to inequality is to express it as a strictly convex, additive function of undiscounted DALYs

$$B = \sum_i \sum_t (\Delta_{it})^\alpha$$

where Δ_{it} is the DALYs suffered by individual i at time t, and $\alpha > 1$. The size of the parameter α will capture the extent of aversion to inter-generational— and inter-individual—inequality.[18] With α large enough, it will no longer be

---

[17] In fact, the 'time paradox' is by no means inevitable. Murray assumes that it will arise as long as the return to investment of the health budget elsewhere is greater than the increase in the cost per DALY averted of an intervention. For if the health budget is invested elsewhere with a return which exceeds the increase in the cost of the intervention, then it will pay to postpone health spending. Note that this argument rests critically on the further assumption that the stream of DALYs in the future will be the same with or without the current health spending. However, failure to invest in health today can significantly increase DALYs in the future—for example, through failure to immunise against communicable diseases or to provide nutritional supplementation. The cost of eliminating these additional DALYs may turn out to be larger than the return to deferring health spending (where the 'return' includes any reduction through improved technology in the cost of preventing DALYs). Hence, one will not 'always choose to put off investing in a health project until the future'.

[18] When $\alpha = 1$ there is no concern for inequality and the criterion reduces to aggregate DALY-minimisation.

cost-effective to defer all expenditure to the future: it will be worth preventing some DALYs now if fewer DALYs arise in the future.

Finally, discounting at 3 per cent in the Murray-*World Development Report 1993* framework implies that we should save the life of a 20-year-old person rather than an infant: more age-weighted and discounted DALYs are prevented in the former case. But does this accord with general intuition? It is the non-monotonic feature of Figures 4 and 5 in Murray (1994: 436 and 441, respectively) and Box Figure 1.3 in World Bank (1993: 26) which jars with our basic intuitions. Discounting, which in itself is totally indefensible in the context of lives and life years, can be shown to compound the problems inherent in age-weighting. Together they comprise the most unappealing features of the DALY formula.

9.2.6. *Sensitivity*

Much is made in Murray et al. (1994) of the extensive sensitivity analysis undertaken on the global burden calculations to the various assumptions concerning unequal age weights, discount rate, and disability-class weights. Two points are relevant here. First, even though changing these parameters may result in small changes to the overall estimates, this does not constitute evidence that the approach is *correct*. Insensitivity to parameter changes can hardly validate a formula! This chapter has raised various concerns about the ethical underpinnings of the DALY approach. These concerns are little affected by any lack of sensitivity of the overall calculations to particular assumptions.

Second, although the overall burden of disease calculation may not be very sensitive to changing crucial parameter values, this in no way indicates that the calculation for individual diseases is not highly sensitive to the underlying assumptions. Evidence from a study of the burden of trachomatous visual impairment (Evans and Ranson 1995) suggests that at the level of specific diseases the calculations are indeed highly sensitive to several of the assumptions in the DALY framework, including the discount rate. It is possible that individual diseases are sensitive in compensating directions, resulting in relative lack of overall sensitivity.

9.2.7. *Whose values?*

There appear to be at least four distinct agents whose values are incorporated in the DALY-minimisation exercise. First, there is a social planner who specifies the exercise—minimising the burden of ill-health—and who determines the DALY function used to measure it. Second, there are a number of other agents whose values are incorporated into the DALY through the parameters of this function: for age-weighting, tuberculosis programme managers (perhaps qua individuals); for disability weights, 'a group of independent experts'; for the discount rate, the authors of the World Bank Disease Control Priorities

Study (Jamison et al. 1993). It is entirely arbitrary to appeal to different agents' values for the different parameters without prior justification or reasoning. Furthermore, it has to be asked why the social planner's objective is to minimise DALYs if individuals themselves have different objectives. And if compelling reasons can be provided for the social planner to override individual preferences and minimise DALYs, why should the social planner rely on individual values for choosing DALY parameters?

Even if it could be argued that individual values should be incorporated in the choice of parameters, a precondition for doing so is that everyone should agree on the form of the DALY function—that is, share a common definition of ill-health. Otherwise, the responses to questions asked in determining parameter values—for example, disability weights or age-weights—will depend on the individual's own conception of ill-health and on his understanding of the purpose for which the estimate is intended. When these differ among individuals the responses provided cannot be compared, let alone averaged.

9.3. RESOURCE ALLOCATION BASED ON THE DALY FRAMEWORK

9.3.1. *General limitations of cost-effectiveness analysis*

There are problems with restricting the framework of health sector analysis and resource allocation to health interventions alone. Many health sector interventions have non-health sector returns, and many non-health sector interventions have health sector returns. Practical examples are easy to construct. For instance, the provision of clean water could, apart from reducing morbidity due to diarrhoeal diseases, also lead to significant economic benefits by reducing the time spent by women in fetching water from distant sources. Evaluating this intervention solely from the health perspective will ignore potentially large non-health sector gains. A non-health sector intervention such as female education, which has been shown to be important in reducing infant mortality and increasing contraceptive use, will reduce DALYs. If mothers' education, or improving water supply and sanitation conditions, generate a bigger 'bang-for-a-buck' than health interventions, then the health budget should be redirected to the ministry of education, or of public utilities. A committed DALY-minimiser should in principle be willing to give over his entire health budget to other ministries! Otherwise, his restricted cost-effectiveness exercise can lead to a seriously suboptimal allocation of resources in the improvement of health outcomes.[19]

---

[19] It is interesting to note the implications of a simple formulaic approach to allocating health-sector resources, such as DALY-minimization. The most cost-effective way to allocate the health budget may be to invest it in a rigorous family planning programme so as to reduce the number of people who can contribute to DALYs. There would be no DALYs if there were no people—a misanthropic implication of the DALY approach! The reverse applies to the metric of QALYs, where a year lived in a state of perfect health receives a weight of unity while death has a weight

Another weakness of cost-effectiveness analysis is that the framework of minimizing DALYs subject to a health budget constraint can be used neither to defend a given budget nor to argue for a different (e.g. larger) one. The cost-effectiveness expert has no basis for commenting on whether the given budget is appropriate. He must remain equally content with a budget which is a half or a tenth the size of his existing budget, since it cannot be compared with 'effectiveness' elsewhere.

9.3.2. *Implications of aggregate DALY-minimisation*

Using the DALY framework for resource allocation may lead to consequences that are at odds with principles of equity. This arises from both the information set that is used in calculating DALYs and the criterion itself, that is, aggregate DALY-minimisation. Broadening the information set to take account of equity will require a substantial re-examination of the DALY-minimisation criterion.[20]

The DALYs prevented by an intervention which extends the life of a disabled person will be less than those prevented for an able-bodied person. For example, a treatment which enables a person in a wheelchair to live another year (without altering the person's existing disability) prevents fewer DALYs than the same treatment given to a perfectly healthy person. This is because, given his existing disability (weighted, say, at a value of $\frac{1}{2}$), he is permanently suffering half a DALY each year. Extending his life by a year thus only averts half a DALY (assuming an age weight of unity and no discounting), whereas extending the life of a perfectly able-bodied person averts a whole DALY.[21] From an ethical point of view it could be forcefully argued that priority should be given to the disadvantaged person rather than to the perfectly healthy person[22]—exactly the opposite of what is implied in using the DALY formula for resource allocation (Anand 1993). Similarly, as discussed in Section 9.2, the age-weighting and discounting schemes of the DALY approach will have implications for resource allocation. They imply preferential treatment of young adults compared with infants or the elderly, and of present generations over future ones.

9.4. CONCLUSION

Whether the purpose to which DALYs are put is measurement of disease burden or resource allocation in the health sector, our contention in this chapter has

of zero. In contrast to DALYs, the criterion of maximising aggregate QALYs may carry with it the implication of *increasing* population size. The elimination of family planning services could in this case both save costs and increase total QALYs.

[20] If the priorities resulting from resource allocation based on the DALY framework happen to identify those diseases which, for example, disproportionately affect the poor, this will be by accident and not by design. There is no built-in concern for equity in the DALY-minimisation exercise.   [21] See Sen (1973); also Lockwood (1988).

[22] Anand (1993) makes such an argument by applying Rawls's Difference Principle in the space of capabilities.

been that the conceptual and technical basis for the metric is flawed. Many of the principles underlying it are at best unclear, and at worst unjustified. While recognising the value of attempting to quantify, by cause, the 'global burden of disease', the DALY framework needs to be modified fundamentally even for this limited purpose. More importantly, the purposes of measuring the quantity of ill-health and of allocating resources must be sharply distinguished— because the information sets appropriate to the two exercises, and the use that is made of some common variables, will be quite different.

Murray (1994: 431) propounds the principle of 'treating like health outcomes as like'. In measuring the disease burden, this principle implies that two people of the same sex, disability status, age, and time period (the variables in his information set) are treated similarly. The appeal of any principle of treating like health outcomes as like must rest on how exactly it characterises 'likeness'. The dimensions used to define likeness will depend on the purpose at hand. In quantifying ill-health, it could indeed be plausibly argued that people of the same sex and disability status, *independent of other characteristics*, should be treated similarly. However, in resource allocation (or even in measuring the 'true' burden of disease), it is not equitable to treat *similarly* people of the same sex and disability status who *differ* in critical characteristics such as wealth or access to publicly-provided services. By being blind to variables other than those included in the DALY information set, the principle lacks cutting power and cannot possibly provide a 'plausible treatment of equity' (1994: 431).

At best the principle of treating like health outcomes as like will be innocuous: obviously we would wish to treat those of the same sex, disability status, age, and time period lived, *ceteris paribus*, similarly. Likewise, *ceteris paribus*, we would also wish to treat similarly those who have the same colour of eyes or hair. However, the principle does not invoke a *ceteris paribus* clause in characterising 'likeness' along dimensions outside the restricted DALY information set. Hence at worst, by failing to distinguish relevant differences between individuals (e.g. in their socio-economic circumstances) the principle ceases to be acceptable.

The principle itself is silent about the treatment of people who are *unlike* along the dimensions that it uses to define likeness. But the DALY framework, through age-weighting and discounting, values life years lived by people of different ages and generations differently. In measuring the burden of disease or in allocating resources, we see no reason why a life year lived by a young or old person should be valued less than that lived by a person in the middle age-groups, or why a life year lived by someone in the next generation should count for less than that by a person in this generation.

Finally, resource allocation that is based on the criterion of aggregate DALY-minimisation can lead to perverse outcomes. Using the DALY information set the criterion implies that, all other things equal, for a given illness episode fewer resources should be allocated to a disabled person compared to an able-bodied one, or to a young or elderly person compared to one in the middle age-groups. This is a consequence of using the particular disability status and age-weighting schemes incorporated in the DALY formula.

In our view, equity must play a central role in public-sector resource allocation. This requires giving priority to the claims of the disadvantaged—for example, the poor and the disabled. As we have shown in this chapter, the DALY approach either ignores equity or runs directly counter to it.

References

Anand, S. (1993). 'Inequality Between and Within Nations', *mimeo*, Center for Population and Development Studies, Harvard University, Cambridge, MA, March.

Anand, S. and A. K. Sen (2000). 'Human Development and Economic Sustainability', *World Development*, 28 (12) December: 2029–49.

Bobadilla, J.-L. and P. Cowley (1995). 'Designing and Implementing Packages of Essential Health Services', *Journal of International Development*, 7: 543–54.

Collins, J. R. (1992). 'Explaining the Gender Gap—Why do Women Live Longer than Men?', unpublished Long Essay for the Honours Degree in Human Sciences, University of Oxford, June.

Evans, T. G. and M. K. Ranson (1995). 'The Global Burden of Trachomatous Visual Impairment: II. Assessing Burden', *International Ophthalmology*, 19: 271–80.

Foege, W. (1994). 'Preventive Medicine and Public Health', *Journal of the American Medical Association*, 271: 1704–05.

Harrod, R. F. (1948). *Towards a Dynamic Economics*. London: Macmillan.

Holden, C. (1987). 'Why do Women Live Longer than Men?', *Science*, 238: 158–60.

Jamison, D. T., W. H. Mosley, A. R. Measham, and J.-L. Bobadilla. (1993). *Disease Control Priorities in Developing Countries*. Oxford: Oxford University Press.

Lockwood, M. (1988). 'Quality of Life and Resource Allocation', in J. M. Bell and S. Mendus (eds.), *Philosophy and Medical Welfare*. Cambridge: Cambridge University Press, pp. 33–55.

Murray, C. J. L. (1994). 'Quantifying the Burden of Disease: the Technical Basis for Disability-Adjusted Life Years', *Bulletin of the World Health Organization*, 72: 429–45.

——, A. D. Lopez, and D. T. Jamison (1994). 'Global Burden of Disease in 1990: Summary Results, Sensitivity Analysis and Future Directions', *Bulletin of the World Health Organization*, 72: 495–509.

Pigou, A. C. (1932). *The Economics of Welfare*, 4th edn. London: Macmillan.

Sen, A. K. (1973). *On Economic Inequality*. Oxford: Clarendon Press.

——(1979). 'Personal Utilities and Public Judgements: or What's Wrong with Welfare Economics?', *Economic Journal*, 89: 537–58.

——(1985). *Commodities and Capabilities*. Amsterdam: North-Holland.

Waldron, I. (1983). 'The Role of Genetic and Biological Factors in Sex Differences in Mortality', in A. D. Lopez and L. T. Ruzicka (eds.), *Sex Differentials in Mortality: Trends, Determinants and Consequences*. Canberra: Australian National University, Department of Demography, pp. 141–64.

World Bank (1993). *World Development Report 1993: Investing in Health*. New York and Oxford: Oxford University Press.

10

Ethical Issues in the Use of Cost Effectiveness Analysis for the Prioritisation of Health Care Resources

DAN W. BROCK

Resources to improve health are and always have been scarce, in the sense that health must compete with other desirable social goals like education and personal security for resources.[1] It is not possible to provide all the resources to health, including health care and health care research, that might provide some positive health benefits without great and unacceptable sacrifices in other important social goods. This should go without saying, and in other areas of social expenditures resource scarcity is not denied, but in health care many people mistakenly persist in denying this fact. It follows from resource scarcity that some form of health care rationing is unavoidable, where by rationing I mean some means of allocating health care resources that denies to some persons some potentially beneficial health care. That rationing may take many forms. In most countries with a national health system it is done through some form of global budgeting for health care. In the United States much rationing is by ability to pay, but in both public programmes like the Oregon Medicaid programme and in many private managed care plans more systematic efforts to prioritise health care resources have been carried out.

This chapter draws heavily on my 'Considerations of Equity in Relation to Prioritization and Allocation of Health Care Resources', in *Ethics, Equity and Health For All* Z. Bankowski, J. H. Bryant, and J. Gallagher (eds.), Geneva: CIOMS (1997) and 'Ethical Issues in the Development of Summary Measures of Population Health States', in *Summarizing Population Health: Directions for the Development and Application of Population Metrics*, Washington, DC: National Academy Press (1998).

[1] Interventions that would improve health should be understood broadly, and in particular extend substantially beyond health care. It is widely agreed that other factors such as improved sanitation and economic conditions have contributed more to the health gains of the past century than has health care. However, in this chapter I shall largely confine myself to health care interventions.

To many health policy analysts it is an unquestioned, and so generally unde-fended, assumption that in the face of limited health care resources, those resources should be allocated so as to maximise the health benefits they produce, measured by either the aggregate health status or disease burden of a popula-tion. Cost effectiveness analysis (CEA) that compares the aggregate health benefits secured from a given resource expenditure devoted to alternative health interventions is the standard analytic tool for determining how to max-imise the health benefits from limited resources. Natural, even self-evident, as this maximisation standard may appear to many health policy analysts and economists, it assumes a utilitarian or consequentialist moral standard, and more specifically a standard of distributive justice, and the utilitarian account of distributive justice is widely and I believe correctly taken to be utilitarian-ism's most problematic feature.

Cost effectiveness analysis comparing alternative health interventions in the quality-adjusted life years (QALYs) produced from a given level of resources constitutes a quantitative method for prioritising different interventions to improve health. There are many unresolved technical and methodological issues in QALYs and CEA, none of which will be my concern here. My con-cern will be instead with the ethical issues in the construction and use of CEAs for the prioritisation of health care resources. The specific issues that I shall briefly discuss below all constitute potential ethical criticisms of CEA as a nor-mative standard, specifically criticisms concerning justice or equity, and so one might hope concerns for justice or equity could be integrated into these quan-titative methodologies. There are at least two reasons, however, for caution, at least in the near term, about the possibility of integrating some of these ethi-cal concerns into cost effectiveness models and analyses. First, although a great deal of work in economics and health policy has gone into the development and validation of measures of health status and the burdens of disease, as well as of cost effectiveness methodologies, much less work has been done on how to integrate concerns of ethics and equity into cost effectiveness measures, although I shall mention one means of doing so later. The theoretical and methodological work necessary to do so remains largely undone. Second, each of the issues of ethics and equity that I take up below remain controversial. Since no clear consensus exists about how each should be treated, there is in turn no consensus about what qualifications or constraints they might justify placing on the cost effectiveness goal of maximising health.

This second difficulty is not likely to be solely a near term limitation, awaiting further work on the ethical issues that I will identify. Instead, most of these issues represent deep divisions in normative ethical theory and in the ethical beliefs of ordinary people; I believe they are likely a permanent fact of ethical life. As I understand and shall present these ethical issues, in most cases there is not a single plausible answer to them. Even from within the standpoint of a particular ethical theory or ethical view, these issues' complexity means that different answers may be appropriate for a particular issue in the different contexts in which CEAs are used. Thus, what is necessary at this point is work developing more clearly and precisely the nature of the issues at stake, the alternative plausible positions on them together with the arguments for and against those positions. Until much more of this work is done, we will not know how deep the conflicts go and the degree to which any can be resolved.

Norman Daniels and James Sabin have recently argued that because ethical theories and theories of justice are indeterminate and/or in conflict on some of these issues, we must turn to fair procedures to arrive at practical solutions to them for health policy (Daniels and Sabin 1997: 303–50). As practical policy matters that need resolution now they are no doubt correct, and a single quantitative measure or model of equity and justice for health care resource prioritisation is certainly not possible now, if it will ever be. But that is not to deny that much important work remains to be done on the substantive issues of equity in health care, and that work should inform the deliberations of those taking part in the fair procedures that we will need to reach practical resolutions and compromises on these issues in real time. What then are some of the main issues of equity raised by cost effectiveness approaches to resource allocation of health care?

10.1. FIRST ISSUE: HOW SHOULD STATES OF HEALTH AND DISABILITY BE EVALUATED?

Any CEA in health care requires some summary measure of the health benefits of interventions designed to improve the health status and reduce the burden of disease of a given population. Early summary measures of the health status of populations and of the benefits of health interventions often assessed only a single variable, such as life expectancy or infant mortality. The usefulness of life expectancy or infant mortality rates is clearly very limited, however, since they give us information about only one of the aims of health interventions, extending life or preventing premature loss of life, and they provide only limited information about that aim. They give us no information about another, at least as important, aim of health interventions, to improve or protect the quality of life by treating or preventing suffering and disability.

Multi-attribute measures like the Sickness Impact Profile (Bergner et al. 1981: 787–805) and the SF 36 (Ware and Sherbourne 1992: 473–83) provide measures of different aspects of overall health related quality of life (HRQL) on which a particular population can be mapped, and an intervention assessed for its impact on these different components of health, or HRQL. Since these measures do not assign different relative value or importance to the different aspects or attributes of HRQL, they do not provide a single overall summary measure of HRQL. Thus, if one of two populations or health interventions scores higher in some respect(s) but lower in others, no conclusion can be drawn about whether the overall HRQL of one population, or from one intervention, is better than the other. Much quantitative based resource prioritization requires a methodology that combines in a single measure the two broad kinds of benefits produced by health interventions—extension of length of life and improvements in the quality of life (Brock 1992).

Typical summary measures of the benefits over time of health interventions that combine and assign relative value to these two kinds of benefits include QALYs and disability-adjusted life years (DALYs). Measures like QALYs and DALYs require a measure of the health status of individuals and in turn of populations at different points in time, such as the health utilities index (HUI) (Torrance et al. 1992) and the quality of well-being scale (QWB) (Kaplan and Anderson, 1988: 203–35), so as to be able to measure the health benefits in terms of changes in HRQL and length of life produced by different health interventions. The construction of any measure like the HUI or QWB requires a two-step process: first, different states of disability or conditions limiting HRQL are described; second, different relative values or utilities are assigned to those different conditions.

The determination of a person's or group's different health related conditions in terms of the various areas of function on the HUI or QWB both before and after a particular health intervention is an empirical question, which should be answered by appeal to relevant data regarding the burden of a particular disease and the reduction in that burden that a particular health intervention can be expected to produce. Needless to say, often the relevant data are highly imperfect, but that is a problem to be addressed largely by generating better data, not by ethical analysis.

The second step of assigning different relative values or utilities to the different areas and levels of function described by a measure like the HUI is typically done by soliciting people's preferences for life with the various functional limitations. This raises the fundamental question of whose preferences should be used to determine the relative value of life with different limitations in function and how they should be obtained. The developers of the DALY used the preferences of expert health professionals, in part for the practical reason that they are more knowledgeable about the nature of different health states, but the degree to which various conditions reduce overall HRQL is not a matter to be settled by professional expertise. Moreover, health professionals may have systematic biases that skew their value judgements about quality of life from those of ordinary persons. Other measures like the HUI and QWB use the value judgements of a random group of ordinary citizens to evaluate different states of disability or limitations in function.

A central issue concerning whose evaluations of different states of disability or functional limitation should be used arises from the typical responses of individuals to becoming disabled: adaptation, that is improving one's functional performance through learning and skills development, coping, that is altering one's expectations for performance so as to reduce the self-perceived gap between them and one's actual performance; and adjustment, that is altering one's life plans to give greater importance to activities in which performance is not diminished by disability (Murray 1996). The result is that the disabled who have gone through these processes often report less distress and limitation of opportunity and a higher quality of life with their disability than the non-disabled in evaluating the same condition. If the evaluations of disability states by the non-disabled are used for ranking different states of health and disability, then disabilities will be ranked as more serious health needs, but these rankings are open to the charge that they are distorted by the ignorance of the evaluators of what it is like to live with the conditions in question. Moreover, those valuations will assign less value to extending the lives of persons with disabilities. If the evaluations of the disabled themselves are used, however, the rankings are open to the charge that they reflect a different distortion by unjustifiably underestimating the burden of the disability because of the process of adaptation, coping, and adjustment that the disabled person has undergone. Moreover, they will assign less value to prevention or rehabilitation for disability because of the results of this process. The problem here is to determine an appropriate evaluative standpoint for ranking the importance of different disabilities which avoids these potential distortions (Brock 1995: 159–84).

Since the preferences for different states of disability or HRQL used to determine their relative values should be informed preferences, it is natural to think that the preferences of those who actually experience the disabilities should be used. Because they should have a more informed understanding of what it is actually like to live with the particular disability in question, we can hope to avoid uninformed evaluations. But this is to miss the deeper nature of the problem caused by adaptation, coping, and adjustment to disabilities.

Fundamental to understanding the difficulty posed by adaptation, coping, and adjustment to disabilities for preference evaluation of HRQL with various disabilities is that neither the non-disabled nor the disabled need have made any mistake in their different evaluations of quality of life with that disability. They arrive at different evaluations of the quality of life with that disability because they use different evaluative standpoints as a result of the disabled person's adaptation, coping, and adjustment. Disabled persons who have undergone this process can look back and see that before they became disabled they too would have evaluated the quality of life with that disability as non-disabled people now do. But this provides no basis for concluding that their pre-disability evaluation of the quality of life with that disability was mistaken, and so in turn no basis for discounting or discarding it because mistaken. The problem that I call the perspectives problem is that the non-disabled and the disabled evaluate the quality of life with the disability from two different evaluative perspectives, neither of which is mistaken. It might seem tempting to use the non-disabled's preferences for assessing the importance of prevention or rehabilitation programmes, but the disabled's preferences for assessing the importance of life-sustaining treatments for the disabled, but this ignores the necessity of a single unified perspective in order to compare the relative benefits from, and prioritise, the full range of different health interventions.

Moreover, what weight to give to the results of coping with one's condition may depend on the causes of that condition, for example, disease or injury that are no one's fault as opposed to unjust social conditions. Most measures of HRQL include some measure of subjective satisfaction or distress, a factor that is importantly influenced by people's expectations. In a society which has long practised systematic discrimination against women, for example, women may not be dissatisfied with their unjustly disadvantaged state, including the health differences that result from that discrimination. The fact that victims are sufficiently oppressed that they accept an injustice as natural and cope with it by reducing their expectations and adjusting their life plans should not make its effects less serious, as measures of HRQL with a subjective satisfaction or distress component would imply.

When measures like the HUI or QWB are applied across different economic, ethnic, cultural, and social groups, the meaningful states of health and disability and their importance in different groups may vary greatly; for example, in a setting in which most work is manual labour limitations in physical functioning will have greater importance than it does in a setting in which most individuals are engaged in non-physical, knowledge-based occupations, where certain cognitive disabilities are of greater importance. Different evaluations of health conditions and disabilities seem to be necessary for groups with significantly different relative needs for different functional abilities, but then cross-group comparisons of health and disability, and of the relative value of health interventions, in those different groups will not be possible. The health programme benefits will have been measured on two different and apparently incommensurable valuational scales. These differences will be magnified when summary measures of population health are employed for international comparisons across very disparate countries.

Some of this variability of perspective may be avoided by a focus on the evaluation of disability instead of handicap, as these are traditionally distinguished, such as in the 1980 International Classification of Impairments, Disabilities and Handicaps (ICIDHWHO 1980). The ICIDH understands disabilities as 'any restriction or lack (resulting from an impairment) of ability to perform an activity in the manner or within the range considered normal for a human being', whereas handicap is 'a disadvantage for a given individual, resulting from an impairment or disability, that limits or prevents the fulfilment of a role that is normal (depending on age, sex, and social and cultural factors) for that individual'. There will be greater variability between individuals, groups, and cultures in the relative importance of handicaps than of disabilities since handicaps take account of differences in individuals' roles and social conditions that disabilities do not. But it is problematic whether these differences should be ignored in prioritising health resources for individuals, groups, and societies, that is, whether disabilities or handicaps are the correct focus for evaluation.

10.2. SECOND ISSUE: DO ALL QALYS COUNT EQUALLY?

QALYs standardly assume that an additional year of life has the same value regardless of the age of the person who receives it, assuming that the different life years are of comparable quality. A year of life extension for an infant, a forty-year-old, and an eighty-year-old all have the same value in QALYs produced, and in turn in a cost effectiveness analysis using QALYs, assuming no difference in the quality of the year of life extension. This is compatible, of course, with using age-based quality adjustments for interventions affecting groups of different age patients to reflect differences in the average quality of life of those different groups; for example, if average quality of life in a group of patients of average age eighty-five is less than that of patients of average age twenty-five, a year of life extension for the twenty-five-year-old would have greater value in QALYs than would a year of life extension for the eighty-five-year-old.

In the World Bank Study, *World Development Report 1993; Investing in Health* (World Bank 1993), the alternative DALY measure was developed to measure the burden of disease in reducing life expectancy and quality of life. Probably the most important ethical difference between QALYs and DALYs is that DALYs assign different value to a year of life extension of the same quality, depending on the age at which an individual receives it; specifically, life extension for individuals during their adult productive work years is assigned greater value than a similar period of life extension for infants and young children or the elderly. The principal justification offered for this feature of DALYs was the different social roles that individuals typically occupy at different ages and the typical emotional, physical, and financial dependence of the very young and the elderly on individuals in their productive work years (Murray 1994).

This justification of age-based differences in the value of life extension implicitly adopts an ethically problematic social perspective on the value of health care interventions that extend life, or maintain or restore function, that is, an evaluation of the benefits *to others* of extending an individual's life, or maintaining or restoring his or her function, in addition to the benefit to that individual of doing so. This social perspective is in conflict with the usual focus in clinical decision-making and treatment only on the benefits to the individuals who receive the health care interventions in question. Typical practice in health policy and public health contexts is more ambiguous on this point, since there benefits to others besides the direct recipient of the intervention are sometimes given substantial weight in the evaluation and justification of health programmes; for example, treatment programmes for substance abuse are argued to merit high priority because of their benefits in reductions in lost work days and in harmful effects on the substance abusers' family members. This social perspective is ethically problematic because it gives weight to differences between individuals in their social and economic value to others; in so doing, it discriminates against persons with fewer dependents and social ties, which arguably is not ethically relevant in health care resource allocation. The social perspective justifying the DALY measure is therefore ethically problematic, in a way the alternative QALY measure is not, if the value of health benefits for individuals should focus on the value to the individuals treated of the health benefits, not on the social value for others of treating those persons. The ethical difficulty here is briefly explored further in the section below on what costs and benefits should count in a CEA.

Giving different value to life extension at different ages, however, might be justified ethically if done for different reasons. For example, Norman Daniels has argued that because everyone can expect to pass through the different stages of the life span, giving different value to a year of life extension at different stages in the life span need not unjustly discriminate against individuals in the way giving different weight to life extension for members of different racial, ethnic, or gender groups would unjustly discriminate (Daniels 1988). Each individual can expect to pass through all the life stages in which life extension is given different value, but is a member of only one race, ethnic group, and gender. Thus, all persons are treated the same at comparable stages of their lives regarding the value of extending their lives, and so the use of DALYs would not constitute unjust age discrimination comparable to gender, ethnic or racial discrimination.

Moreover, individuals, and in turn their society, might choose to give lesser weight to a year of life extension beyond the normal life span than to a year of life extension before one has reached the normal life span based on a conception of what equality of opportunity requires, or on what Alan Williams calls the 'fair innings' argument (Williams 1997: 117–32). People's plans of life and central long term projects will typically be constructed to fit within the normal life span, and so the completion of these central projects will typically require reaching, but not living beyond, the normal life span (Daniels 1988; Brock 1989).

10.3. THIRD ISSUE: WHAT COSTS AND BENEFITS SHOULD COUNT IN COST EFFECTIVENESS ANALYSES OF HEALTH PROGRAMMES?

It is widely agreed that cost effectiveness analyses in health should reflect the direct health benefits for individuals of their medical treatment, such as improving renal function or reducing joint swelling, and of public health programmes, such as reducing the incidence of infectious diseases through vaccination programmes. The direct costs of medical treatment and public health programmes, such as the costs of health care professionals' time and of medical equipment and supplies, should also be reflected. But medical and public health interventions typically also have indirect non-health benefits and costs. For example, some disease and illness principally affects adults during their working years, thereby incurring significant economic costs in lost work days associated with the disease or illness, whereas other disease and illness principally affects either young children, such as some infectious diseases, or the elderly, such as

Alzheimer's dementia, who in each case are not typically employed and so do not incur lost wages or lost work time from illness. Should an indirect economic burden of disease of this sort be given weight in a cost effectiveness analysis used to prioritise between different health interventions? (Brock 2003).

From an economic perspective, as well as from a broad utilitarian moral perspective, indirect non-health benefits and costs are real benefits and costs of disease and of efforts to treat or prevent it, even if not direct health benefits and direct treatment costs; they should be reflected in the overall cost effectiveness accounting of how to use scarce health resources so as to produce the maximum aggregate benefit. A possible moral argument for ignoring these indirect non-health costs and benefits in health resource prioritisation is grounded in a conception of the moral equality of persons. Giving priority to the treatment of one group of patients over another because treating the first group would produce indirect non-health benefits for others (e.g. other family members who were dependent on these patients) or would reduce indirect economic costs to others (e.g. the employers of these patients who incur less lost work time) could be argued to fail to treat each group of patients with the equal moral concern and respect that all people deserve; in particular, doing so would fail to give equal moral concern and weight to each person's health care needs. Instead, giving lower priority to the second group of patients simply because they are not a means to the indirect non-health benefits or cost savings produced by treating the first group of patients gives the second group of patients and their health care needs lower priority simply because they are not a means to these indirect non-health benefits or cost savings to others. It would violate the Kantian moral injunction against treating people solely as means for the benefit of others.

In public policy we often use a notion of 'separate spheres', which in this case could be used to argue that the purpose of health care and of public health is health and the reduction of disease, and so only these goals and effects should guide health care and public health programmes (Walzer 1983; Kamm 1993). There are obvious practical grounds for the separate spheres view from the difficulty of fully determining and calculating indirect benefits and costs. But the Kantian moral argument could serve as a principled moral basis for ignoring indirect benefits and costs in a cost effectiveness analysis to be used to prioritise health resources and interventions that serve different individuals or groups.

10.4. FOURTH ISSUE: SHOULD DISCOUNT RATES BE APPLIED TO HEALTH CARE BENEFITS?

It is both standard and recommended practice in cost effectiveness analyses, within health care and elsewhere, to assume a time preference by applying a discount rate to both the benefits and costs of different programmes under evaluation, although the reasons for doing so and the proper rate of discount are controversial (Gold 1996: chapter 7). It is important to separate clearly the ethical issue about whether health benefits should be discounted from other economic considerations for discounting, as well as to be clear why the issue is important for health policy. It is not ethically controversial that a discount rate should be applied to economic costs and economic benefits; a dollar received today is worth more than a dollar received ten years from now because we have its use for those ten years, and there is a similar economic advantage in delaying the incurring of economic costs. The ethical issue is whether a discount rate should be applied directly to changes in life extension and well-being or health. Is an improvement in well-being, such as a specific period of life extension, a reduction in suffering, or an improvement in function, extending, say, for one year of substantially less value if it occurs twenty years from now than if it occurs next year?

Future benefits are appropriately discounted when they are more uncertain than proximate benefits. Proximate benefits, such as restoration of an individual's function, also are of more value than distant benefits if they make possible a longer period of, and thus larger, benefit by occurring sooner. But neither of these considerations require the use of a discount rate—they will be taken account of in the measurement of expected benefits of alternative interventions. The ethical question is whether an improvement in an individual's well-being is of lesser value if it occurs in the distant future than if it occurs in the immediate future, simply and only because it occurs later in time. This is a controversial issue in the literature on social discounting and my own view is that no adequate ethical justification has been offered for applying a discount rate directly to changes in health and well-being, though I cannot pursue the justifications offered by proponents of discounting here. The avoidance of paradoxes that arise when no discount rate is applied or when different discount rates are applied to costs and benefits, has influenced many economists to support use of the same discount rate for costs and benefits (Keeler and Cretin 1983: 300–6), but I believe these are properly dealt with not through discounting, but rather through directly addressing the ethical issues they raise, usually about equity between different generations.

The policy importance of this issue is relatively straightforward in the prioritization of health care interventions. Many health care and public health programmes take significantly different lengths of time to produce their benefits. Applying a discount rate to those benefits leads to an unwarranted priority to programmes producing benefits more rapidly. It results in a programme that produces benefits in health and well-being say twenty years into the future being given lower priority than an alternative health care programme that produces substantially less overall improvement in health and well-being, but produces that improvement much sooner. Many public health and preventive interventions, for example, vaccination programmes and changes in unhealthy behaviour, reap their health benefits years into the future. If those benefits are unjustifiably discounted, they will be given lower priority than alternative programmes that produce fewer aggregate benefits. The result is a health policy that produces fewer overall health benefits over time than could have been produced with the same resources.

10.5. FIFTH ISSUE: WHAT LIFE EXPECTANCIES SHOULD BE USED FOR CALCULATING THE BENEFITS OF LIFE SAVING INTERVENTIONS?

In calculating QALYs it is standard practice to take account of differences in the average ages and in turn life expectancies of patients served by different health care programmes; for example, a treatment for a life-threatening childhood disease would produce more QALYs than a comparable treatment for a life-threatening disease affecting primarily the elderly. Similarly, accurate estimates of the expected QALYs from different interventions would adjust for differences in the average life expectancies of patients caused by diseases other than those treated by the interventions; for example, an intervention that improved the quality of life of patients with cystic fibrosis, who have a much lower than average life expectancy as a result of their disease, would produce fewer QALYs than an intervention with a comparable improvement in lifetime quality of life for patients with average life expectancies undiminished by disease. This latter case raises difficult issues about discrimination against people with disabilities that I take up later. But there are other differences in the life expectancies of different groups that an accurate estimate of QALYs produced by health interventions serving those groups would seemingly have to reflect; for example, there are significant differences in the life expectancies between different genders, racial and ethnic groups, and socio-economic groups within most countries. Internationally, the differences in life expectancies between different countries are often much larger. Should these differences affect calculations of the QALYs gained by health care and public health interventions that extend life or improve quality of life? An accurate estimate of the additional life years actually produced by those interventions should not ignore differences in life expectancies that the health care interventions will not affect, but the result will be that it is less valuable to save the life of a poor person in an underdeveloped country than a rich person in a developed country.

The differences in life expectancies between different racial, ethnic, and socio-economic groups within a single country, as well as the very large differences between life expectancies in economically developed and poor countries, are often principally the result of unjust conditions and deprivations suffered by those with lower life expectancies. It would seem only to compound those injustices to give less value to interventions that save lives or improve quality of life for groups with lower life expectancies caused by the unjust conditions and deprivations from which they suffer. Differences in life expectancies between the genders, on the other hand, are believed to rest in significant part on biological differences, not on unjust social conditions. Whether the biologically based component of gender differences in life expectancies should be reflected in measures like QALYs or DALYs is more controversial. For example, on the one hand, the lower life expectancy of men does not result from any independent injustice, but, on the other hand, it is explicit public policy and required by law in the United States to ignore this gender-based difference in most calculations of pension benefits and annuity costs so as to avoid gender discrimination. The developers of the DALY explicitly chose to use a single uniform measure of life expectancy (except for the biological component of the gender difference), specifically that observed in Japan which has the highest national life expectancy, to measure gains from life saving interventions. They justified their choice in explicitly ethical terms as conforming to a principle of 'treating like events as like', although the reasoning was not pursued in any detail (Murray 1994: 7). How this issue is treated can have a substantial impact on the priorities that result from the cost effectiveness analysis, especially at the international level where country differences tend often to be greater than group differences within specific countries.

Each of the preceding five ethical issues can be considered issues in the *construction* of a cost-effectiveness analysis in health care. The other issues I want to briefly note can be considered issues in the *use* of cost effectiveness analysis in health resource prioritisation. They are each issues of distributive justice or equity raised by the fact that a cost effectiveness analysis is insensitive to the distribution of health benefits and of the costs of producing them. Yet people's beliefs about equity and justice directly affect the relative priority they assign to different health interventions. One standard response to this point is that a CEA can only be an aid to policy-making in general, and health resource prioritisation in particular, and that policy makers must take account of considerations of equity in final policy decisions and choices. But as with the ethical issues in the construction of CEAs, much work remains to be done to clarify and assess alternative positions on these issues of equity so the policy choices on them can at least be better informed, even if they remain controversial. Here, there is only space to state four of the main equity issues in the use of CEAs and some of the principal ethical considerations supporting different positions on them (Daniels 1993: 224–33). After doing that, I shall mention an alternative quantitative methodology that, unlike CEA, incorporates considerations of equity within the quantitative analysis.

10.6. SIXTH ISSUE: WHAT PRIORITY SHOULD BE GIVEN TO THE SICKEST OR WORST OFF?

It is a commonplace that most theories of distributive justice require some special concern for those who are worst off or most disadvantaged (Brock 2002); for example, it is often said that the justice of a society can be measured by how it treats its least well-off members. In the context of health care allocation and the prioritisation of health interventions, the worst off with regard to need for the good being distributed might reasonably be thought to be the sickest patients. In many cases, the sickest will be given priority by a CEA comparing treating them as opposed to less sick patients; the sickest have greater possible improvements in HRQL because they begin from a lower HRQL, and so, for example, in comparing fully effective treatments those for the sickest will produce the greater benefits. But in other cases giving priority to the sickest will require a sacrifice in aggregate health benefits. An abstract example makes the point most concisely. Suppose Group A patients have a very serious disease that leaves them with a health utility level of 0.25 as measured by the HUI, and this would be raised only to 0.45 with the best available treatment because no treatment is very effective for their disease; for example, patients with severe chronic obstructive pulmonary disease or with severe chronic schizophrenia that is largely resistant to standard pharmacological treatments. A similar number of Group B patients have a health utility level of 0.60 because they have a considerably less serious disease, but since treatment for their disease is more effective, although no more costly, it would raise their health utility level to 0.90; for example, patients with asthma, or with milder forms of pulmonary disease or schizophrenia that both leave them less disabled without treatment and are more responsive to treatment. Should we give priority to treating Group B because doing so would produce a 50 per cent greater aggregate health benefit at the same cost, as the CEA standard implies, or to treating Group A who are the sickest? In some empirical studies, both ordinary people and health professionals prefer to sacrifice some aggregate health benefits in order to treat the sickest patients, although the degree of sacrifice they are prepared to make is variable and not statistically reliable (Nord 1993: 227–38).

One difficulty raised by this issue is determining what weight to give to this particular aspect of equity—concern for the worst off. Virtually no one would prefer to treat the sickest, no matter how costly their treatment and how small the benefit to them of doing so, and no matter how beneficial and inexpensive treatment for the less sick might be. However, there seems no objective, principled basis for determining how much priority to give the sickest, that is, how much aggregate health benefits should be sacrificed in order to treat or give priority to the sickest. Instead, the most one can say is that most people and many theories of distributive justice have a concern both for maximising overall benefits with scarce health resources and for helping the worst off or sickest, but there is a large range of indeterminacy regarding the proper tradeoff between these two concerns when they are in conflict.

One issue in understanding this concern for the worst off important for health care priorities is whether it should focus on who is worst off at a point in time or instead over an extended period of time, such as a lifetime. When choosing between patients to receive a scarce resource, such as in organ transplantation, it is often plausible to focus on lifetime well-being, since otherwise we may give priority to the patient who is worst off at the time the distributive choice is made, but whose lifetime level of well-being is far higher than the other patient. Frances Kamm has defended a notion of need in this context according to which the neediest patient is the patient whose life will have gone worst if he or she does not get the scarce resource, such as an organ transplant (Kamm 1993: chapter 8). However, some justifications for giving priority to the worst off may support focusing on the sickest here and now.

What are the ethical justifications for giving priority to the worst off? I can mention only two possibilities here. One is that we must give priority to the worst off in order to avoid increasing the already unjustified disadvantage or inequality they suffer relative to those better off. But it is worth noting that a concern for the worst off is not always the same as a concern to produce equality in outcomes. In the example above of Groups A and B, equality could be achieved by what Derek Parfit has called 'levelling down', that is by bringing B's health utility level down to that of A's instead raising A's level up to that of B (Parfit 1991). If equity here is equivalent to equality in outcomes, then if it were not possible to raise A's level above 0.40 with treatment, equity would seem to support not treating Group B and letting their condition deteriorate until it reached the lower level of Group A. The fact that no one would defend doing this suggests that this aspect of our notion of equity or justice is best captured by the idea of giving priority to improving the condition of the worst off, rather than by a simple concern for equality in outcomes. A different justification for giving priority to treating the sickest, offered by some participants in Nord's research, is that it would be subjectively more important to the sickest to obtain treatment, even if the health benefits they receive from treatment are less than those that would go to the less sick; this justification might support focusing on who is worst off at the point in time at which the decision about who to treat is made, not whose lifetime well-being will be lowest (Nord 1993: 227–38).

One further issue concerning the priority to the worst off should be mentioned. In the context of health resource prioritisation in health policy it seems natural to understand the worst off as the sickest. But this may not always be correct. At the most fundamental ethical level in our general theories of equity and distributive justice, our concern should be for those who are overall or all things considered worst off, and they will not always be the sickest. It could be argued that giving priority to the worst off in health resource prioritisation sometimes requires giving priority to those with the lowest levels of overall well-being, even at some cost to aggregate health benefits produced *and* at the cost of not treating sicker persons whose overall well-being is much higher. A preference for health interventions that raise the level of well-being of those who are worst off in overall well-being, instead of giving priority to the sickest, might be justified in order not to increase the unjustified disadvantage suffered by those with the lowest overall level of well-being. If, instead, the priority to the worst off in health resource prioritisation should focus only on health states and so on the sickest, a justification of this narrowed focus is needed.

10.7. SEVENTH ISSUE: WHEN SHOULD SMALL BENEFITS TO A LARGE NUMBER OF PERSONS RECEIVE PRIORITY OVER LARGE BENEFITS TO A SMALL NUMBER OF PERSONS?

Cost effectiveness and utilitarian standards require minimising the aggregate burden of disease and maximising the aggregate health of a population without regard to the resulting distribution of disease and health, or *who* gets what benefits. The issue about priority to the worst off focuses on who gets the benefits. A different issue concerns *what* benefits different individuals get. Some would argue that health benefits are often qualitatively different and so cannot all be compared on a single scale like the HUI, or in turn by a single measure like QALYs, but that is not the issue of concern now. In its most general form the issue about aggregation concerns what ethical limits there are, if any, on aggregating together different size benefits for different persons in comparing and prioritising different health interventions; CEA accepts no such limits. There are many forms in which this issue can arise which cannot be pursued here (Kamm 1993: Part II), but the version that has received the most attention, and which Daniels has called the aggregation problem, is when, if ever, large benefits to a few individuals should take priority over greater aggregate benefits to a different and much larger group of individuals, each one of whom receives only a small benefit. This issue arises when a very serious disease or condition for those affected that is also very costly to prevent or treat is compared with a much more prevalent disease or condition that both has a very small impact on each individual affected and is very inexpensive to treat or prevent in any one individual. Applying cost effectiveness or utilitarian standards, preventing or treating the very prevalent but low impact disease or condition at a given cost will receive higher priority when doing so produces greater aggregate benefits than using the same funds to treat or prevent the disease or condition that has a very great impact on each individual affected. The example that received considerable attention in the United States arose in the Oregon Medicaid priority setting process where capping teeth for exposed pulp was ranked just above an appendectomy for acute appendicitis, a potentially life-threatening condition. Because an appendectomy was estimated to be about 150 times as expensive as capping a tooth for exposed pulp, the aggregate benefit of capping a tooth for 150 patients was judged to be greater than the benefit of an appendectomy for one patient. Since Medicaid coverage decisions were to be made according to the list of treatment/condition pairs ranked in terms of their relative cost effectiveness, it could have turned out, depending on the overall level of resources available to the Medicaid programme, that tooth capping would have been covered but appendectomies not covered.

This result, and other less extreme cases like it, was highly counterintuitive and unacceptable to most people, whose intuitive rankings of the relative importance or priority of health interventions are based on one-to-one comparisons, for example, of one tooth capped as opposed to one appendectomy performed. In the face of these results Oregon made a fundamental change in its prioritisation methodology, abandoning the cost effectiveness standard in favour of a standard that did not take account of differences in costs. This was not a minor problem requiring tinkering at the margins of the CEA standard, but a fundamental challenge to it and so required a fundamental revision in it.

Yet, it is by no means clear that no such aggregation can be ethically justified. The very case that precipitated Oregon's Medicaid revision was a twelve-year-old boy in need of a bone marrow transplant as the only effective chance to save his life. Oregon denied coverage under its Medicaid programme on the grounds that it could do greater good by using its limited resources to improve prenatal care for pregnant women, in this case giving higher priority to small benefits to many over a potentially much larger benefit to a few. Moreover, many public policy choices appear to give higher priority to small benefits to many over even life-saving benefits to a few; for example, governments in the United States support public parks used by tens or hundreds of thousands of persons, while reducing funding for public hospitals resulting in quite predictable loss of life.

The cost effectiveness or utilitarian standard that permits unlimited aggregation of benefits might be defended by distinguishing between the clinical context in which physicians treat individual patients and the public health and health policy context in which health resource allocation decisions are made that will affect different groups in the population. In the clinical context, physicians forced to prioritise between individual patients typically will first treat the patient who will suffer the more serious consequences without treatment, or who will benefit the most from treatment, even if doing so will prevent her treating a larger number of less seriously ill patients. But from a public health or health policy perspective, it could be argued that the potential overall or aggregate effects of alternative interventions on population health is the appropriate perspective. However, the Oregon experience makes clear that even when allocating public resources for interventions to improve the health of a population it is ethically controversial whether always giving priority to producing the maximum aggregate benefits, even when that is done by giving small benefits to many at the cost of forgoing large benefits to a few, is justified.

Just as with the problem of what priority to give to the worst off, part of the complexity of the aggregation problem is that for most people some, but not all, cases of aggregation are ethically acceptable and equitable. The theoretical problem then is to develop a principled account of when, and for what reasons, different forms of aggregation satisfy requirements of equity and when they do not (Kamm 1993). There is no consensus on this issue either among ordinary persons or within the literature of health policy or ethics and political philosophy. As with the problem about priority to the worst off, the complexities of this issue have received relatively little attention in bioethics and moral and political philosophy, and there is much difficult but important work to be done.

10.8. EIGHTH ISSUE: THE CONFLICT BETWEEN FAIR CHANCES AND BEST OUTCOMES

The third ethical issue in the use of CEA for health resource utilisation that I will mention here has been characterised as the conflict between fair chances and best outcomes (Daniels 1993: 224–33). The conflict is most pressing when the health intervention is life saving and not all those whose lives are threatened can be saved, but it arises as well when threats are only to individuals' health and well-being. In the context of health care, this issue first received attention in organ transplantation where there is a scarcity of life-saving organs such as hearts and lungs resulting in thousands of deaths each year of patients on waiting lists for an organ for transplant; an abstract example from transplantation can illustrate the issue most clearly and succinctly (Brock 1988).

Suppose two patients are each in need of a heart transplant to prevent imminent death, but there is only one heart available for transplant. Patient A has a life expectancy with a transplant of ten years and patient B has a life expectancy with a transplant of nine years (of course, precise estimates of this sort are not possible, but the point is that there is a small difference in the expected benefits to be gained depending on which patient gets the scarce organ), with no difference in their expected quality of life. Maximising health benefits or QALYs, as a CEA standard requires, favours giving the organ to patient A, but patient B might argue that it is unfair to give her no chance to receive the scarce heart. Just as much as A, she needs the heart transplant for life itself and will lose everything, that is her life, if she does not receive it. It is unfair, B might argue, to give the organ to A because the quite small increment in expected benefits from doing so is too small to justly determine who lives and who dies. Instead, she argues, each of them should receive a fair chance of getting the organ and having their health needs met; in this case, that might be done by giving each an equal chance of receiving the transplant through some form of random selection between them, or by a weighted lottery that gives the patient who would benefit more some greater likelihood of being selected to receive the organ, but still gives the patient who would benefit less some significant chance of getting it instead (Broome 1984: 38–55; Brock 1988; Kamm 1993: Part III).

Most prioritisation and rationing choices arise not from physical scarcity of the needed health resource, as in organ transplantation, but from economic scarcity, limits in the money society devotes to health care. Will this issue of equity arise in health resource prioritisation and allocation choices forced by economic scarcity? Two considerations will often mitigate the force of the ethical conflict between fair chances and best outcomes there. First, allocation of resources in health care is typically not an all or nothing choice, as in the case of selecting recipients for scarce organs, but is usually a matter of the relative priority for funding to be given to different health programmes or interventions.

That one health programme A promises a small gain in aggregate health benefits over a competing programme B need not entail that A is fully funded and B receives no funding, but only that A should receive higher priority for, or a higher level of, funding than B. Persons with the disease or condition that A treats will have a somewhat higher probability of being successfully treated than will those who have the disease or condition that B treats; in the case of prevention, those at risk of A will have a somewhat higher probability of successful prevention than will those at risk of B. When there is significant resource scarcity this will involve some sacrifice in aggregate health benefits that might have been produced by always preferring the more cost effective alternative. But doing so means that individuals who are served by B have no complaint that the small difference in expected benefits between programmes A and B unfairly prevents them from having their health needs met at all. Instead, the small difference in expected benefits between programmes A and B need only result in a comparably small difference in the resources devoted to A and B; it is not obvious that this is unfair to those patients served by B, whose needs are somewhat less well served than patients in programme A because of B's lower priority and level of funding.

The second consideration that may mitigate some of the conflict between fair chances and best outcomes in health resource prioritisation forced by economic scarcity is that often, probably usually, the diseases and health problems to be treated or prevented are not directly life threatening, but instead only impact on individuals' quality of life, and often for only a limited period of time. In these cases, the difference in health benefits between individuals who receive a needed health intervention that is given a higher priority and individuals who do not receive a needed health intervention because their condition is given lower priority, is much less, making the unfairness arguably less compelling.

These two considerations may mitigate, but they do not fully avoid, the conflict between fair chances and best outcomes in prioritisation decisions about health interventions forced by economic scarcity. When a more cost effective health programme is developed for one population instead of a different less cost effective health programme for a different population, individuals who would have been served by the second programme will have a complaint that they did not have a fair chance to have their needs served only because of a small gain in the benefits that are produced by the first programme. The fair chances versus best outcome conflict will arise in prioritising health interventions in health policy; how this conflict can be equitably resolved is complex, controversial, and unclear.

10.9. NINTH ISSUE: DOES USE OF CEA TO SET HEALTH CARE PRIORITIES UNJUSTLY DISCRIMINATE AGAINST THE DISABLED?

In several contexts using CEA to set health care priorities will result in assigning lower priority to both life extending and quality of life improving treatment for disabled rather than non-disabled persons with the same health care needs (Brock 1995: 159–84; 2000: 223–35). Here are five such contexts. First, since already disabled persons have a lower HRQL from their disability than non-disabled persons, treatment that extends their life for a given number of years produces fewer QALYs than the same treatment that extends the life of a non-disabled person for the same number of years. Second, if two groups of patients with the same HRQL have the same need for a life sustaining or quality of life improving treatment, but one will be restored to normal function and the other will be left with a resultant disability, more QALYs will be produced by treating the first group. Third, persons with disabilities often have a lower life expectancy because of their disability than otherwise similar non-disabled persons. As a result, treatments that prevent loss of life or produce lifetime improvements in quality of life will produce fewer QALYs when given to disabled than to non-disabled persons with the same health care needs. Fourth, disabilities often act as comorbid conditions making a treatment less beneficial in QALYs produced for disabled than for non-disabled persons with the same health care needs. Fifth, the presence of a disability can make treatment of disabled persons more difficult and so more costly than for non-disabled persons with the same health care needs; the result is a lower cost effectiveness ratio for treating the disabled persons.

In each of the five cases above, disabled persons have the same medical and health care need as non-disabled persons, and so the same claim to treatment on the basis of their needs. But treating the disabled person will produce less benefit, that is, fewer QALYs, *because of their disability* than treating the non-disabled. Thus, their disability is the reason for their receiving lower priority for treatment. This at least arguably fails to give equal moral concern to disabled persons' health care needs and is unjust discrimination against them on grounds of their disability. Indeed, United States Health and Human Services Secretary Louis Sullivan denied Oregon's initial request for a waiver of federal regulations for its proposed revisions to its Medicaid plan on the grounds that Oregon's method of prioritisation of services was in violation of the Americans with Disabilities Act (ADA).[2] Sullivan cited some of the five kinds of cases I noted above in support of that position, and Oregon in turn made essentially ad hoc revisions in its ranking to avoid the putative violation of the ADA.

Disabled persons charge that in cases like the first I cited above concerning life saving treatment, the implication of use of CEA to prioritise health care is that saving their lives, and so their lives themselves, have less value than non-disabled persons' lives. They quite plausibly find that implication of CEA threatening and unjust. There are means of avoiding these problems about discrimination against persons with disabilities, but they involve abandoning fundamental features of CEAs. For example, one response to the first case cited

---

[2] Unpublished letter from Secretary of Health and Human Services, Louis Sullivan, to Oregon Governor, Barbara Roberts, 3 August 1992.

above would be to give equal value to a year of life extension, whatever the quality of that life, so long as it is acceptable to the person whose life it is (Kamm 1993: Part I). But that has problematic implications too since, for example, a small percentage of persons in surveys say they would want their lives sustained even if they were in a persistent vegetative state. I cannot pursue the issues further here, but I believe the problem of whether CEA unjustly discriminates against the disabled is a deep and unresolved difficulty for use of CEA and QALYs to prioritise health care.

The sixth, seventh, and eighth issues above all raise possible criticisms of the maximisation standard embodied in CEA; in each case, the claim is that equity requires attention to the distribution of health benefits and costs to distinct individuals. Steadfast utilitarians or consequentialists will reject the criticisms and hold fast to the maximisation standard. But most people will accept some departure from the maximisation standard of CEA; there are two broad strategies for how to do so. The first and probably most common is to propose CEA as an aid to policy-makers who must make prioritisation and allocation choices in health care, but then to remind those policy-makers that they must take account of these considerations of equity as well in their decision-making; this may be, but usually is not, accompanied by some guidance about alternative substantive positions, and reasons in support of them, on the equity issues. Moreover, some use of CEA in health policy and health programme evaluation does not raise these last three issues of equity; for example, CEA of alternative treatments that each have uniform but different benefits for a group of patients with a particular medical condition. And outside of a CEA, either QALYs or DALYs can be used for evaluating alternative interventions, or for monitoring changes over time in health status or the burdens of disease, in a given group or population.

The second strategy for responding to concerns about equity seeks to develop a quantitative tool that measures the specific weight people give to different equity concerns in comparing interventions that raise issues of distributive justice because they serve different individuals or benefit individuals differently. The most prominent and promising example is the 'person trade-off' approach which explicitly asks people how many outcomes of one kind they consider equivalent in social value to X outcomes of another kind, where the outcomes are for different groups of individuals (Nord 1999). For example, people can be asked, as in our earlier example, to compare treatment A for very severely ill patients who are at 0.25 on the HUI without treatment and who can be raised only to 0.45 with treatment, with treatment B of less severely ill patients who are at 0.60 and can be raised to 0.90 with treatment; filled out detailed examples, of course, will make the comparisons more understandable. Respondents are then asked how many patients treated with A would be equivalent in social value to treating 100 patients with B. Answers to questions of this form will tell us in quantitative terms how much importance people give to treating the sickest when doing so conflicts with maximising aggregate health benefits.

The person tradeoff approach is designed to permit people to incorporate concerns for equity or distributive justice into their judgements about the social value of alternative health programmes. There has been relatively little exploration and use of this methodology in health care evaluation in comparison with the mass of methodological work on and studies of aggregate QALYs and CEAs, in part because many health policy analysts and health economists assume, often with little or no argument, that the social value of health programmes is the sum of the individual utilities produced by the programme. As I noted in the introduction to the chapter, the early stage we are now at in the development and use of the person tradeoff approach is a reason for caution at the present time about using it to settle issues of equity in health resource prioritisation. While the utilitarian assumption in CEA is rejected in most philosophical work on distributive justice, as well as in the preferences most ordinary people express for different health outcomes and programmes, I also noted in the introduction a second more important reason for caution about bringing considerations of equity into health policy decision-making through a quantitative methodology like the person tradeoff methodology— the issues of distributive justice that must be addressed by equitable health resource prioritisation represent deep and long-standing divisions in moral and political philosophy about which there is not now, and may never be, anything approaching consensus. There is a strong case to be made, though I cannot pursue it here, that important value conflicts about justice of this sort should be addressed in public, democratic political processes, or in fair, participatory, and accountable procedures within private institutions like managed care organisations (Daniels and Sabin 1997: 303–50). The person tradeoff method can be a useful aid to those deliberative decision-making processes in providing more structure and precision to different people's views about equity in health care resource prioritisation and tradeoffs, but it is not a substitute for that deliberation. Despite these briefly noted reservations, I do emphasise that for purposes of resource prioritisation and allocation, the person tradeoff approach is the proper perspective, in comparison with CEA, because it correctly reflects that the choices are typically about how health benefits and costs are distributed to different individuals.

10.10. CONCLUSION

I have distinguished above nine distinct issues about equity and justice that arise in the construction and use of cost effectiveness analysis to minimise the burdens of disease and to maximise health outcomes. In each case the concern for equity is in my view valid and warrants some constraints on a goal of unqualified maximisation of health outcomes. There has not been space here to pursue at all fully any of these nine issues regarding equity and justice— each is complex, controversial, and important. In each case, my point has been that there are important ethical and value choices to be made in constructing and using the measures; the choices are not merely technical, empirical, or economic, but moral and value choices as well. Each requires explicit attention by health policy-makers using CEA. In a few cases I have indicated my own view about how the potential conflict between equity and utilitarian maximisation might be resolved, but in other cases I have simply summarised briefly some arguments for giving the particular concern about equity some weight when it conflicts with maximisation of utility. For some of these issues, the literature and research is at a relatively early stage and one cannot be confident about how the issues should be resolved or even about the range of plausible positions and supporting reasons on them. However, this is not grounds for ignoring the issues, but instead for getting to work on them and for ensuring that they receive explicit attention and deliberation in decisions about health resource prioritisation and allocation.

References

Bergner, M., R. A. Bobbitt, W. B. Carter, and B. S. Gibson (1981). 'The Sickness Impact Profile: Development and Final Revision of a Health Status Measure', *Medical Care*, 19: 787–805.

Brock, D. W. (1988). 'Ethical Issues in Recipient Selection for Organ Transplantation', in D. Mathieu (ed.), *Organ Substitution Technology: Ethical, Legal, and Public Policy Issues*. Boulder and London: Westview Press.

—— (1989). 'Justice, Health Care, and the Elderly', *Philosophy & Public Affairs*, 18(3): 297–312.

—— (1992). 'Quality of Life Measures in Health Care and Medical Ethics', in A. Sen and M. Nussbaum (eds.), *The Quality of Life*. Oxford: Oxford University Press.

—— (1995). 'Justice and ADA: Does Prioritizing and Rationing Health Care Discriminate Against the Disabled?' *Social Theory and Policy*, 12: 159–84.

—— (2000). 'Health Care Resource Prioritization and Discrimination Against Persons With Disabilities', in L. Francis and A. Silvers (eds.), *Americans With Disabilities*. New York: Routledge.

—— (2002). 'Priority to the Worst Off in Health Care Resource Prioritization', in M. Battin, R. Rhodes, and A. Silvers (eds.), *Medicine and Social Justice*. New York: Oxford University Press.

—— (2003). 'Separate Spheres and Indirect Benefits,' *Cost-Effectiveness and Resource Allocation* 1: 4.

Broome, J. (1984). 'Selecting People Randomly', *Ethics*, 95: 38–55.

Daniels, N. (1988). *Am I My Parents' Keeper? An Essay on Justice Between the Young and the Old*. New York: Oxford University Press.

—— (1993). 'Rationing Fairly: Programmatic Considerations', *Bioethics*, 7(2–3): 224–33.

—— and J. Sabin (1997). 'Limits to Health Care: Fair Procedures, Democratic Deliberation, and the Legitimacy Problem for Insurers', *Philosophy and Public Affairs*, 26(4): 303–50.

Gold, M. R. et al. (1996). *Cost-Effectiveness in Health and Medicine*. New York: Oxford University Press, chapter 7.

Kamm, F. M. (1993). *Morality/Mortality. Volume One. Death and Whom to Save From It*. Oxford: Oxford University Press.

Kaplan, R. M. and J. P. Anderson (1988). 'A General Health Policy Model: Update and Applications', *Health Services Research*, June 23: 203–35.

Keeler, E. B. and S. Cretin (1983). 'Discounting of Life-Saving and Other Non-Monetary Effects', *Management Science*, 29: 300–6.

Murray, C. J. L. (1994). 'Quantifying the Burden of Disease: The Technical Basis for Disability-Adjusted Life Years', in C. J. L. Murray and A. D. Lopez (eds.), *Global Comparative Assessments in the Health Sector: Disease Burden, Expenditures and Intervention Packages*. Geneva: World Health Organization.

Murray, C. J. L. (1996). 'Rethinking DALYs', in *The Global Burden of Disease: A Comprehensive Assessment of Mortality and Disability From Disease, Injuries, and Risk Factors in 1990 and Projected to 2020*. Geneva: World Health Organization.

Nord, E. (1993). 'The Trade-Off Between Severity of Illness and Treatment Effect in Cost-Value Analysis of Health Care', *Health Policy*, 24: 227–38.

—— (1999). *Cost-Value Analysis in Health Care: Making Sense of QALYs*. New York: Cambridge University Press.

Parfit, D. (1991). 'Equality or Priority', *The Lindley Lecture*. Copyright: Department of Philosophy, University of Kansas.

Torrance, G. W. et al. (1992). 'Multi Attribute Preference Functions for a Comprehensive Health Status Classification System', *Working Paper No. 92–18*. Hamilton, Ontario: McMaster University, Center for Health Economics and Policy Analysis.

Walzer, M. (1983). *Spheres of Justice*. New York: Basic Books.

Ware, J. E. and D. C. Sherbourne (1992). 'The MOS 36-item Short Form Health Survey', *Medical Care*, 30: 473–83.

WHO (World Health Organization) (1980). *International Classification of Impairments, Disabilities and Handicaps*. Geneva: World Health Organization.

Williams, A. (1997). 'Intergenerational Equity: An Exploration of the "Fair Innings" Argument', *Health Economics*, 6(2): 117–32.

World Bank (1993). *World Development Report 1993: Investing in Health*. New York and Oxford: Oxford University Press.

11

Deciding Whom to Help, Health-Adjusted Life Years and Disabilities

FRANCES M. KAMM

In this chapter, I discuss how to allocate scarce resources related to health. In particular, I am concerned with health care resources. I discuss microallocation problems, for example, giving a health care resource to one person rather than another, and also macroallocation problems, for example, allocating money to production of one health care service or product rather than another. In Section 11.1, I describe the possible theoretical foundations for assigning weights to some factors and not to others when allocating.[1] Ultimately, I present in outline a decision procedure for allocating. In Section 11.2, I consider several problems that arise in allocating resources using quality- and disability-adjusted life years (QALYs and DALYs) if we take seriously principles of allocation presented in Section 11.1. One such problem is whether to treat the disabled as equal candidates with the non-disabled for scarce life-saving resources. I first offer the Principle of Irrelevant Goods as an explanation of why the disabled and non-disabled should be treated equally. In Section 11.3, I consider the possibility that in some cases, ignoring the Principle of Irrelevant Goods would not necessarily involve invidious discrimination. I try to offer an alternative principle, the Principle of Irrelevant Identity, that distinguishes discriminatory from nondiscriminatory conduct.

11.1. BRIEF OVERVIEW OF MORAL ISSUES IN ALLOCATION

Suppose we are dealing with two-way conflict cases between potential recipients of a scarce resource. When there are an equal number of people in conflict who stand to lose the same if not aided and gain the same if aided (and all other morally relevant factors, such as how badly off each will be, are the same),

---

[1] Section 1, for the most part, summarises and tries to make more accessible some points I made in detail elsewhere (Kamm 1993). Parts are excerpted from Kamm (2000).

fairness dictates giving each side an equal chance for the resource by using a random decision procedure.

But there may be a conflict situation in which different numbers of relevantly similar people are on either side and they stand to lose and gain the same thing. The following Aggregation Argument for Best Outcomes applied in a micro life-and-death case tells us that it is a better outcome if more are helped: (1) It is worse for both B and C to die than for only B to die; (2) A world in which A dies and B survives is just as bad, from an impartial point of view, as a world in which B dies and A survives. Given (2), we can substitute A for B on one side of the moral equation in (1) and get that it is worse if B and C die than if A dies.

But even if it would be a worse outcome from an impartial perspective that B and C die than that A dies, that does not necessarily mean that it is right for us to save B and C rather than A. We cannot automatically assume it is morally permissible to produce the best outcome, for doing so may violate justice or fairness.

Here is an argument against its being unjust or unfair to save the greater number in this case. The Balancing Argument claims that in a conflict, justice demands that in this case each person on one side should have his or her interests balanced against those of one person on the opposing side; those that are not balanced out in the larger group help determine that the larger group should be saved. On this view, justice does not here conflict with producing the most good.

How might we extend these principles to conflicts when the individuals are not equally needy? Consider a case where the interests of two people, conflict, B and C, with the interests of one, A. The potential loss (ten years of life) of A is equal to the potential loss of B, and they will both be equally badly off (dead). The potential loss and bad fate of the second person of the pair is not very significant, for example, his sore throat will not be cured. To take away A's 50 per cent chance of having ten years of life rather than death in order to increase overall good produced by saving B and gaining the marginal benefit of a sore throat cure fails to show adequate respect for A who could be saved. This is because from his or her *personal point of view*, he or she is not indifferent between his or her being the one getting to live the ten years and someone else getting it. This form of reasoning I am here using to justify *not* maximising the good gives equal consideration from an impartial point of view to each individual's partial point of view, so it combines objective and subjective perspectives. Hence, I call it *Sobjectivity*. It accounts for why we should give fair chances. It also implies that certain extra goods (like the throat cure) can sometimes be morally irrelevant; I call this the Principle of Irrelevant Good. Whether a good is irrelevant is context dependent. Curing a sore throat is morally irrelevant when others' lives are at stake, but not when others' earaches are. The Sore Throat Case shows that we must refine the claim that what we owe each person is to balance her interests against the equal interests of an opposing person and let the remainder help determine the outcome. Sometimes the remainder is not determinative. Further, so long as the loss and the fate that person A or person B can avoid is as described, *no number of the small losses occurring in a great number of different people should be aggregated on B's side* so as to outweigh A's equal chance of avoiding the large loss.

But suppose the additional lesser loss is someone's losing a leg. We should save a person's life when he can then live ten years rather than save someone else's leg when these are the *only* morally relevant choices. However, perhaps it is permissible to together save one person's life and a second person's leg rather than to give a third person an equal chance at having his life saved. This might be because only one life will be saved no matter what we do and the loss of a leg is a large loss. This would be evidence that giving someone *his equal chance for life* should not receive as much weight from the impartial point of view as saving a life when we would otherwise save no one.

So far, I have been discussing decision procedures that are consistent with what philosophers call 'pairwise comparison'. That is, we check to see that for everyone who will be badly off on one side that there is someone who will be equally badly off on the other side before we consider weighing in those who will be less badly off to determine which side gets aided. This is one way of being sure we help the worst off people first (at least when we can make a significant difference to their fate). But it is possible that principles which involve such pairwise comparison are requirements of fairness in choosing whom to aid only in micro situations (e.g. in the emergency room). To make *macro* decisions, for example, whether to invest in research to cure a disease that will kill a few people or research to cure a disease that will only wither an arm in many, we might have another principle. It permits aggregation of significant (though not insignificant) bad fates to many people to outweigh even worse fates in a few, even though no individual person in the larger group will be as badly off as each individual in the smaller group will be. As such, it does not give absolute priority to helping the worst off. As the Principle of Irrelevant Goods emphasised, whether a lesser bad fate is significant, and hence whether its occurrence in many people is aggregatable, is judged relative to the nature of the worse fate. Hence, determining if a lesser bad fate is aggregatable over many is context-dependent. On this view, the important point is that whether a fate should be aggregated over people to weigh against a worse fate in others is *not* merely a function of how many people suffer it, but also of how bad it is relative to the size of the worse fate. There are no number of headaches such that we should prevent them rather than certainly save a few lives.

Notice this may seem to raise a problem of intransitivity: relative to n, y is a significantly lesser bad fate. So at the macro level, it may be better to prevent many people from y than to save a few from n. But relative to y, z is a significant lesser bad fate, and so it would be better to save a *great* many from z *rather than save* many from y. But suppose all three sets—those suffering n, y and z—are present together and transitivity of 'better than' holds. Then it seems it would be better to save a great many suffering z than a few suffering n. Yet, it may be that relative to n, z is not a significant less bad fate, since 'significant' is context relative and so is not transitive.

My suggestion for dealing with this problem is as follows: if we can save a few suffering from *n*, we may save many from suffering *y* instead, but we should not go so far as to save a great many from suffering *z*. (This is so on the continuing assumption that the people are alike in all morally relevant respects besides these different fates.) This is true, even though if some suffering *n* were not present, we should save a great many from *z* rather than save many from *y*. This is because which outcome is better and what we should do can be dependent on the alternatives we can bring about.

A theory of the fair distribution of scarce resources should also tell us if certain characteristics that one candidate for the resources has to a greater degree than another are morally relevant to deciding who gets the resource. I call this the problem of allocation when there is *intrapersonal aggregation*, because one candidate has characteristics the other has *plus* more. We have already considered principles that apply when the additional goods we can achieve, if we help one of the worse off people, are *distributed over* several people. The question arises whether we can revise these principles to apply when additional goods we can achieve are *concentrated* in one person rather than another.

A system I suggest for evaluating candidates for a resource who differ intrapersonally starts off with only three factors—need, urgency, and outcome—but it could add other factors later. Urgency is here defined as how badly off someone's life will go if he is not helped. 'Need' is here defined as how badly someone's life *will have gone* if he is not helped. 'Outcome' is here defined as the difference in expected outcome produced by the resource relative to the expected outcome if one is not helped; that is, the benefit someone will get from the resource. The neediest people may not be the most urgent. Suppose C will die in a month at age sixty-five unless helped *now* and D will die in a year at age twenty unless helped *now*. I suggest that, other things being equal between them, D is less urgent but needier, since one's life will have gone much worse if one dies at 20 rather than at 65. (This does not mean we should always help the neediest; for example, if we could only extend the younger life to age twenty-two but could give the sixty-five-year-old ten years more, this would be a reason to help the sixty-five-year-old.)

(Notice that there is a different sense of urgency in which both C and D are equally urgent, namely they require care just as soon—*now*—in order to be helped.[2] I have chosen to use 'urgent' to refer to how bad one's prospects are; I shall use 'urgent-C' (short for 'urgent care') if necessary to refer to how soon treatment is needed.)

In thinking about how urgent or needy someone is, or how good an outcome is, we must think how badly or well will life go, or have gone, *in what ways*? In microallocation of health services, I believe we should be concerned with the *health*-way rather than overall well-being (including economic and

---

[2] As pointed out to me by Derek Parfit.

cultural factors). This means that at the micro level, health is treated as a separate sphere of justice.[3] So, if E would be in worse health than F, the fact that F would be economically much worse off than E is not a reason to say F is more urgent than E is and treat F with the health care resource. But suppose E's health overall has been painlessly much worse than F's in his life (e.g. limited mobility), but F now faces a lot of pain and E just a little. It is possible that we should consider all *dissimilar* aspects of ill health and help E, so that he will not have had to lead a much worse life healthwise than F. On the other hand, since we can only help E's future in a small way and can do nothing to undo his past, the much greater good we can do for F's future may be determinative. (Some may find the judgement that we should help E more convincing when we ignore E's past but decide based on the fact that he but not F *will* also have limited mobility *in the future*. Some may think it correct to consider only how much pain each will have in the future or will have had overall, since some part of this pain is the aspect of well-being we can affect now.)

By contrast, at the macro level, when deciding whether to invest in providing one health service or another, it might be that we should make an *all-things-considered judgement* about how well-off people have been or will be. That is, the way in which people have and will fare in health may be considered together with the way they have or will fare economically and culturally. This means health would not be treated as a *separate sphere of justice* at the macro level. This has important implications for the very idea of 'health equity'. Suppose, for example, that we can invest in curing a disease that causes the poor to die at age seventy or a disease that causes the rich to die at age sixty. If we care about equality, we might chose to invest in the former, since having a nicer life might compensate the rich for having a shorter one; things will be overall more equal if the poor at least live longer, so long as their lives are worth living. So, *equity of health—getting the just or fair amount of it—is not inconsistent with inequality of (prospect) for it.*

The alternative is to treat health as a separate sphere, even at the macro level, in the way we treat liberal freedoms. We would not consider a person who lacked a right to free speech that others had to be adequately compensated by the fact that he has more money than they have. If health is a separate sphere, we would have to compare how people are doing just along the health dimension separately, even at the macro level.

Let us return to need in the microallocation context. To consider how much weight to give to need, we hold the two other factors of outcome and urgency constant and imagine two candidates who differ only in neediness. One argument for taking differential need into account is fairness: give to those who, if not helped, will have had less of the good (e.g. life) that our resource can provide (at least if they are equal on other health dimensions) before giving to those who will have had more of it even if they are not helped. Fairness

---

[3] For the idea of separate spheres of justice, see Walzer (1983).

is a value that depends on comparisons between people. But even if we do not compare candidates, it can simply be of greater moral value to give a certain unit of life to a person who has had less of life.

But need will matter more the more absolutely and comparatively needy a candidate is, and some differences in need may be governed by a Principle of Irrelevant Need, which implies that relative to a context, some differences in need are morally irrelevant. This is especially so when each candidate is absolutely needy, a big gain for each is at stake, and if the needier person is helped he will wind up having more of the good (e.g. a longer life) than the person who was originally less needy than he. Need may also play a different role depending on whether life is at stake or quality of life is at stake, for a low quality of life can be less bad for someone than his dying. When it is, we deprive the needy of less if we do not give them priority when quality of life is at stake, and of more if we do not give them priority when life is at stake.

Suppose there is conflict between helping the neediest and helping the most urgent (where we are giving the same benefit). I claim that when there is true scarcity, it can be more important to help the neediest than the urgent. If scarcity is only temporary, the urgent-C should be helped first, since the others will be helped eventually anyway.[4]

Still, there are constraints on the relevance of need in a correct theory of distribution. For example, giving a resource to the person who will have had less overall of the good it can provide may be impermissible if it fails to respect the rights of each person. Consider another context: if two people have a human right to free speech, how long someone's right has already been respected may be irrelevant in deciding whom to help retain free speech. If having health or life for a number of years were a human right, it might not be appropriate to ration resources on the basis of the degree to which people's rights have already been met or on the basis of whether they had more of other goods. On this view, how much life one had already would not be a reason for rationing on the basis of age, so long as one had not reached the level guaranteed by right. (There might still be other indirect reasons for rationing on the basis of age, for example, if the goods possible at a certain age were not very valuable to the person who will receive them.)

Now we come to outcome. Some might consider all effects of a resource for determining outcome. I suggest, at least in micro contexts: (1) Effects on third parties whom a resource helps only indirectly should be given less weight than its direct effects, even though these are effects on health. For example, if we face a choice between saving a doctor and a teacher, the fact that the doctor will be irreplaceable in saving lives should not mean that all the lives he will save are counted on his side against the teacher. (Hence, this goes beyond the view that health effects belong to a separate sphere.) It might be suggested that this is true because the person who is not selected for aid when he does not

---

[4] In Kamm (1993) I did not distinguish urgency from urgency-C when I claimed that in temporary scarcity, the urgent should be treated before the needier.

positively affect others is being inappropriately evaluated from only an instrumental point of view, and not also as an end-in-himself. But consider the following case: we have a scarce resource to distribute and if we give it to A, he can then also carry it to another person, C, who needs our resource. B cannot do this. In this case, it is permissible, I think, to select A over B, excluding B since he cannot be instrumentally useful. This is because it helps us to better serve those who directly need our resource. Hence (surprisingly), it seems it is not essentially distinguishing persons on the basis of their instrumental role that determines if our behaviour is objectionable, but whether we are using our resource for its best direct effects. (2) Some differences in outcome between candidates may be irrelevant because achieving them is not the goal of the particular 'sphere' which controls the resource (e.g. that only one potential recipient in the health care sphere will write a novel if he receives a scarce drug should not count in favour of his getting it).

Other differences in expected outcome between candidates may be covered by the Principle of Irrelevant Goods, even if they are relevant to the sphere. For example, relative to the fact that each person stands to avoid death and live for ten years, that one person can get a somewhat better quality of life or an additional year of life should not determine who is helped, given that each wants what he or she can get. One explanation for this is that *what both are capable of achieving (ten years) is the part of the outcome about which each reasonably cares most in the context*, and each wants to be the one to survive. The extra good is frosting on the cake. The fact that someone might accept an additional risk of death (as in surgery) to achieve the 'cake plus frosting' for himself or herself does not necessarily imply that it is correct to impose an additional risk of death on one person so that another person, who stands to get the greater good, has a greater chance to live.

However, in life and death decisions, any *significant* difference between two people in expected life years may play a role in selecting whom to help. This result is analogous to the claim that if we could save x's life or else y's plus z's leg, we should do the latter. Still, because the large additional benefit would be concentrated in the same person who would already be benefited by having her life saved for at least the same period as the other candidate, it should count for less in determining who gets the resource than it does when the additional benefit is distributed to a third person. This is on account of fairness and the diminishing moral value of providing an additional benefit to someone who would already be greatly benefited. Large differences in expected quality of life among candidates for a resource may also count in situations where improving quality of life is the point of the resource.

Between the irrelevant differences in goods and those that are large enough to outweigh other factors might be differences in outcome that should be treated by giving people chances in proportion to the good of the differential outcome.

What if taking care of the neediest or most urgent conflicts with producing the best relevant difference in outcome? Rather than always favouring the worst off, we might assign multiplicative factors in accord with need and urgency by which we multiply the expected outcome of the neediest and urgent. These factors represent the greater moral significance of a given outcome going to the neediest (or most urgent), but the non-neediest could still get a resource if his or her expected differential outcome was very large. Furthermore, doing a significant amount to raise those who are very badly off in absolute terms to an appropriate minimal level of well-being might have lexical priority over even an enormous improvement in those already better off.

My views on outcome, need, and urgency can be summarised in an *outcome modification procedure for allocation*. We first assign points for each candidate's differential expected outcome. We then check the absolute level of need and urgency of candidates. If some are below a certain minimal level of well-being and the good we can do would significantly raise them toward the minimal level, these receive the resource. For those above this minimal level of well-being, we assign multiplicative factors for their need and urgency in accordance with the moral importance of those factors relative to each other and relative to outcome. We multiply the outcome points by these factors. The candidate with a sufficiently high point score gets the resource. If the difference is too small to be morally relevant, we give equal chances. If it is in between, chances in proportion to the score might be suitable.[5]

11.2. SOME REASONS FOR IGNORING DISABILITY WHEN ALLOCATING

QALYs and DALYs are used to measure the impact illness has on someone in terms of both morbidity and mortality; they also measure the impact of care on someone in terms of reducing both morbidity and mortality. The theory is that we can do more than merely count the number of years that will (we expect) be gained as a result of health intervention. We also count how good these years will be. (Note that even counting years is a step beyond merely considering whether a life has been saved but not considering *for how long it will be saved*.) So we may multiply the number of years of life by the quality or disability of each year. Alternatively, we may determine how effective aid is by considering how badly someone's life would have gone—or as it is said how disabled he would have been—without the intervention. In this way, we see how much reduction in such disabled years we produce by the intervention. We aim to increase QALYs and decrease DALYs.[6]

---

[5] Perhaps this can still be only a rough guide where more than two options are present. This could be because what we ought to do is a function of what the alternatives are, and so it may not always be right to produce what gives the higher score. For example, in the case I discussed on pp. 227–8 involving one person who will lose n, many who will lose x and yet more who will lose z, I argue that we should help prevent z rather than x if it were only a choice between x and z, but should help x if it were a choice between all three.

[6] The reduction of DALYs should not, of course, be taken to mean that we merely eliminate the person with many DALYs.

How would the use of DALYs bear on the allocation of health resources to disabled people (who, I assume, have physical impairments)? DALYs evaluation of their lives could make it clear that their lives are worse than the lives of the non-disabled, and so health resources should be directed to curing or compensating for their impairment. But if we cannot cure, so that their lives are still higher on DALYs ratings, how will they fare in the competition with the non-disabled for other health care resources? Even if we cure their other illnesses or save their lives, we cannot thereby produce a person with as low a rating for DALYs as if we treat the non-disabled. Our outcomes can never be as good, holding other factors constant. If it is not, in general, unfair to consider outcomes in deciding where to allocate resources, is it permissible to 'discriminate' in such decisions against the disabled? This is the issue with which I shall be concerned.

Consider the following scenario: one person is on island A, and another person is on island B. They share all the same properties, except that one just recently lost a hand and the other did not. We can save the life of either one but not both. Each will be as badly off as the other if we do not help him (dead). But if we help the person without the hand, we do not reduce the badness (the DALYs) as much. (Call this the Islands Case.) I think it is morally wrong to decide whom to aid on this ground. We cannot rely on the principle of giving weight to the worst off to account for this conclusion, since each would, by hypothesis, be as badly off as the other if not aided. However, the Principle of Irrelevant Goods, which I described in Section 11.1, can account for the right decision.

The explanation of the principle in the Islands Case may be the same as described earlier: what both people are capable of achieving is the part of the outcome about which each reasonably cares most, or put differently, what is reasonably held to be most important to each person can be had by either— long life saved with good quality of life. Furthermore, we should take seriously from an *objective* point of view the fact that each person, from his *subjective* perspective, wants to be the one to survive. Fairness may require, therefore, that we not deprive either of his equal chance for the great good of extended survival for the sake of having the additional benefit of a hand in one person. This benefit is irrelevant in this context, though perhaps not in another. This is especially true when that one person who would get the additional benefit is someone who would already be getting the other great benefit of additional life. (That is, it is a case of a good concentrated in one of the two rather than dispersed over a third person.) I shall call this the Major Part Argument.

On the basis of this case, we can see that it is compatible with recognising that not having a hand makes a life worse and makes an outcome worse to think that, relative to the question of whose life we should save, it could be a morally irrelevant consideration. Hence, targeting funds to replace a missing hand because life without it is worse than life with it is not inconsistent with giving equal weight to save the lives of the disabled and the non-disabled. This is contrary to what a simple use of DALYs in distributing scarce resources would predict.

I applied the Principle of Irrelevant Goods to the Islands Case as an explanation of why we ought not to decide whose life to save in that case on the basis of the fact that one person is disabled and the other is not. Does the principle, however, truly account for the range of our judgements about when disabilities should make a difference to whom we help?

Consider a case involving a larger disability. We must choose between saving the life of a paraplegic (QALYs 0.5) and a person who would be saved to a perfectly healthy life (QALYs 1). Suppose we agree that the paraplegic is living a worse life than a non-paralysed person who merely has to wear glasses. Hence, if the issue were whether to give him resources to cure his paraplegia or to provide some other equally costly services to cure nearsightedness, we should treat the paraplegic. That is, we move someone up from 0.5 (given some significant change) before we move someone from 0.999 up to 1. This is consistent with the claim that when the two people's lives are at stake, the difference in their expected quality of life can be morally irrelevant in deciding whom to aid. That is, when the prospect each faces is to fall to 0, it is a significant good merely to achieve 0.5, and perhaps a person should not be deprived of the equal chance he wants to get that merely because someone else could achieve that plus an additional benefit.

Why might this be so? Can we say, in this case, as we could in the Islands Case, that what each gets is the *major part of what both* stand to get, and the difference is frosting on the cake? No, for if one person can be saved to perfect health and this difference is (assumed to be) equivalent to another 0.5, this means that 0.5 is *not* the major part of 1. Of course, one must have traversed from 0 to 0.5 before he can go further, so 0.5 is a prior good in that sense, But we cannot say that there is diminishing marginal good in going further than 0.5, if reaching the top is specifically ranked as twice as good as being at 0.5.[7] Certainly, it would be reasonable to take a much larger risk of falling from 0.5 to 0 in order to achieve a life ranked at 1, than it would be reasonable to take to go from 0.5 to 0.6 (achieving mere frosting on the cake).

An alternative explanation is that it may be morally more important to give someone the basic goods that help him avoid the worst evils and *make a life one worth living* than to give him the goods which admittedly double the value of his life. Analogously, it may be *morally* more important to give someone their first $500 than to give them whatever amount of additional money doubles the monetary value of their life. Hence, without claiming that a life QALY-rated at 1 provides less than twice the good as one ranked at 0.5, we can claim that moving someone from 0 to 0.5 is *morally* more important than moving him from 0.5 to 1. Another way of putting this point might be that it is having a life worth

---

[7] This is compatible with its taking many more goods or avoidance of evils to go from 0.5 to 1 than it took to go from 0 to 0.5. At this level, there may be diminishing marginal good. This is analogous to its taking only $500 to reach level 0.5 of well-being, but $1,500 to reach to level 1 of well-being, because once one has $500, it takes much more than an additional $500 to make one twice as well-off.

living that is of crucial significance, and if paraplegics can have this, they have all that is relevant to deciding who lives. Hence, I call this alternative argument for giving the disabled and non-disabled equal chances the Moral Importance Argument.

Another argument for ignoring the move from 0.5 to 1 is as follows: suppose one can only have 0.5 and not 1, and the alternative is 0 (death), which is very bad. One may reasonably want 0.5 as much as one would want 1 if one could have it. So, for example, given that 0.5 is all that one can have and 0 is very bad, one might reasonably do as much to achieve 0.5 (e.g. spend as much money, suffer as much) as one would do to achieve 1 if one could have it. This is consistent with the willingness to even risk losing 0.5 and falling to 0 for a chance at 1. That is, the fact that one would risk 0 to get 1 does not show that one would be more likely to risk 0 in other pursuits (e.g. risky activities such as skiing) because one would only be losing a life rated 0.5 instead of 1. Notice that some lives are worth living (e.g. an additional three conscious and happy months of life), but are not goods sufficient to make it reasonable for the person who would live it to sacrifice as much to save it as to save a long life rated 1.[8] So, in this argument, it is not merely having a life worth living that is crucial. I call this the Sufficient Only Option Argument.

What it implies is that when 0.5 by itself is compared with 0, it is worth x (some sacrifice), and when 1 by itself is compared with 0, it too is worth x. This suggests that relative to 0, $0.5 = 1$. But that does not mean that 0.5 is equivalent to 1 *per se*. For example, we could give up 0.5 for 1 and also risk going from 0.5 to 0 to get 1. This argument may seem to generate an intransitivity, that is, $x = 0.5$, $x = 1$, $-(0.5 = 1)$, but it is explicable because of the effects of different contexts in which different alternatives for action are available.

Notice that the Sufficient Only Option Argument implies that a paraplegic could reasonably choose to risk death in order to get a better life as a non-paralysed person though he will not care about this life any more than he cares about the life he already has. This shows that 'if one can have only x, one cares about it as much as one would care about y if one had it' is not equivalent to 'one cares to have x as much as one cares to have y'. All this may seem paradoxical, yet I think it is true.[9] (I have said—and those who wish to employ QALYs and DALYs note that the data show—that disabled individuals might be willing to risk losing life years for improved quality of life or reduced disabilities). So, for example, suppose each person in a society is willing to take a 5 per cent risk of death (thereby risking losing, let us say, twenty years of life) in order to have a 95 per cent chance of being cured of paraplegia. From such data—which we can refer to as individual welfare functions—some would like to derive implications for society as a whole—deriving a social

[8] I owe this point to David Sussman.
[9] I thank Susan Wolf, David Sussman, and other members of Philamore for discussion of this point.

welfare function. So some might think that the above data from the individual cases would validate the conclusion that as a society, it is permissible to allow five people to die so that ninety-five people can be cured of paralysis when the 100 are otherwise relevantly similar for moral purposes. But is this a correct argument for tradeoffs between people? When an individual takes a chance, no one may die and he may benefit. Indeed, he takes the risk hoping this is so. And when each person in the society thinks of the gamble in his case, he may also imagine that he will not die and hope to benefit. But in the group, some people will certainly die (given that it is large enough) and others will be benefited. Each person hopes that this death will be someone else's. Perhaps these are morally significant reasons not to derive the social welfare function from the combination of individual welfare functions. It might be argued that we will get the morally wrong principle of social justice, if we think that *ex ante* reasoning behind a veil of ignorance involves each person thinking of himself as having a possibility of occupying each outcome-position—for example, ninety-five chances to be one of the healthy, and five to be one of the sick. Rather, behind a veil of ignorance each person should take seriously the fates of the persons who will actually occupy each of the outcome-positions, including death. I leave the issue unreasolved here.

If either the Sufficient Only Option or the Moral Importance Argument is true, the Principle of Irrelevant Goods is supported and can be used to argue for not discriminating in allocation against those with large disabilities, even if the Major Part Argument does not apply.

These results of the Principle of Irrelevant Goods are consistent with what is sometimes understood as the correct account of a nondiscriminatory policy: If a treatment whose aim is to correct a particular problem is equally successful in a disabled and non-disabled person, the difference in outcome due to the disability is irrelevant. Call this the Treatment Aim Principle. But the Principle of Irrelevant Goods also implies that some differences in the degree to which a particular problem is treated could be morally irrelevant and that successful treatment of the problem in someone who cannot have a sufficient good outcome (e.g. he is permanently comatose) is ruled out.

But notice, if the Principle of Irrelevant Goods says we should not prefer saving an unparalysed person to a paraplegic person (other things being equal), it would imply that we should not prefer saving a paraplegic, who, as a side effect of life-saving treatment, will also be able to walk again, as opposed to a paraplegic who will just as successfully be saved but will remain paraplegic. That is, if we rely on the Principle of Irrelevant Goods to argue for giving equal status to significantly disabled and non-disabled candidates, it also implies no role for big differences in expected outcome among equally disabled candidates. It also implies no role for such differences in outcome between equally non-disabled candidates—so if one unparalysed person would become paraplegic if we saved his life but another would not, this should make no difference in whom we choose to save. (Call these Switch Cases.) Is this correct?

11.3. TAKING ACCOUNT OF DISABILITY WITHOUT DISCRIMINATING

These last examples raise the following possibility: (1) Sometimes a sizeable extra good, x, that we can produce in the outcome if we treat one person rather than another, can be morally relevant in deciding whom to help. (2) Yet, it also might be suggested that if candidates for treatment who present themselves already have this difference, x, between them, and this is why it shows up in the outcome we can produce, it should be morally irrelevant to deciding whom we treat. The *Principle of Irrelevant Goods* cannot account for the simultaneous truth of (1) and (2), when non-treatment would result in the same fate in each candidate in (1) and (2) (e.g. death or dialysis).

What proponents of the view involving claims (1) and (2) need is a principle that will explain why the fact that a person is disabled should be irrelevant in deciding whom to help and if it were relevant this would be (invidiously) discriminatory against the disabled, but the presence of a disability or non-disability in an outcome can sometimes be morally relevant and non-discriminatory in deciding whom to help. Call this the *Asymmetry Problem*. A principle that explains it would say why it is permissible to save in a forced choice the life of the paraplegic who will, through the procedure that saves him, become non-paraplegic and not treat the non-paraplegic who would, through the procedure that saves him, become paraplegic. The principle that explains it would also offer a different understanding of discrimination from the Treatment Aim Principle. For even when we could successfully treat each patient for what the treatment aims at, one would be preferred. Even someone who thought the difference, x, in outcomes should never matter might be interested in seeing if we can distinguish a *discrimination objection* to counting x from a more general objection to counting such a difference in outcomes based on the Principle of Irrelevant Goods. My claim will be that sometimes, even if we violated the Principle of Irrelevant Goods (and the Treatment Aim Principle), we would not be engaged in discriminatory conduct. Our conduct might be wrong but not because it involved discrimination.

It is important to realise that the Asymmetry Problem does not depend on another asymmetry which is sometimes discussed, that is, the fact that prior to being disabled, people rate the disabled state as much worse than people do who are disabled. It might be thought that it is because the disabled person who comes for treatment rates his life equal to the non-disabled but the non-disabled rates the same disability in his future as very bad that the Asymmetry Problem arises, at least when treatment would make a non-disabled candidate disabled.[10] But this is not so. For purposes of argument, *I am holding constant the negative value of the disability in those already disabled and those who*

---

[10] This explanation would not help with the case in which the paraplegic will become non-paralysed.

will be newly disabled. I am assuming that the life of the already-disabled is worse than the life of the non-disabled, other things equal—that is *the reason why* a new disability should be avoided—and yet it could be wrong to treat differently the non-disabled and the already disabled.

A principle that can account for the responses I have described in the preceding cases can be referred to as the Causative Principle. It tells us to decide which people to help based only on the difference we can make to their situations, not on the difference they bring to the situation. More precisely, the Causative Principle is concerned with the differential effectiveness of our treatment for avoiding the less-valued state or producing the more valued state. It tells us to ignore differences that arise in any other way, whether because the less-valued state inheres in the person, or will arise because of what inheres in him, or even will arise from causes outside of him other than the treatment. (For example, if we know a criminal will do something to one unparalysed person to make him paraplegic if he lives, we should ignore it. For convenience, I will just say it tells us to ignore who the people are.) The Causative Principle can be combined with a limited use of the Principle of Irrelevant Goods in that some relatively small differences we cause are still morally irrelevant.

A proposed justification for the Causative Principle is that when outcomes are affected by who a person is and/or by what we do, counting only effects of what we do is consistent with respect for persons, at least so long as the effect is significant. Counting the difference the people themselves bring is not consistent with respect for persons, except when the difference involves a life below a certain minimum (e.g. not worth living, not worth taking risks for). We can reasonably value paraplegia less than non-paraplegia as a state, and count it when we produce it, without treating a person who is already in the state differently. This is like hating the sin, but not the sinner. Admittedly, though, valuing the non-paraplegic state more than the paraplegic state can have a worse consequence for one person (whom we care about equally) than for another. For if we use these values to choose whom to aid when we cause the difference, rather than giving people an equal chance at treatment, the one who will become or remain paraplegic (in the two types of Switch Cases) will definitely not be saved in the contest. (This contrasts with disvaluing the paraplegic state and so choosing *not to create* a paraplegic person. Here no person will exist who can be negatively affected by our choice.) The Causative Principle implies that we are entitled to seek better outcomes when we can cause them; when we do so, we are not being unfair, as we would be if we merely took advantage of what is indepnedent of our doing.

The previous discussion implicitly gestures towards *three possible understandings of (invidious) discriminatory conduct*. The *first* possible understanding tells us that acting in any way on the differential value attributed to being abled or being disabled is discriminatory. But this would imply that common surgeries undertaken to cure people of paraplegia are discriminatory conduct if we perform them because we think it is better to be unparalysed than paralysed. I believe we should reject the first suggestion. The *second* possible understanding tells us that acting on the differential value attributed to being abled or disabled when this makes the person who would be disabled worse off than he might otherwise have been (in a coin toss) is discriminatory. This understanding of discrimination would rule out the Causative Principle. If we think this is wrong, we could endorse a *third* possible understanding of discrimination: It is discriminatory to act on the differential value attributed to being abled or disabled, when this makes the disabled worse off than he might have been because of what he is or would be independent of what we do. (I shall add to this third understanding below and so consider this a tentative formulation.)

However, a problem arises for the Causative Principle. Suppose that if we save the paraplegic, we will also cure his paralysis, whereas if we save an unparalysed person we will just save his life there being no paralysis to cure. Here the outcomes are the same, but *we* produce a significantly larger difference if we treat the paraplegic person than if we treat the nonparalysed person. Our treatment is, in that sense, more effective with him. The Causative Principle, as presented above, therefore, tells us in a forced choice to save the paralysed person rather than the unparalysed. However, I think this is the wrong conclusion and there is no good reason for favouring one over the other, since the final outcomes are the same.

We would also do more harm in the life of an unparalysed person if we save her when we also cause her to be paralysed than we would do to an already paralysed person in saving him. The Causative Principle here tells us to favour treating the paralysed person, but I think there is no moral reason to do this, since the final outcomes are the same.

What can we substitute for the Causative Principle that accounts for all the cases? Here is a suggestion: The important point is that what the person is (consisting not only in what he is now but what he would become due to causes independent of us if he survives) should not determine whether he is saved, so long as the outcome that can come about through helping him is significant (e.g. a life for which it is reasonable to take important risks rather than saving someone already in a permanent coma). This does not mean that the differential outcome does not matter, only that we do not let the differences in what the person is independent of the change we make make a difference. This has two implications. When the outcomes expected in different individuals are different, to pay attention to anything but the causative difference we make would be to make the difference in them affect our decision whom to aid. Hence, we can abstract from who they are by attending to the causative component. Alternatively, we can imaginatively add the good property that one party is missing to his outcome (or subtract the good property the other party has from his outcome). But when the outcome we expect in different individuals is the *same*, to attend only to the causative difference we make (from how they were or would have been independent of us if alive) *results in the differences in who they are playing a role*. That is, when the bottom line is the same, paying attention to the difference we make is an indirect way of treating people differently on the basis of who they are. For if we need to do less to reach a given bottom line, that implies the person had more to begin with, and so the Causative Principle would say that we should not treat equally someone who had more to begin with. It holds against the person who is non-disabled the fact that he is non-disabled, since this is what makes there be less of a difference that we make in his being alive and non-disabled. If we do not want who the person is to count against or for him when outcomes are the same, we could add into our calculation the disability condition to one person who actually lacks it or take it away in our calculation from the other who actually has it. Then the causative difference we make would be the same in each. But we achieve the same result by just attending to the fact that the outcomes are the same.

Hence, treating persons so that who they are (their personal identity, but also more generally, what will happen to them independent of the change we make) does not count for or against them is the dominant point. This only sometimes commits us to the subsidiary Causative Principle. I shall describe the dominant point as the Principle of Irrelevant Identity.

It might be suggested that abstracting from the differences in what people are and will have independent of what we do for them is also one way of avoiding what I shall call *linkage*. Linkage means that what happens to me at t1 affects what will happen at t2. It accounts for those who have, getting more and those who do not have, not getting. If we wish, for example, to limit the bad further effects of some underserved bad thing having happened to someone, we could abstract from the immediate difference in persons made by that bad event and behave as though that difference were not there when making allocation decisions (so long as we can still provide a life that is sufficiently good).

There is reason to doubt, however, that the Principle of Irrelevant Identity is really a non-linkage principle. This is because distinguishing between what the person is, and what results we will produce abstracted from what he is should not, I believe, prevent our attending to results that occur *due to what he is*. We should, if we wish not to discriminate invidiously, abstract from the disability he brings to the treatment situation as a *component of his life*, not from its *causal* role. So, for example, suppose that if we save a haemophiliac, he will remain haemophilic and live five years, but if we save a non-haemophiliac, he will remain non-haemophiliac and live for ten years. Assume they are alike in all other morally relevant respects. Even if the fewer years alive we can expect from the haemophiliac are entirely due to the fact that he is haemophilic, it need not be discriminatory to take them into account in the allocation decision. This is linkage. Yet, taking account of haemophilia's effects (its causal role) on life span is consistent with not attending to the intrinsic properties of haemophilia (its role as a component in the lived life, for example, needing blood products, being in more pain, and whatever else characterises the life of the haemophiliac during the years he lives) in deciding how to allocate.[11] Obviously, to make this

---

[11] How long someone will live is not a quality of a life such that someone might say we are discriminating against the short-lived, at least when we are deciding so as to determine whether there will be 'long' or short life.

account work, more would have to be done to distinguish the characteristics of a condition from its effects. One cannot just identify effects as those things not distinctive to that condition (e.g. not living long has many causes), because characteristics nondistinctive of a condition can be intrinsic to it.

The distinction between the purely causal role and the component role of the properties the person's life has independent of what we do to him is also crucial in answering one potential objection to the Principle of Irrelevant Identity.[12] It may be said, if our treatment cures paraplegia in addition to saving a life only in P1, it must because of some difference between P1 and P2, for example, an allergic reaction in P2 blocking a cure. Therefore, to let the difference in outcome count makes the difference between people count, and is that not contrary to the Principle of Irrelevant Identity? But, I would argue, there can be a moral difference between counting against someone the allergy's intrinsic properties as a *component* of the life and counting its *causal* role. Only the former constitutes discrimination on grounds of the allergy; it would be treating people differently because we dislike allergies per se. That we are not holding the disability against someone as a component of the lived life is further reinforced by considering a case where something that we agree *improves* a life when considered as its component has a bad effect. For example, suppose hardiness adds positively to a life, and yet hardiness is constituted by a protein that interacts badly with our life-saving treatment and so causes paraplegia. Ignoring hardiness as a good component and so not discriminating in favour of the hardy would be consistent with attending to its purely causal role. Deciding not to help the hardier person because of the causal effects of hardiness would not constitute discrimination against him on grounds of his hardiness.

Given this distinction between causal and component role, we can revise the third understanding of discrimination that I described above (p. 239), so that it is consistent with the Principle of Irrelevant Identity: It is invidiously discriminatory to act on the differential component value attributed to being abled or disabled when this makes the disabled or abled worse off than he might have been because of what he is or would be independent of what we do.

Can we summarise this discussion of principles as a decision procedure? Here is one attempt:

1. Check the level to which you can bring someone relative to another.
2. Check to see if, in reaching this level, counting anyone's starting point (or factor other than what we do) would make it work (as a component feature) in favour of or against him relative to others.
3. If the answer to (2) is no, deciding whom to help by differences in level of well being will not involve discrimination.
4. If nondiscrimination is all that matters morally (i.e. if nondiscrimination alone stands in the way of producing best outcomes), decide by (1), (2), and (3).

---

[12] The objection was raised by Douglas MacLean and John Broome.

This leaves it open that differences in outcome should not matter because they are morally irrelevant goods. Indeed, my conclusion is that while it may be wrong to ignore the Principle of Irrelevant Goods, doing so may not always involve discrimination. Hence, some complaints on behalf of the disabled may have to appeal to the Principal of Irrelevant Goods rather than to discrimination.[13,14,15]

References

Kamm, F. M. (1993). *Morality/Mortality. Volume One. Death and Whom to Save From It.* Oxford: Oxford University Press.

——(2000). 'Nonconsequentialism,' in H. Lafollette (ed.), *Blackwell's Guide to Ethical Theory.* Oxford: Blackwell.

——(2002). 'Health and Equity,' in Murray, C. J. L. et al. (eds.) *Summary Measures of Population Health: Concepts, Ethics, Measurement and Applications.* Geneva: World Health Organization, pp. 685–706.

——'Disability, Discrimination, and Irrelevant Goods' in *Fairness and Goodness,* forthcoming.

Walzer, Michael (1983). *Spheres of Justice.* New York: Basic Books.

[13] A problem that we must be prepared for in using the Causative Principle and the Principle of Irrelevant Identity in accounting for the judgements I have described in this article is apparent intransitivity in choices. This is because my discussion implies that it is nondiscriminatory to prefer a paraplegic candidate (P) who will become unparalysed (U) to one who will not (i.e. $(P \rightarrow U) > (P \rightarrow P)$). Nondiscrimination requires giving equal chances to a paraplegic candidate who will remain that way in a contest with an unparalysed candidate who will remain that way (i.e. $(P \rightarrow P) = (U \rightarrow U)$), not favouring a paralysed candidate who will become unparalysed over someone all along unparalysed, implying that $\neg [(P \rightarrow U) > (U \rightarrow U)]$. In other words, it is permissible for A not to be chosen over C, even though it is nondiscriminatory to pick A over B, and B must be treated as equal to C. These apparent intransitivities, however, really raise no deep problem, as the choices are fully explicable on a pairwise basis. Because the pairwise options give rise to different factors that determine our choice, we should not expect transitivity. What should we do when the three people present themselves to us at once? My sense is that nondiscrimination requires us to toss a coin between $(P \rightarrow U)$ and $(U \rightarrow U)$, even though, if the coin favours $(U \rightarrow U)$, this will mean that he is selected over $(P \rightarrow P)$. This is nondiscriminatory in the context because $(P \rightarrow P)$ has been eliminated as a candidate not by $(U \rightarrow U)$ but by $(P \rightarrow U)$.

[14] This article is one of a series. For further discussion expanding on what has been said here, see 'Health and Equity', in C. J. L. Murray et al. (Kamm 2002), and 'Disability, Discrimination, and Irrelevant Goods' in *Fairness and Goodness* (Kamm, forthcoming). In the latter I also suggest the Treat Similarity Principle which permits selecting for treatment by disfavoring a component property that is similar to a property it is the aim of the treatment to eliminate.

[15] For comments, I am grateful to Sudhir Anand, D. Brock, N. Daniels, C. Murray, D. Wikler, and the members of the Health Equity Group at the Harvard Center for Population and Development Studies and the Fairness and Goodness Group at the WHO.

12

The Value of Living Longer

JOHN BROOME

12.1. LONGEVITY AND DISTRIBUTIONS OF WELL-BEING

Longevity is an important aspect of health. Anyone who wants to measure the health of a population will need to take it into account. But there are special difficulties about doing so. This chapter explains why.

Measuring health is one thing and valuing health is another. Which should we aim at? I assume we are interested in a person's health as a component of her well-being. Well-being consists of various different sorts of goods, such as health, comfortable living, freedom from oppression, and so on. So we are interested in health as one good thing to be set alongside others. We are therefore interested in how good it is, which means we are interested in its value. This chapter is about valuing health—measuring the value of health—rather than measuring the quantity of health. Specifically, it is about the value of longevity.

To set a value on longevity is an aspect of a general problem in the theory of value: the problem of aggregating good or well-being.[1] Let us concentrate on a particular country. Each person who lives in this country is born at some time, dies at some time, and at each time during his or her life enjoys some degree of well-being. Figure 12.1 is a schematic illustration of the country's progress. Time is measured horizontally in the diagram. Stacked up vertically is a series of horizontal lines. Each is the horizontal axis of a little graph, which shows the progress of a single person's well-being through his or her life. In these graphs, well-being is measured vertically. A person's graph starts at the time he or she is born, and ends at the time he or she dies. One of the lines has no graph on it, for a reason that will appear later in this section. In sum, this diagram shows how well-being is distributed in the country, across people and across time.

The problem of valuation, looked at in the most general way, is to set a value on distributions like this. We are trying to judge how well off is a country's population, and this must be determined by the well-being of each person at each time. So we need to *aggregate* well-being across a distribution; we need

[1] The problem of aggregating good is discussed in my *Weighing Goods* (1991) and *Weighing Lives* (2004).

People

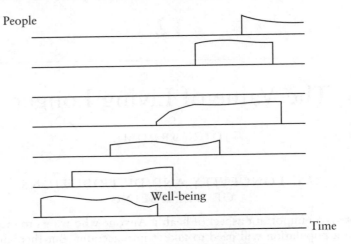

Well-being

Time

Figure 12.1. *A distribution of well-being*

to take the well-being of each person at each time, and put all those quantities of well-being together to determine how good is the distribution as a whole.

In practice, rather than calculating the absolute goodness of a single distribution, we shall be more interested in making comparisons between distributions, to see which is better than which, and how much better. When things change, we need to know whether the change is beneficial or harmful, and the size of the benefit or harm. In this chapter I am interested particularly in changes that increase or decrease the lengths of people's lives, to measure the overall harm or benefit that results.

Unfortunately, we cannot entirely isolate this single question of longevity. For one thing, in valuing longevity, we shall have to be guided by the principles that govern aggregation in general, and we need to keep in mind what those principles are. Also, there is one fact about longevity that we particularly cannot ignore. Changing the lengths of people's lives generally changes the number of people who are born. For example, as death rates fall and people live longer, they tend to have fewer children. Consequently, we cannot ignore changes in the country's population when we try to value longevity.

Figure 12.2 illustrates the general problem of comparison. It shows two alternative distributions of well-being. People mostly live longer in one than in the other. One of the alternatives also has a larger population than the other, so some people exist in one who do not exist in the other. Each person is allocated a horizontal line in the diagram; corresponding lines in the two halves of the diagram represent the same person. So when a person lives in one alternative and not the other, his or her line is left blank on one side of the diagram.

The problem of comparison is to determine which of two distributions like this is better overall. This chapter is about those aspects of this problem that have to do with the length of people's lives.

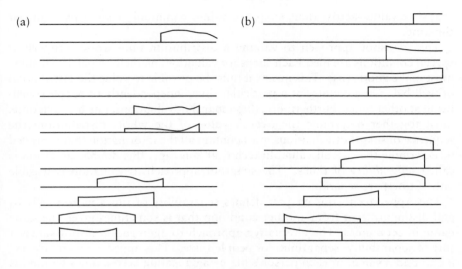

Figure 12.2. *Two alternative distributions of well-being*

12.2. AGGREGATION AND SEPARABILITY

We need to take a whole distribution of well-being, and aggregate across time and across people, to arrive at an overall value. There are different ways we might set about doing that. We might hope to do it in two steps, aggregating across people as one step and across times as another. We might take these steps in either order. One approach is to start by aggregating across people, doing so for each time separately, and then to aggregate across times. In this approach, the first step values the state of the country at each time. The second takes all these values arrived at in the first step—one for each time—and aggregates them across times. An alternative approach is first to set a value on each person's overall well-being, by aggregating across times within the person's life. Then the second step is to take all these values arrived at in the first step, one for each person, and aggregate them across people.

The first of these approaches involves setting a value, at each time, on everybody's well-being taken together. Let us call this a 'snapshot' valuation, because it is made for a single moment in time, and let us call this first approach to valuing a distribution 'the snapshot approach'. To make a snapshot valuation, it is as though we photograph a diagram like Figure 12.1 through a narrow vertical slit, which only reveals the distribution of well-being at a single time. Snapshot valuations are implicit in a great deal of our thinking about the progress of a country—for example, its progress in health. We talk about how a country's health improves from year to year, or perhaps how the inequality in its health increases. In doing this, we set a value on the state of the country at each time, and watch this value develop as time passes. So even if we are not intending to take the second step of aggregating the snapshot values across time, snapshot values commonly have a place in our thinking.

The snapshot approach to valuing a distribution only works properly if special conditions are met. Each snapshot valuation, made for a particular time, must make good sense. This means it must be possible to value the distribution of well-being in a country at a particular time, independently of people's well-being at other times. Furthermore, these snapshot valuations, one for each time, must together determine the overall value of the whole distribution: the sequence of snapshot valuations must contain all the information that is needed to determine the overall value. In technical language, this double condition is called *separability* of times.[2] The snapshot approach to valuation is feasible only if times are separable.

The Appendix to this chapter defines separability of times more precisely, and distinguishes it from another condition that is sometimes given the same name in economics. The alternative approach to aggregation also assumes a sort of separability: separability of people's lives. This approach starts by trying to find a value for each person's life by aggregating across times within his or her life. It is as though we look at the diagram through a horizontal slit. Then as a second step we aggregate across people. I shall call this the 'people approach' to aggregation. It will work properly only if a person's life can be valued independently of other people's well-being, and if the separate values for each person's life together determine the overall value of the distribution. This double condition is called separability of lives.[3]

It is plausible that lives are separable. It is implied by something I call 'the principle of personal good'.[4] This principle is formally parallel to the well-known Pareto principle, but it is expressed in terms of what is good for people—people's well-being—rather than their preferences. The principle of personal good says that the value of a distribution of well-being depends only on the well-being of the individual people. To put it another way, overall goodness is a function of individuals' well-being. This implies we can value a distribution by first calculating each individual's well-being—aggregating across times in his or her life—and then calculating overall goodness on the basis of these amounts. So it implies separability of lives. Since the principle of personal good is very plausible,[5] separability of lives is plausible. This means the people approach to aggregation could be successful.

On the other hand, separability of times is not a plausible assumption, so the snapshot approach is dubious. At least, separability of times implicitly commits us to much more than most of us would be willing to accept.

---

[2] Technically, it is *weak* separability. Separability and its implications are explained in *Weighing Goods* (1991: chapter 4). See also Appendix to this chapter.

[3] I make a distinction between separability of lives and a stronger condition I call separability of people. The distinction is explained in *Weighing Lives* (2004: chapter 8) but is not important for this chapter.   [4] *Weighing Lives* (2004: chapter 8).

[5] To be sure, there are objections to it, which are discussed in *Weighing Goods* (1991: chapters 8 and 9).

My principal aim in this chapter is to make this point. It means we cannot legitimately make snapshot valuations of health.

12.3. THE OBJECTION TO SEPARABILITY OF TIMES

To see why times are not separable, think first about the example shown in Figure 12.3. It shows two alternative distributions of well-being that are to be compared. In each, exactly two people are alive at each time. All the people who live in either alternative have the same constant level of well-being throughout their lives. The difference between the distributions is that each person in (a) lives longer than each person in (b) (twice as long, as I have constructed the example).

The example is very stylised, in that the population is only two, and people live completely uniform lives. Still, it captures some of the features of a typical 'demographic transition'. In a typical demographic transition, a country starts from a stable population with a high birth rate and a high death rate. Then the birth and death rates drop, and eventually the country arrives at another stable population, with lower rates. Figure 12.3 shows two possible states of a country, each with a stable population. The birth and death rates are high in the second and low in the first. So it is a stylised picture of a country after and before a demographic transition. One unrealistic aspect is that the population at any time is the same in both states: just two people. In practice, when a country passes through a demographic transition, its death rate falls before its birth rate. The result is that by the time its population reaches a new stable state, it is much larger. The example misses this feature, but it does represent another important feature of a transition: afterwards, people live longer.

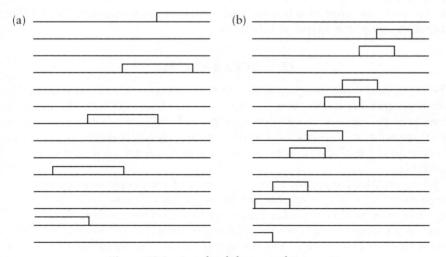

Figure 12.3. *A stylised demographic transition*

Which of the two distributions is better? Let us try to compare them using the snapshot method. The method starts by comparing them time by time. We take each particular time on its own and without reference to any other time, and compare the values of the two distributions at that time. When we do this for any particular time, we see that the two distributions are identical at that time in terms of well-being. Each has two people alive, and each of those people has the same well-being. So we have to conclude that the two alternatives are equally good at that time. We must reach the same conclusion for every time. If times were separable, these snapshot comparisons would fully determine the comparative value of the two distributions. We would therefore be forced to conclude that the distributions, viewed as a whole, are equally good. That would be the consequence of separability of times.

We could not escape this conclusion by looking at the moments of birth and death. In my example, each person comes into existence at midnight; before midnight he or she does not exist and at midnight or later he or she does exist. Each person also goes out of existence at midnight; before midnight he or she exists and at midnight or later he or she does not exist. Consequently, there are no momentary overlaps when three people are alive, and no momentary gaps when only one person is alive.

So if times were separable, we would be forced to conclude that the two distributions in Figure 12.3 are equally good. Yet, that is surely wrong. Intuition suggests that longevity is valuable and consequently that Figure 12.3(a) is better than Figure 12.3(b), because in Figure 12.3(a) each person has a longer life. (Section 12.4 examines the basis of this intuition.) Therefore, times are not separable.

The example shows what is wrong with separability of times. For a person to live a longer life is a good thing. Yet the length of a person's life is not something that shows up when we look at times separately. It is a feature of his or her life that only appears when we take a span of times together. So its value cannot show up in a snapshot valuation.

12.4. SEPARATISM

The objection I made to separability is that (a) in Figure 12.3 is better than (b), which separability denies. But the basis of this claim was only the intuitive thought that longevity is valuable. One possible response to the objection is simply to reject it. This is a hard-headed, intuitively implausible response, but it is possible. I shall call it 'separatism'. Separatism is the view that times are separable.

When we take a snapshot of the well-being of the people in a country at a single time—surveying a vertical line in one of my diagrams—we see a lot of little pieces of well-being, each belonging to a different person. A snapshot does not allow us to see how these pieces are connected in a horizontal direction with other pieces; we do not see how pieces are packaged together within individual lives. That is why the length of people's lives does not appear in a snapshot valuation. But the horizontal packaging of lives seems intuitively to make a real difference to value; longevity seems a good thing, for instance. The separatist denies this.

Separatism implies that horizontal connections make no difference. All that matters is the little pieces of well-being that appear at each time, not their packaging in lives. Consequently, longevity is not valuable. At least, it is valuable in one way but not another. Other things being equal, prolonging a person's life adds pieces of well-being to the distribution of well-being, and a separatist values those pieces. In that way, he or she values longevity. However, he or she gives no value to the fact that those pieces are joined on to a life that already exists, to make a longer life. Suppose a person were to die and a new person appear in his or her place and enjoy the same well-being. From the separatist point of view, that would be just as good as the first person's continuing to live would be. In *that* way, a separatist does not value longevity. He or she gives no more value to a long life than to several short lives that together make up the same period of time.

In Figure 12.3, the same total amount of time is lived in (a) as in (b). But in (a) it is apportioned to fewer longer lives, and in (b) to more shorter lives. A separatist values both options equally, because he or she does not care how the living is divided among lives.

The separatist view that horizontal connections make no difference is an extreme version of the view that personal identity does not matter, which was propounded by Derek Parfit in Part III of *Reasons and Persons* (1984). Parfit arrives at his own less extreme view on metaphysical grounds. Some further philosophical arguments might bring us to the stronger conclusion that times are indeed separable.[6] I shall not review the arguments here. I only want to suggest that separatism could be given some philosophical basis, despite its implausibility.

The simplest example of a separatist theory of value may be called 'complete utilitarianism'. A complete utilitarian thinks that the value of a distribution is simply the total of all the well-being enjoyed at any time by anyone. To arrive at an overall value, we simply add well-being across the whole distribution—across people and across times. One distribution is better than another if and only if it has a greater total of well-being. A complete utilitarian does not care in any way about how well-being is distributed. For one thing, he or she does not care how it is packaged into individual lives. All that matters is well-being; who gets well-being is irrelevant.

Although separatism might receive a philosophical defence, I shall continue to reject it on grounds of its implausibility. From now on in this chapter, I shall assume it is false.

---

[6] *Weighing Goods* (1991: chapter 11), contains a discussion of a related strong assumption of temporal separability.

12.5. DISPERSING VALUE

I have argued that times are not plausibly separable. But those who measure health will not give up snapshot valuations so easily. Apart from the tough separatist defence, there is a more pragmatic way of trying to preserve separability in the face of the objection I have raised.

I said the value of longevity does not show up when we look at times separately, but only when we take a span of times together. Consequently, it does not show up in snapshot valuations. However, one component of a person's well-being at any time is his or her health. His or her health in turn consists of several components: functioning limbs, freedom from pain, and so on. A person's longevity is one component of his or her health, so we might simply include it along with the other components at every time. We might say that someone who has a longer expectation of life is in this respect healthier at every time than someone who has a shorter expectation. So we might include his or her expectation of life within his or her health at each time, and hence within his or her well-being at each time. If we do that, when we make a snapshot valuation at any time, the person's longevity will show up in the snapshot. In this way, we might make times separable, and snapshot valuations legitimate.

I want to keep the term 'separatism' for the hard-headed view that gives no value to longevity. So I do not count this new idea as a version of separatism, even though it supports separability. It is an example of a strategy within the theory of value that I call the 'dispersion' of value. For the sake of comparison, I shall mention a different application of dispersion, before assessing how successfully it copes with longevity.

The different application provides a defence of separability of lives, rather than separability of times. Separability of lives can seem to be threatened by the value of equality. I explained earlier that separability of lives is a consequence of the principle of personal good. According to this principle, the value of a distribution of well-being depends solely on the well-being of individual people. But many people think equality of well-being has value: a more equal distribution of well-being is better than a less equal one. One might think this value cannot belong to any individual person, because it depends on a relation between people: specifically on the difference between some people's well-being and others'. It seems we first need to determine how well-off each person is before we can see how equal the distribution is. Consequently, the value of equality must be a purely social value, separate from each individual's well-being. So one might think, and the thought threatens separability of lives.

This argument about equality is investigated in chapter 9 of my *Weighing Goods*. I argue there that if equality is indeed a good thing, it is so because it is good for individual people. Conversely, if inequality is a bad thing, it is so because it is bad for individual people. The badness of inequality is not a separate negative value beyond people's own well-being. It is part of people's well-being itself. This argument is an example of dispersion. At first, equality seems to be a separate, social value that cannot be captured within the well-being of individuals. But I took this apparently social value and dispersed it among the individuals. I argued it actually belongs to the individuals separately, despite first appearances.

An essential part of the strategy of dispersion is to justify it.[7] Take any value that apparently does not belong to people as individuals, so it seems to contradict separability of lives. Let it be biodiversity, say—suppose biodiversity is valuable. A theorist could always disperse this value in a formal way by arbitrarily dividing it into parts and allocating each part to a person. He or she could then say that each person's allocated part was a component of that person's well-being. But this would not be a sound move unless the theorist could demonstrate that biodiversity was indeed part of the person's well-being. This demonstration needs to be made for the specific value that is in question. In the case of biodiversity, it might or might not be convincing. In the case of equality, I hope I justified dispersion successfully by producing an account of the value of equality in terms of fairness, which made it definitely an individual value.

Unless an instance of dispersion is shown to be genuine in this way, it will be no help with aggregation. If we know the aggregate value of a distribution, we can always disperse the value arbitrarily to people. But to do that, we would have to know the aggregate value first. Since we are trying to find aggregate value, this arbitrary manoeuvre would be pointless. On the other hand, if the value is genuinely a part of each individual's well-being, we should be able to assess each person's share of it independently, and then include these shares in an aggregation across people.

12.6. DISPERSING THE VALUE OF LONGEVITY

Now back to our original problem, and separability of times. On the face of it, the value of longevity does not appear at individual times. But we could attribute it to individual times by treating it as part of a person's health at each time. That is to say, we take this value, and disperse it to individual times. In this way, perhaps we can make the value of longevity separable between times. That is the strategy.

If we knew the aggregate value of a distribution, including the value of longevity, we could arbitrarily divide it up and disperse it among the times separately. There are many arbitrary ways of dispersing the aggregate in such a way that the dispersed parts could be re-aggregated to reach the correct result. But as I say, an arbitrary dispersion is not enough, because it will not help with aggregation. The dispersion must be justified.

I doubt that dispersing the value of longevity across time could be justified. It seems to me that longevity is genuinely a value that does not appear at any

---

[7] See the discussion of dispersion in *Weighing Goods*, (1991: 191–2).

particular time in a person's life; it is genuinely a feature of the life taken as a whole. But to give dispersion a chance, I shall waive this general scepticism about justification. The value of longevity might be divided up among times in various ways, and I shall examine some of them, without insisting that they be fully justified in advance. I shall ask only that they are not entirely arbitrary; they must make some sort of sense. I shall show that, quite apart from the matter of justification, they do not do what they need to do. They do not succeed in properly capturing the value of longevity.

This argument against dispersion will not be conclusive. I cannot rule out the possibility that someone might invent a convincing and successful way of dispersing the value of longevity. I can only say that the methods of dispersion I can think of fail. I shall also be able to explain why they fail, and this strengthens my argument. The explanation of why these particular methods fail can be generalised. It explains why dispersion in general can be expected to fail. So by the end of this section, we shall have good grounds for rejecting dispersion.

Take Figure 12.4 as an example. It is a diagram of my usual sort, showing graphs of people's well-being. It shows well-being *without* taking account of life expectancy. That is to say, it does not include any dispersed value that we might attribute to longevity and add into the people's well-being at a time. The diagram shows two alternatives as usual. In both of them, two people are alive at each time, and their well-being apart from longevity is at the same constant level throughout their lives. In (a), everyone lives for two years. In (b), some people live for three years and others for one.

Distribution (a) is surely better than (b). In (a), everyone lives for two years. In (b), three-quarters of the people live for only one year and the remaining quarter

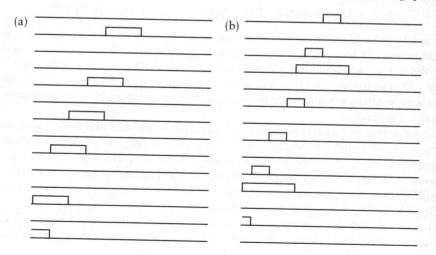

Figure 12.4. *Another example*

live for three years. In (a), people's lifetimes are on average two years; in (b), they are on average one and a half years. (The average lifetime of the people *who are alive at any particular time* is two years, but that is a different matter.) If we care about longevity, therefore, we will definitely favour the first alternative. This conclusion does not depend on caring specifically about the average. Look at it this way. In (a), each period of twelve years lived is lived by six people. In (b), each period of twelve years lived is lived by eight people. So the same period of life is divided among more people in (b). If we value people's longevity in any way, we will certainly favour (a).

There is plausibly a further consideration in favour of (a): equality. People's lives are equally long in (a) but unequally long in (b). If we value equality, that will give us reason to count (a) better. But it is a quite separate reason from the value of longevity. It stems from the value of equality in longevity rather than from the value of longevity itself. My example has the feature that the value of longevity is correlated with the value of equality in longevity. This is unfortunate, because it muddies the argument, but I cannot eliminate it. Unfortunately, it is inequality in lifetimes that causes dispersion to fail, but in a way that is independent of the value of equality itself; I shall explain why at the end of this section. So instead, I propose to isolate the value of longevity by ignoring any value that equality may have. For the sake of argument, then, let us assume equality has no value.

I say (a) is better than (b), on grounds of longevity. Not everyone would agree. If you value only the total amount of well-being, independently of whom it comes to, or how it is packaged into lives, then you will think the two distributions in Figure 12.4 are equally good. Both have the same amount of well-being altogether. Your view is then the one I called complete utilitarianism. It implies separatism, and it gives no value to longevity. If you take this view, you already believe times are separable, without dispersion. You think dispersion makes no contribution to separability, because separability is correct anyway. In this section, I am not addressing you. I am addressing people who think longevity is valuable, but nevertheless hope to preserve separability of times by means of dispersion.

These people will want to reproduce the conclusion that (a) is better than (b). They are hoping to do so by means of snapshot valuations, taking each time separately and comparing the distributions at that time. They want to bring longevity into the calculation by dispersing its value.

They need to disperse it in some way that is not purely arbitrary—a way that makes some sense. Let us start with the simplest way. Let us treat a person's expectation of life as a component of his or her well-being at every time in his or her life; we add a component for each person's longevity into the person's well-being at each time. So now a person's well-being is more than is shown in Figure 12.4. As well as the well-being shown in the diagram, each person has an extra component of well-being at every time in his or her life, given by the length of his or her life. This component remains constant throughout life. What happens to our valuation of the distributions when we add in this extra component?

We first have to make snapshot valuations at each time; we have to compare the two distributions at each time separately. The two distributions in Figure 12.3 were identical at each time, so the comparison between them was easy. But the two distributions in Figure 12.4 are not identical at each time, so there is a further complication. In each distribution, two people are alive at each time, but they do not have the same well-being once we take longevity into account. In order to compare the distributions at each time, we have to aggregate together the well-beings of the two people who are alive at that time. I have not yet said how we might do that.

The natural way is simply to add their well-beings together. If equality is valuable, adding may not be the right way to aggregate across people. But I have set aside the value of equality, and I know no other objection to adding. So that is how I shall proceed.

We have two components of the people's well-beings to add together, at each time. First we add up their well-beings apart from longevity, which are shown in Figure 12.4. Here, we find both distributions have the same total, so there is nothing to choose between them on that account. Then we add the second component, longevity. It turns out there is also nothing to choose between the distributions on grounds of total longevity either. The two people alive at each time in (a) each have a life expectancy of two years. So their total life expectancy is four years. The two people alive in (b) have life expectancies of, respectively, one and three years. Their total life expectancy is four years too. At each time, then, total life expectancy is the same in both distributions.

The conclusion is that the two distributions are equally good at every time, even taking longevity into account. Consequently, when we come to aggregate the snapshot values across times to reach an overall evaluation, the two distributions will be equally good overall. We reach this conclusion even when we try to disperse the value of longevity across times. We shall also reach the same conclusion if we disperse the value of longevity in a different way. I have been taking the length of a person's life as a component of his or her well-being throughout his or her life. This component remains constant throughout his or her life. An alternative is to take his or her *future* life expectancy as a component of his or her well-being. This too is a way of dispersing value that makes some sense. The result is more complicated, because the aggregate of people's future life expectancies varies over time. (The calculation is easy to do, and I shall not spell it out.) Still, the same conclusion emerges when we aggregate across time. This sort of dispersion also gives no reason to favour (a) over (b).

Yet, if longevity is valuable, (a) is better than (b). So dispersion seems unable to capture adequately the value of longevity. If we try to distribute the value of longevity to times, so as to make it consistent with separability, we will get the wrong conclusions about value.

This is not just bad luck. We can see the source of the difficulty from the example. Longer-lived people live for longer. Therefore, if we make snapshot valuation at individual times, each longer-lived person appears in our valuations more often than a shorter-lived person does. So longer-lived people get counted more often in the snapshot route to aggregation. This gives the result an incorrect bias. I do not see how the strategy of dispersion can get around this problem.

The bias only arises when some people live longer lives than others. This explains why inequality of lifetimes cannot be eliminated from my example.

So I think dispersion will be unsuccessful in rescuing separability of times. The only way we could justify separability is by embracing the implausible doctrine of separatism. This means denying the value of longevity. Rather than that, we shall have to abandon the snapshot approach to aggregation.

12.7. CAUSAL DATING

If longevity is valuable, times are not separable. Consequently, trying to value a country's health at any particular time, taking account of longevity, is doomed to failure. The reason, to put it in a nutshell, is that the benefit of living longer cannot be pinned down to a date. Indeed, the conclusion I have reached goes further than this. We simply cannot assume times are separable at all, in any context where the lengths of people's lives are not fixed. Separability of times is a bad assumption, in measuring health or in any other context.

This is a pity. We might very naturally want to trace a country's progress in combating disease or improving life expectancy. To do this, it would be nice to have a sequence of dated valuations, to see how they change over time. It turns out that snapshot valuations are not available to make up such a sequence. However, there may be an alternative way of making dated valuations; we might attach a date to harms and benefits in a different way. Because times are not separable, we cannot always identify a date when a harm or benefit *occurs*. However, we may be able to date it according to when it is *caused*.

The cause of a harm or benefit may occur at a different date from the harm or benefit it causes. A leak of radiation may do no harm to anyone for many years, but in due course people may suffer from it. The cause is the leak, which occurs at some date; the harm occurs at a later date. It may also happen that a cause can be given a date, whereas the harm or benefit it causes cannot be tied down to any particular date. That will be so if a cause extends or shortens people's lives. We know by now that the good or harm of extending or shortening lives cannot itself be dated. But the cause of this good or harm might be datable. For example, the cause might be an epidemic or a vaccination programme, which occurs at an identifiable date.

This gives us the idea I call 'causal dating': we date harms and benefits by the date of their causes. For example, we might use causal dating for the 'burden' that disease imposes on the population of a country—the harm it does. We might calculate a sequence of dated burdens. Each would be a valuation of the harm caused by disease-in-a-particular-year. It would not be the-harm-in-a-particular-year caused by disease.

Let us think of disease as the cause and ill health as the effect. So causal dating seems natural if we are measuring the burden of disease, whereas it would be less natural in a measure of health. Christopher Murray seems to have causal dating in mind when he proposes 'disability-adjusted life years' (DALYs) as a measure of the burden of disease.[8] Take an example. Suppose an infectious disease strikes a person and leaves him or her disabled. The harm done by the disease continues through all the years the person's disability lasts, but the cause of the harm should be dated to the time when the disease strikes. This is how Murray dates it,[9] and this is why I think he is aiming at causal dating. I think this is an appropriate aim.

However, he does not put this aim into effect consistently, as another example shows. Suppose an infectious disease leaves a person disabled, and also weakens his or her constitution so that he or she eventually dies prematurely. Both the harm of the disability and the harm of the premature death should be dated to the time of the disease. But Murray would date the harm of the death to the date when the death itself occurs.

Indeed, I doubt that causal dating even *could* be consistently put into effect. Causal dating is not the subject of this chapter, and I cannot investigate it thoroughly here, but I shall mention a serious difficulty that I see with it. Nothing I have said so far stands against it, because it does not require separability of times, but it has different difficulties of its own. They are not in the realm of ethics, like those that defeat snapshot valuations. They are metaphysical problems associated with causation. It is hard to connect causes and effects in the way causal dating requires, when several causes operate. I shall explain why.

At first sight, you might think the benefit or harm caused by an event is the difference between the value of what happens given that the event occurs and the value of what would have happened had the event not occurred. Let us call this difference the 'counterfactual' measure of the harm or benefit. Suppose we want to evaluate the harm caused by an epidemic. We would apply the counterfactual measure as follows. Given that the epidemic occurs, there will be a particular distribution of well-being in the country. If the epidemic had not occurred, there would have been a different distribution. This gives us a comparison to make like the one shown in Figure 12.2: a comparison between two two-dimensional distributions of well-being. We know we cannot make this comparison through the snapshot approach; we cannot compare the distributions time by time. Nevertheless, each distribution has some overall value. In principle at least, we should be able to compare their values by some other method than the snapshot one. The difference between their values is the counterfactual measure of the harm caused by the epidemic.

---

[8] See his 'Quantifying the burden of disease'.
[9] See the section on 'Incidence versus prevalence perspectives' on pp. 431–2.

That is how we might try to identify the harm caused by an epidemic. But actually this counterfactual measure may not be correct. Implicitly, it takes for granted a counterfactual analysis of causation, which has well-known problems. One is the problem of overdetermination. Sometimes an effect that is actually caused by one event would have been caused by a different event had the first event not occurred. Then the effect is said to be overdetermined. The counterfactual measure of harms will not correctly identify overdetermined harms.

Here is an example. Suppose an epidemic strikes a country in two successive years. An epidemic of this particular sort always kills one-tenth of the population. Suppose the country's population is initially 1,000,000. Suppose no births occur in these years, and no deaths from causes other than the epidemics. The first epidemic kills 100,000 people, leaving 900,000 alive when the second epidemic strikes. The second epidemic then kills 90,000 people. The total number of deaths is 190,000. If the first epidemic had not occurred, 1,000,000 people would have survived into the second year. 100,000 would then have died. So the difference between the actual number of deaths and the number there would have been had the first epidemic not occurred is 90,000. This is the counterfactual measure of the harm caused by the first epidemic. However, the number of deaths caused by the first epidemic is 100,000, not 90,000. The counterfactual measure is incorrect.

As it happens, the counterfactual measure of the deaths caused by the second epidemic is correct: 90,000. Adding together the counterfactual measures for the two epidemics gives us 180,000 deaths altogether, whereas there were actually 190,000. So the problem with the counterfactual measure is not merely that it allocates effects to the wrong causes. It also miscalculates the total of effects. If we tried to use it in this example for the causal dating of harms, we would not simply give the wrong date to particular harms. We would get the wrong total of harms.

In this particular example, our intuitions about causation can correct the error of the counterfactual measure; we know which deaths were caused by the two epidemics. So we might succeed in causal dating of the harms by other means. But in other examples intuition fails too. For example, it fails when there is joint causation. Suppose an epidemic in one year kills nobody, but weakens the population. Suppose that, consequently, a second epidemic in the next year kills 100,000, whereas without the first epidemic it would have killed no one. The 100,000 deaths are caused by the two epidemics together, but we have no intuitive guidance in allocating them to the two separately. Consequently, we have no guidance in dividing the deaths between the two years, for the purposes of causal dating.

I do not know how causal dating could be applied to this second example. The counterfactual measure is useless. If the first epidemic had not occurred, there would have been no deaths. Actually there are 100,000. So according to the counterfactual measure, the first epidemic kills 100,000 people. So does the second, for parallel reasons. Both these conclusions are evidently false.

In practice, diseases often act as joint causes, and their effects are often overdetermined. Just one example: a persisting disease may cause gradually increasing disability in a person and eventually kill him or her after many years. I do not know how all the harms caused by this disease—the death and the various levels of disability—should be assigned a date of causation. Difficulties like this make me doubt that causal dating is a viable method in practice for monitoring changes in the burden of disease.

12.8. DECISION-MAKING

I have concluded that, once the lengths of people's lives are in question, we cannot construct a dated sequence of valuations for the state of a country's health. How much of a loss is this?

It is not so bad. We can still value and compare distributions of well-being. We cannot do it by the snapshot approach; we cannot evaluate the state of a country's health in snapshot fashion, at a particular time. But we can still evaluate two-dimensional distributions—distributions of well-being across people and across time—as a whole.

I said in Section 12.2 that separability of lives is plausible. This gives us the people approach as a feasible route to aggregation: first aggregate across times within each person's life; then aggregate across people. I do not suggest aggregation is easy by the people approach. But at least it is not ruled out from the start, as the snapshot approach is ruled out. There may be other feasible approaches too.

If it works, an alternative route to aggregation—the people approach or some other—will allow us to value and compare distributions as a whole. This is all we need for the practical purpose of making decisions. Suppose we have to decide some practical question, perhaps whether to institute a new health programme or what level of carbon tax to impose. In principle, we can evaluate the two-dimensional distributions of well-being that will result from each of the available alternatives, and determine which is the best. That is a sufficient basis for the decision. If we institute some programme, we cannot break down the harms and benefits it does into a sequence of harms and benefits at particular times. But to decide the value of the programme, we do not need this breakdown. Dated valuations are not needed in practice.

For instance, take the first of my epidemic examples from Section 12.7. Suppose we are wondering whether to spend some money in order to prevent the first of the two epidemics. What is the benefit of doing so? It is the difference between the number of deaths that will take place if the epidemic occurs and the number that will take place if the epidemic does not occur. This number is 90,000. It is what I called in Section 12.7 the 'counterfactual measure' of the epidemic's effects. I explained in Section 12.7 that the counterfactual measure is actually incorrect as a measure of the effects, because the epidemic actually causes 100,000 deaths. Nevertheless, the counterfactual measure is exactly what is needed for decision-making: the benefit of preventing the first epidemic is indeed 90,000 lives saved.

The difficulties raised in this chapter are difficulties for the dating of harms and benefits. They mean we cannot present the progress of a country's health in a particular manner that would be attractive and easy to understand. But they need not interfere with our practical decision-making.

References

Broome, John (1991). *Weighing Goods*. Oxford: Blackwell.
——(2004)*Weighing Lives*. Oxford: Oxford University Press.
Murray, Christopher (1994). 'Quantifying the Burden of Disease: the Technical Basis for Disability-Adjusted Life Years', *Bulletin of the World Health Organization*, 72: 429–5.
Parfit, Derek (1984). *Reasons and Persons*. Oxford: Oxford University Press.

APPENDIX

A Note on Separability.

Separability is a formal notion that has various applications. Economists often use it in a way that is different from mine. This appendix aims to avert misunderstanding amongst economists, by adding some more explanation and some notation. In particular, it distinguishes my assumption that times are separable from a quite different assumption that may be given the same name.

If a person p is alive at a time t, let $g_p{}^t$ be his or her well-being at that time, which I take to be represented by a real number. If p is not alive at t, let $g_p{}^t$ have a non-numerical value that I shall designate as Ω. Ω is simply a notational device that indicates a person's non-existence at a particular time. Since $g_p{}^t$ does not always stand for well-being, I call it p's 'condition' at t.

In Section 12.1, I assumed that the overall value of a distribution depends only on people's conditions at all times. That is to say:

$$G = v(g_1{}^1, g_1{}^2, \ldots, g_1{}^T, g_2{}^1, g_2{}^2, \ldots, g_2{}^T, \ldots, g_P{}^1, g_P{}^2, \ldots, g_P{}^T),$$

where G is the overall value of the distribution, which is represented by a real number. (In this section, assume for simplicity that we are dealing with a finite number of people and times.)

My assumption that times are separable is the assumption that this function can be expressed in the form:

$$G = \bar{v}\,(v^1(g_1{}^1, g_2{}^1, \ldots, g_P{}^1), v^2(g_1{}^2, g_2{}^2, \ldots, g_P{}^2), \ldots, v^T(g_1{}^T, g_2{}^T, \ldots, g_P{}^T)),$$

where each function $v^t(\cdot)$ is real-valued and $\bar{v}\,(\cdot)$ is increasing in all its arguments. To make the nature of the assumption more explicit, we might call it 'intertemporal separability of well-being' or more accurately 'intertemporal separability of conditions'.

The assumption that lives are separable is the assumption that the function can be expressed in the form

$$G = \underline{v}(v_1(g_1{}^1, g_1{}^2, \ldots, g_1{}^T), v_2(g_2{}^1, g_2{}^2, \ldots, g_2{}^T), \ldots, v_P(g_P{}^1, g_P{}^2, \ldots, g_P{}^T)),$$

where each function $v_p(\cdot)$ is real valued except possibly if p never exists, and $\underline{v}(\cdot)$ is increasing in all its arguments.[10]

Those are formalisations of the assumptions I mentioned in Section 2. Now I need to distinguish a different assumption. It plays no part in this chapter, but it must be distinguished from those that do.

A person's well-being at each time he or she is alive will be determined by events of various sorts: the diseases that afflict him or her, the medical care he or she receives, his or her education, the health of the family, the food he or she eats, and so on. Economists often think of the relevant events as 'consumptions'. In truth, this category is too narrow, since people's well-being is determined by much more than just consumptions. However, because it is convenient for what I need to say, I shall treat all relevant events as consumptions too. So I assume for the sake of argument that a person's well-being at each time he or she is alive will be determined by consumptions. But for the moment I do not assume it is determined only by his or her own consumptions at that particular time.

Unlike an event in general, a consumption has the convenient feature that it belongs to a person at a time. Let $c_p{}^t$ be the vector of consumptions of person p at time t. (Presumably it will be a zero vector at times when the person does not exist.) I am assuming that each person's well-being at each time he or she is alive is determined by consumptions. I have also assumed that overall value G is determined by each person's condition at each time. So G is determined by each person's consumption at each time, that is

$$G = w(c_1{}^1, c_1{}^2, \ldots, c_1{}^T, c_2{}^1, c_2{}^2, \ldots, c_2{}^T, \ldots c_P{}^1, c_P{}^2, \ldots, c_P{}^T).$$

An assumption that might be called 'intertemporal separability of consumptions' is

$$G = \bar{w}(w^1(c_1{}^1, c_2{}^1, \ldots, c_P{}^1), w^2(c_1{}^2, c_2{}^2, \ldots, c_P{}^2), \ldots, w^T(c_1{}^T, c_2{}^T, \ldots, c_P{}^T)),$$

This is obviously false. In determining people's well-being, there are obviously strong interactions between consumptions at different times. The value of your reading a book at some time is influenced by your education; the value to you of a tetanus injection depends on when you previously had one; and so on. The assumption of intertemporal separability of consumptions is too implausible to be taken seriously. That is why it plays no part in this chapter.

But intertemporal separability of conditions is not so obviously false; it deserves to be taken seriously. This chapter aims to show it is indeed false, nevertheless. In the text, I call it simply 'separability of times'. In this appendix I have distinguished it from intertemporal separability of consumption.

---

[10] Separability of people is the same assumption except that each v_p must always be real.

PART V

EQUITY AND CONFLICTING PERSPECTIVES ON HEALTH EVALUATION

13

Health Achievement and Equity: External and Internal Perspectives

AMARTYA SEN

13.1. INTRODUCTION

Judgements of health equity as well as aggregative achievements in health care are inescapably dependent on the *assessment* of individual states of health. There are, however, many complex issues in evaluating the state of health of a person. One of the major complexities arises from the fact that the person's own understanding of his or her health may not be congruent with the appraisal of a medical expert. More generally, there is a conceptual contrast between the 'internal' view of health, as seen by the person in question, and 'external' views that others may take of the person's state of health. The contrast goes well beyond incidental differences between two assessments, and can reflect different ideas as to what can be understood as 'good health' of a person.

There is also a disciplinary contrast between the methodological inclinations of 'observation-oriented' subjects (economics is a prime example of this) and 'perception-oriented' studies (often favoured by anthropologists). Public health officials often have no option but to rely on external observations, and in this sense they typically tend to fall on the same side of the divide as economists do. The perceptions of the patients and of persons in general are often hard to access. But there is a substantial issue of epistemology—and ultimately of ethics as well—involved in this choice, and if the 'internal' or 'perception-oriented' views were to be judged to be superior, the methods of health assessment for public policy may have to be appropriately reoriented.

Anthropologists have provided interesting and important investigations of seeing illness and health in an 'internal' perspective: not as observed by a doctor or an outside expert, but by the patient himself or herself. The observation-oriented view of illness and health tends to be, typically, rather detached from *self-perception*, with greater reliance on *externally observed medical statistics*.

The author is grateful for the comments of Sudhir Anand, Arthur Kleinman, and others participating in the Health Equity Workshop at Harvard University in November 1998. An earlier version of the paper was presented at the Bologna Symposium on 'Health & Illness: Metaphors for Life and Society', 24–7 October 1998.

The choice is often determined somewhat arbitrarily by the relative simplicity of easily measurable statistics, which in this case takes the form of data emerging from external observations. But that is not a good enough reason to opt in that direction. There are ways of 'getting at' perceptual information—questionnaires have been a mainstay of the social sciences for a long time—and the enterprise of information-gathering can certainly be redirected *if* the 'internal' view were to be established as being epistemically superior to external observations. The conceptual debate, thus, has major policy implications.

It is this choice that I want to scrutinise and examine in this chapter. I shall examine some insights and understandings that have emerged from works in anthropology, and then examine their bearing on the analysis of health and health care in general. I shall argue that those inclined to be predisposed to take an 'external' or 'observation-oriented' view (economists and the usual public health statisticians, among them) can indeed profit from the anthropological perspective. However, I shall also argue that there are excellent reasons for not overturning the traditional 'external' perspective altogether in favour of new insights from anthropological arguments in favour of 'internal' judgements. There is a strong case for continuing to rely on 'observation-oriented' statistics (done with appropriate scrutiny and analysis), with systematic supplementation by 'perception-oriented' information. In the last analysis, the case for making extensive use of 'external' assessment does not rest on the relative simplicity of observational statistics, but on its epistemic relevance.

13.2. INTERNAL VIEW OF HEALTH: SUFFERING AND MORBIDITY

In initiating the Bologna Symposium on 'Health and Illness: Metaphors for Life and Society', in October 1998, the President of the Symposium, Dr Manfredo Pace, said:

The title of the Symposium stems from the belief that illness and pain are rooted in the person and accompany him/her throughout his/her life (1998).

Dr Pace is a medical practitioner of distinction—and the Medical Director of *Ospedale Maggiore* and *Bellaria*—rather than an anthropologist. But the basic idea and understanding from which he derives the theme of the conference have very clear anthropological connections. The subject of anthropology is the 'person' in his or her own setting and seen from the person's own perspective, in so far as we can understand that perspective. In this sense, the motivation for the important Bologna conference was rooted in a basic anthropological enlightenment.

All of us who are interested in understanding health and illness have reasons to be grateful to anthropologists for the work they have done in this area and the illumination that their works have provided. In recent years, the specialized subject of medical anthropology has been particularly active and rich in terms of academic research and findings (well illustrated, for example, by the major contributions of Arthur Kleinman and his colleagues).[1] There are a great many insights in these works that are of substantial importance for understanding the nature of illness, for considering health policy, and for enriching economic analysis of resource allocation. To illustrate (with a specific focus on what economists may learn from these works), I shall consider two particular examples.

First, these works bring out the importance of seeing *suffering* as a central feature of illness. No mechanically observed medical statistics can provide an adequate understanding of this dimension of bad health, since pain—as Wittgenstein had noted—is a matter of self-perception. If you *feel* pain, you do *have* pain, and if you *do not feel* pain, then no external observer can sensibly reject the view that you *do not have* pain. In dealing with this aspect of illness, the empirical material on which health planners, economic allocators, and cost-benefit analysts frequently rely may, thus, be fundamentally deficient. There is need to draw on the rich discernment provided by the less easy but ultimately more rewarding anthropological investigation of these matters.

Second, in getting a grip on what counts as illness, how it arises and how healing can be done, any kind of exclusive reliance on externally observed clinical symptoms and remedial connections cannot but be at least partly deceptive. If 'illness and pain are rooted in the person' (as Dr Pace identifies), then the kind of detached statistics on which economists and medical statisticians frequently rely may have to be very seriously supplemented by more involved scrutiny of how people comprehend and appreciate what is happening to them and to their near ones, and also the social influences that affect these realisations. Again, the economist has to seek the assistance of the anthropologist in completing his or her work.

13.3. LIMITATIONS OF THE INTERNAL VIEW

I could add other examples, but these two illustrate the kind of help that economists and policy makers can fruitfully obtain from anthropological works and practice. I want now to turn in the other direction. It is also important, I believe, not to reject the 'external' view altogether, when seeking supplementation from anthropological works and their 'internalist' analysis. It is a question of balance, and I now want to be more defensive of the view from outside—the kind of view that comes more naturally to economists, inclined as they are to look for external observations.

When the external and the internal views diverge, there are important cases in which the external view has a cogency and reach that may not be equally present in the internal view. The internal view of the patient is not only

---

[1] Arthur Kleinman (1980, 1986, 1988, 1995). See also Kleinman et al. (1997).

informed by knowledge to which others do not have access, but it is also *limited* by the social experience of the person in interpreting what is happening and why. A person reared in a community with a great many diseases may tend to take certain symptoms as 'normal' when they are clinically preventable. Also, a person with little access to medical care and little education on medical matters can take certain bodily conditions as inescapable even when they are thoroughly amenable to effective medical treatment. Thus the internal view may also be informationally limited in a very serious way, even though the informational limitation comes here from a different direction compared with restrictions that apply to the external view.

The dependence on contingent social experience can be a very big limitation in the epistemology of the internal view and has a direct bearing on the reach of mainstream anthropological approaches. Let me illustrate the issue with an example: consider the different states of India, which have very diverse medical conditions, mortality rates, educational achievements, and so on. The state of Kerala has the highest level of longevity (a life expectancy of seventy-four years—seventy-six for women), in comparison with the Indian average of 64 years. But it also has incomparably the highest rate of reported morbidity. Even when we make age-specific comparisons, Kerala has remarkably higher rates of reported illnesses than any other Indian state, so that the difference is not just a reflection of the higher age pattern of the Kerala population. At the other end, the low-longevity states in India such as Bihar (with life expectancy much below that of the Indian average) also have much *lower* rates of reported morbidity. Do we accept self-perceived assessment of health as a criterion of good and bad health, and declare Bihar as being blessed with much higher achievement of health than Kerala? Or do we go by the evidence of mortality rates, confirmed by professional assessment by medical practitioners, to take exactly the opposite view?

Aside from the decisional question involved in the choice over this dichotomy of evidence, there is also the explanatory question as to why this dichotomy arises. It does seem apparently odd that a population—like that of Kerala—where self-perceived illness and disease are so rampant, and which uses so much medical care, should be exactly the population that lives the longest and escapes premature mortality so successfully. To disentangle the picture, what is needed is not so much to ignore self-perceptions. In fact, quite the contrary. Rather, we have to see that the population of Kerala with its very high literacy rate and with the most extensive public health facilities in the country is in a much better position to diagnose and perceive particular illnesses and do something about them than the population of other states in India.

Furthermore, seeking medical attention is not only a reflection of the *awareness* of health condition, it is also a way of *achieving remedy* (one goes to the doctor to *get* medical help rather than to influence medical statistics). The illiterate and medically ill-served population of Bihar may have little perception of illness, but that is no indication that there is little illness to perceive. There is no real mystery here once the positional conditions are woven into the interpretation of medical statistics.[2]

The possibility that this is a likely explanation of the dissonance between (1) the perceived morbidity rates; and (2) observed mortality rates, is supported also by comparing the reported morbidity rates in Kerala and India, on the one hand, and in the United States, on the other. These comparisons have been made by Lincoln Chen and Christopher Murray (1992). In disease by disease comparison, it turns out that while Kerala has much higher reported morbidity rates for most illnesses than the rest of India, the United States has *even higher* rates for the same illnesses. A summary picture is presented in diagram 1. Thus, if we insist on going by self-reported morbidity, we would have to conclude that the United States is the least healthy in this comparison, followed by Kerala, with the rest of India enjoying the highest level of health (led by the states most backward in health care and education, such as Bihar and Uttar Pradesh).

The approach for which I have tried to argue invokes the notion of 'positional objectivity', seeing the perception of reality in terms of the observers' 'position' in relation to the things being observed.[3] There is need for socially situating the statistics of self-perception of illness, taking note of the connection between self-perception, on the one hand, and levels of education and public health facilities, on the other. In analysing equity in the allocation of health care, it would be, in this analysis, a great mistake to take low perception of morbidity as positive evidence of good health status. A more credible picture can be constructed through combining diagnostic investigations of medical practitioners with the statistics of mortality and causes of death, supplemented by social analysis in trying to make sense of reported perception of morbidity (particularly by linking it *both* with the privileged information of self-perception, on the one hand, and with the limits of actual social experience related to health care, education, and other social parameters, on the other).

I have argued for this approach elsewhere and will not try to defend it further here.[4] In the context of the subject matter of the Bologna symposium, I would simultaneously emphasise both (1) the illumination provided by self-perception of health and illness; and (2) its basic epistemological limitation. We can disagree on what relative importance to place respectively on the positive and the negative aspects of self-evaluational information. Much would also depend on the exact focus of our inquiry and the motivation underlying it. Arguments can perhaps be found for attaching primary importance to self-perception of illness if our focus is particularly on the psychology of suffering,

[2] On this see Sen (1993).

[3] The general feature of positionality of observations and the concept of objectivity from a positional perspective are discussed in my paper 'Positional Objectivity' (1993).

[4] In addition to 'Positional Objectivity' (1993), the approach is also discussed and used in my paper 'Objectivity and Position: Assessment of Health and Well-being' (Sen 1994). In the same volume, Arthur Kleinman's article offers a defence of his very different approach.

anxiety, and the sense of healing. However, our focus can also be, instead, on more clinical aspects of medical prognosis and possible mortality, and on the choice of intervention, including medication or surgery, in which case the need to go beyond self-evaluational information can be very strong.

13.4. A CONCLUDING REMARK

Just as the external view has limitation, so has the internal perspective. For an adequately informed understanding of illness and health, we need to draw on both approaches. Anthropological works can make the economist and the policy-maker much more informed in some respects, and this illumination is badly needed. However, an exclusive reliance on the 'internal' view can also mislead in very serious ways. There is an important need for being more open and catholic in approach—in the necessity to draw both on internal understanding and on external observation.

What has to be avoided above all is the narrowness and limitation of choosing *either* the internal *or* the external perspective on its own, and rejecting the other. We have to go beyond the self-inflicted injury of methodological narrowness and dogmatism—of either kind. Practical reason demands open-minded epistemology.

References

Chen, Lincoln and Christopher Murray (1992). 'Understanding Morbidity Change', *Population and Development Review*, 18(3): 481–503.

Kleinman, Arthur (1980). *Patients and Healers in the Context of Culture: An Exploration of the Border between Anthropology, Medicine and Psychiatry*. Berkeley: University of California Press.

——(1986). *Social Origins of Disease and Distress*. New Haven: Yale University Press.

——(1988). *The Illness Narrative: Suffering, Healing and the Human Condition*. New York: Basic Books.

——(1995). *Writing at the Margin: Discourse between Anthropology and Medicine*. Berkeley: University of California Press.

——, Veena Das, and M. Lock (eds.) (1997). *Social Suffering*. Berkeley: University of California Press.

Pace, Manfredo (1998). 'Dramas, Dilemmas and Silences of the Twentieth Century', in *Health & Illness: Metaphors for Life and Society*. Bologna: Aula Magna S. Lucia.

Sen, A. (1993). 'Positional Objectivity', *Philosophy and Public Affairs*, 22(2): 126–46.

——(1994). 'Objectivity and Position: Assessment of Health and Well-being', in Lincoln Chen, Arthur Kleinman, and N. Ware (eds.), *Health and Social Change: An International Perspective*. Cambridge, MA: Harvard University Press.

14

Ethics and Experience: An Anthropological Approach to Health Equity

ARTHUR KLEINMAN

14.1. REPRISE OF TANNER LECTURES

This chapter draws from the Tanner Lectures I delivered at Stanford University in April 1998 on 'Experience and Its Moral Modes: Culture, Human Conditions, and Disorder'. I turn to that source in order to set out an anthropological approach to health equity and health rights. But my purpose here is different; I am not concerned with revisiting a critique of ethics that I have already set out in several publications (Kleinman 1995a, 1997), but rather I seek to sketch an anthropological orientation to health equity and health rights that is collaborative with ethics in framing these issues. Only by cobbling together a framework that incorporates both local moral processes in everyday experience and transnational ethical discourse, I have come to believe, can health equity and health rights receive adequate treatment.[1]

For the ethnographer, ordinary experience is the social grounds of human conditions. Experience is the flow of everyday interactions in a local world. Experience is intersubjective. It is made up of the negotiations and contestations among others with whom we are connected. It is perhaps best thought of as a cultural and social *medium* in which collective processes (such as social values and relationships) and subjective states (such as emotions and memory) interfuse. Experience occurs in local worlds: a village, a neighbourhood, networks, families. Local worlds, as we have learned, are not bounded entities but rather are open to many influences that extend from neighbouring localities to global social forces. But no matter how permeable and changing, local

---

[1] In a recent paper, Amartya Sen shows that both 'internal' and 'external' views of health statuses have their uses and limits. They really need to be put together to provide a more valid understanding of this subject. As illness experience (internal evaluation) is to disease pathology (external evaluation) in his paper, so moral processes (local perspectives and practices) might be said to be to ethics (external perspectives and practices). And in this paper, following Amartya Sen's responsive call for a more inclusive account, I shall attempt to put together these two aspects of health values into a more inclusive approach to health equity. (See Amaryta Sen 1998).

worlds are the grounds of human lives, and in those worlds we find ourselves positioned participants who have a history of past relationships; an empirically describable cluster of current statuses, roles, and networks; and an ongoing trajectory of work and family and personal engagements that delimit the future.

What characterises experience is an orientation of overwhelming practicality. The participants in a local world are absorbed in certain things that matter, matter greatly. Those lived values, those things that really matter, may be shared—such as concern over status, resources, survival, and transcendence. But they can also be distinctive owing to the deep cultural and social differences that make local worlds rather different places. What is at stake often varies across historical epochs and cultures. Even in the same local world different things are at stake owing to differences in gender, age cohort, class, ethnicity, religion, and individuality. But that some things really matter and that those things that matter most orient agonistic (and antagonistic) interactions is what gives to each local world its moral conditions. That is to say, at the level of social experience, the moral is defined by local processes concerning lived values that are at stake (Kleinman 1995*b*; Kleinman et al. 1997).

Among the things that matter are dangers, threats to local practices and values. Local worlds are dangerous in several senses. What is at stake for individuals and collectives may be under assault or compromised and nullified, owing to political, economic, institutional, and relational pressures. Suffering is one of those dangers. Whether in the form of trauma from natural or social catastrophe or routinised misery such as deep poverty or contingent misfortune such as illness, suffering (and responses to it) is part of what defines local moral worlds. In the literature of medical anthropology and the history of medicine, much greater popular and professional concern centers on suffering than on health. This may simply be an example of the practical orientation of most people to danger and to the threat it poses to those things that are most at stake. But suffering also concentrates attention on what is at stake, and thereby episodes of suffering become occasions of drama when moral processes become particularly visible.

Seen in this ethnographic light, moral processes differ in a fundamental way from ethical discourse. Whereas moral experience is always about practical engagements in a particular local world, a cultural space that carries political, economic, and psychological specificity—a view from somewhere and actions and reactions that are partisan—ethical discourse is a globally elaborated abstract articulation of and debate over translocal values. It strives for an acontextual universality and objectivity: a view from nowhere. Ethical discourse is generated out of and applied in local worlds, however, so that it gets taken up in moral processes that are inseparable from local relations and conditions. The institutions, relationships, and lived experiences that serve ethical deliberations are themselves grounded, of course, in the moral processes of local worlds. So that in actual practice the distinction has blurred boundaries with overlapping components. But for heuristic purposes it is still useful to draw the distinction between local moral processes that are inseparable from local relations and conditions and ethical discourse that brings, or at least aspires to, a translocal perspective.

To begin with, local worlds may be unethical: that is to say, what is at stake for most participants in a local setting may be condemnable from the perspective of a translocal ethical orientation. Think of the majority of a community of Bosnian Serbs ethnically cleansing their Muslim neighbours or a village of Rwandan Hutu in which nearly all participate in massacring their Tutsi friends and family members. One of the advantages of the distinction between moral processes and ethical discourse is that not only do we see the utility of a translocal perspective when we confront such local horror, but we can see that the local moral world itself contains alternative moral positions (such as that of victims and internal resisters or even public critics in the examples given) into whose structural situations and personal acts of witnessing and resisting ethical commentary can be locally anchored.

But the other side of this duality is that ethics can be (and all-too-frequently are) irrelevant to local moral worlds. Thus, structural positioning of poverty and wealth systematically distributes health and health care resources inequitably as part of what defines the moral reality of a local world. To talk about universal ethical formulations of justice and equity, without beginning with the local moral condition of real people who experience the systematic injustices of higher rates of ill health and fewer health care resources owing to their positioning in local social structures of power is to make those formulations utopian and irrelevant to the local world (Daniels et al. 1999). When, for example, informed consent in bioethics is made into the overriding ethical condition of international health research, say in vaccine trials for HIV in impoverished African villages where few people are literate and there is no equivalent in local knowledge of ideas of randomised controlled trials, placebo controls, or perhaps even individual autonomy in deciding about participation in a community-wide activity, while the systematic injustice in the global economy that has deepened these people's poverty and suffering via structural adjustment programmes and the local conditions of absence of the most basic health care resources to treat AIDS are also absent from ethical discourse, then application of the ethical in the local setting of the moral is highly suspect (cf. Farmer 1999).

For this reason, medical ethics and human rights concerns must be centred in ethnographically informed evaluations in which local knowledge and local moral processes are made as salient as are the issues in global ethical discourse. Indeed, how to take into account and appropriately apply that universalising discourse in local settings needs to be the core question. The relationship between the moral and the ethical should be at the heart of efforts on behalf of health equity. Regrettably, the absence of this issue in much of public health and social development elides the local and in its place creates inauthenticity, mediocentrism, and otiose public health practices. I would go so far as to argue that this is business-as-usual in international approaches to local problems, and is characteristic of many social development and international health projects.

A telling example is to be found in Kevin Carter's haunting photo. The photo was taken up in international efforts to respond to famine that repeatedly has affected Nilotic peoples in the Southern Sudan.

It miscasts suffering from starvation as a phenomenon of nature (note the vulture as icon) owing to crop failure (note the ruins of the stubble field). But in the Southern Sudan, famine is a policy goal of the political violence the state in the Arab North authorises as a means of controlling and punishing the involvement of Nilotic peoples in the South in its decades old civil war. It is not nature but politics that is at issue here. That the humanitarian response called forth responds to the former (the famine as a natural catastrophe) rather than the latter (the famine as a political policy with local victims and global audience) not only confuses cause and effect, but ultimately helps perpetuate the disaster from year to year.

Or think of the gathering discourse on sale of organs by poor people in impoverished local worlds to rich people in technologically advanced societies or even in their own countries (e.g. India). Eliding the social inequality and systematic injustice experienced by the former, and its sources in international political economy, in order to model a transaction as ethically acceptable so long as the specific conditions of buying and selling follow legal regulations is to fail utterly to engage ethical discourse with local moral processes (Cohen 1999). That is a failure to understand social reality as much as it is a failure in framing and resolving value conflicts in society.

14.2. FURTHER RELEVANCE FOR HEALTH EQUITY AND HEALTH RIGHTS

Also in the Tanner Lectures, I examined how ideas of 'human nature' are used to underpin ethical framings as a universal basis for codes, standards, and actions. From an ethnographic and social historical perspective, this approach is highly problematic. To begin with, human nature means very different things to ethical theorists in different epochs and societies. There is no universally accepted theoretical definition of human nature. Nor is there an agreed upon empirical scientific understanding of human nature—from biology or psychology—to authorise ethical claims. In our own era of economic expansion of market models into almost every corner of life and of far-reaching technological consequences of genetic and molecular science, little has been learned to help resolve our understanding of what human nature is about and how it is to be understood as the grounds of ethical claims.

But I have another concern altogether in mind when I critique ideas of human nature. From the data base of ethnography and social history, there is such a tumult of change in cultural representations of human values, in collective human experience, and in definitions of self and feelings of subjectivity that there is no evidence that whatever is claimed to be definingly human is the same in different epochs or cultures. In contrast, there is simply enormous historical and cross-cultural data that there are very different human conditions in the world and that they are undergoing such frequent and substantial change that experiences of what we too often take to be 'existential' human emotions, such as responses to suffering via compassion, witnessing, and engagement, are neither universally found nor routinely elicitable in settings of catastrophe and trauma.

Evidence for this assertion can be marshaled from a variety of sources. The Western and non-Western traditions supply almost endless examples of the most diverse and contradictory and truly extraordinary assertions about human nature. Confucianists argued that human nature was basically good, yet others in the same tradition asserted it was basically bad (Wong 1969; Lau 1970). Adam Smith (1983: 9) asserted that human nature underwrites stronger feelings of tenderness toward children than filial love for parents. The classical Confucian tradition stood for the obverse perspective on innate human values. Even within the modern profession of psychology where one might expect that disciplinarity would protect a much narrower understanding of human nature, schools contend over whether sexual instincts or instincts for power are more basic, whether human nature is genetically based, socialised in infancy, altered in fundamental ways by childhood and adult development, shaped by stress especially trauma, universal or culturally specific, gendered, or so variable across individuals as to convey greater personal diversity than interpersonal consistency. In contradistinction to the last point, the neo-Confucianists, as interpreted by Wei Ming Tu (1979), insisted that the deeper one goes into individual selves, the more one finds universals. Some developmentalists say human nature is differentiated as the child develops, others that it is the other way around: human nature dedifferentiates over time (Shweder 1985). E. O. Wilson (1998), the always provocative sociobiologist, makes the astonishing claim that 'causal explanations of brain activity and evolution, while imperfect, already cover most facts known' about human nature as the basis of moral experience. Convincing evidence in fact is almost nonexistent. Even as careful and sensitive a theorist as Charles Taylor (1989: 8) still avers that there is an inner 'craving which is ineradicable from human life. We have to be rightly placed in relation to the good'. The ethnographic, social historical, biographical and psychotherapeutic literatures include hundreds of studies that suggest how unsupported this and most other assertions about human nature actually are.

Judith Perkins (1995) writing about early Christian communities shows how a suffering self with an entirely new and oppositional view of human nature was advanced by Christian leaders as a political as well as a cultural challenge to Roman commitments to a radically different idea and ideal of human nature. Tzvetan Todorov (1993) charts the remarkable diversity of perspectives in French thought through the ages on human nature. Even on such a seemingly narrow topic as the nature of perpetrators of the Holocaust, historians clash as to whether the human nature of killers is ordinary or atypical, normal or pathological, or a question that religious, moral, or medical suppositions can resolve. Primo Levi (1989), the discerning Holocaust survivor–author, insisted that human nature in the death camp was so fundamentally altered that it became in effect incomparable with how the same individuals behaved in normal times. With such enormous differences, it is prudent to conclude that human nature is a loose and unspecifiable terminology that carries so many meanings that it is better to avoid the term altogether. In fact this is the conclusion of the moral theorist C. A. J. Coady (1992). Emmanuel Levinas (1988), the French moral theorist, responded to this troubling lack of agreement as to what human nature could mean by insisting that all people are individuals who are so different that there is no class of moral beings to which they can be said to belong, rather each is a class unto himself or herself.

14.2.1. *Relevance for health rights*

If the idea of human nature is so problematic as to be unavailing for an empirically grounded moral theory, then health rights (however we construe them) cannot be derived from what has been taken by many to be their ultimate source: namely, a fixed, shared, and knowable 'nature' of persons. What then are we left with?

I see no other way out, but that we must ground this subject of health equity and health rights in the local worlds that I described above as the basis of social experience. Local worlds are, among other things, also the grounds of social experiences of health, suffering and health care. What is at stake for patients, family members, and professional health care providers in particular localities defines one side of health rights and responsibilities: we might call this side, following the ethnographic terminology that I have put to use, moral processes. These same moral processes incarnate the inequities in health status and in the distribution of health care resources that is the source of concerns about health equity and social justice.

The other side is ethical discourse, which, as I have defined it, is universal, or at least aspires to be translocal. But to apply ethical discourse, in this instance concerning equity and rights, we first must ground it in local worlds in at least two senses. First, ethical discourse is appropriated and engaged by members of a local world (cf. Moody-Adams 1997). Indeed, we can think of ethical discourse as itself divided between indigenous ethical meanings that are projected into the transnational discourse on ethics and translocal meanings that are appropriated within the local but come from outside. Second, ethical deliberation about and engagement with particular local realities occur among ethicists who themselves are often members of other worlds, experts who participate in both a foreign locality and a panlocal discourse. Yet, they themselves need to be understood as positioned in their different worlds. That is, ethicists, like health policy planners, bring his or her local world and its moral processes with them into ethical deliberation. And he or she must clarify how that other local background and set of interests positions them with respect to the different local worlds into which they introduce their translocal ethical orientation. That is to say, we must develop transparent strategies to translate ethics into local worlds, and to take into account both global and indigenous ethical points of view.

14.3. THE ETHNOGRAPHIC METHODOLOGY

The upshot is best configured, it seems to me, by employing a vision of ethnography as a means of relating moral processes and ethical discourse. (I am not asserting a hegemonic role for anthropology here; rather I am only proposing that the ethnographic method offers an instructive means of bridging the local and the translocal—which should not be surprising since this is the epistemiological issue at the heart of anthropological enquiry.) The 'universal' claims of health rights and responsibilities emerge from an understanding of local worlds that is both internal (beginning with local realities and local positions on rights and responsibilities) and external (drawing on local uses of international ethical formulations and also on external assessment of the local based in that global ethical formulation). Thus, there is a practical activity of empirical and theoretical scholarship that needs to establish the meaning and implications of rights and responsibilities from actual studies, including comparative studies of local and translocal claims and conditions. This descriptive and interpretive and comparative task fits in well with the work of the ethnographer as I have characterised it in several recent publications (see, e.g. Kleinman 1988: chapter 15, 1995b: 41–69, 95–119; as well as the final section of my Tanner Lectures).

The ethnographic methodology for accomplishing this work can be crudely simplified into the following four steps:

1. The ethnographer first clarifies his or her own moral positioning in his or her lived worlds of work and domestic life. This is a mixture of self-disclosure and self-reflexivity.
2. The ethnographer describes the particularities of the local world he or she has been asked to engage. He or she does so by setting out three sorts of knowledge: (1) knowledge of what is locally at stake for stakeholders concerning the particular instances of health, suffering and health care under consideration; (2) knowledge of how local parties use indigenous or global ethical framings to understand these moral processes in their own world; and (3) knowledge of how the ethnographer himself or herself applies ethical categories to the issue at hand locally. The ethnographer, as

the instrument of interpretation and comparison, then triangulates across these different forms of knowledge to set out a framework for understanding how the intersection of moral processes and ethical discourse in this particular world define the local human conditions of health equity and the local human consequences of health rights and responsibilities. The ethnographer should not seek for a determinative understanding, which usually is illusory and can itself become an obstacle to a serviceable understanding that sustains engagement, but rather should emphasize the process of soliciting and engaging multiple perspectives as the most valid means of relating internal and external approaches.

3. That processual framework, and its specific implications for policies and programmes, then becomes the grounds for community-wide conversations between stakeholders (e.g. laypersons and professionals), out of which will emerge an agenda for practical action. At each level, the ethnographic task is to encompass and incarnate both agonistic and antagonistic framings. It is not the ethnographer's responsibility to resolve these tensions, but rather to clarify and relate them in such a way that they can be better seen and understood and handled by participants. The burden of responsibility of the ethnographer is to make unavoidable the engagement of alternatives that is the grounds of moral and ethical action. The limit of ethnography is that it provides no assurance or means of resolving this prototypical conflict. But the steps I have outlined establish the most favourable conditions for such an outcome. Yet, they also teach that 'good outcomes' may not occur. This tragic sense mixed in with the optimism of a practicable approach is the kind of knowledge ethnography can at its best produce. Of course, like any useful intervention, it too can have untoward effects; and that needs to be taken into account case by case.

14.4. SUICIDE IN CHINA: AN ILLUSTRATION

To illustrate the application of this ethnographic methodology, I will use the case example of suicide in China.

Suicide in China raises important questions concerning health equity and health rights (Lee and Kleinman 2000). This form of social suffering is so widespread that each day more than 870 Chinese kill themselves: at least (and some argue more than) 300,000 deaths per year. The rate of suicide is three times the rate in the United States. Because the reporting system for suicide in India, Indonesia, and other large-scale countries is less adequate, the Chinese data are inflated in the world-wide context. Hence China (which makes up 21 per cent of global population) accounts for 44 per cent of all suicide and more than 50 per cent of all suicides in women. Nonetheless, even if these percentage are reduced by new data from other countries, as they are sure to be in future, suicide in China, and especially among women, is a simply enormous public and social health problem.

Suicide in China notably follows a non-Durkheimian pattern, inasmuch as it is much more common in rural than in urban areas: 70 per cent of China's 1.26 billion people live in rural areas, but 90 per cent of suicides are rural. China is also the only country in which women commit suicide more frequently than men. The rate for rural women is three times the urban rate. There are two peaks in China's statistical profile of suicide: young women (16–26 years of age) and older females and males (over fifty-five years of age with the highest rate for those older than seventy-five). Suicide is the fifth commonest cause of death for Chinese women, and, when measured by disability-adjusted life years (DALYs), it is more costly than heart disease or cancer (see Phillips 1999).

Here are examples of common types of suicide:[2]

Suicide as social escape or resistance in oppressive local worlds: Miss Chen (1) was eighteen years old. Under her parents' arrangement, she was engaged when she was only twelve. Although she was supposed to have been 'in love' with this man for six years, the two of them never spoke to each other. Their relationship consisted only of 'casting a sidelong glance' at each other occasionally. Miss Chen (2) was engaged even earlier, at the innocent age of ten. On growing up, she became very dissatisfied with the prospect of a loveless marriage. Miss Chen (3) was a lively girl who was good at singing and dancing. She too was engaged at an early age, but fell in love instead with a young male actor from the village's theatrical troupe. Although she wanted to break off the engagement, her parents were insistent that she should comply. Being similarly afflicted and feeling much pity for one another, the three girls decided to model a scene in a play by choosing to die together in protest against the arranged marriage. It was two days after they died that people discovered their bodies on a secluded hillside (Lee and Kleinman 2000).

Suicide as an adverse consequence of economic reform in China that has undermined family solidarity, filial values and the status of ageing people: A sixty-year-old illiterate rural man with three daughters and two sons, all of whom were married, was forced to live alone. None of his children wanted to support him. They quarrelled over the responsibility of caring for him and complained that he simply 'ate the bread of idleness' (*chi bai shi*). Following another quarrel, he ingested pesticide and killed himself (Li and Wan 1987).

Suicide as a response to increasingly inadequate and inequitable health care in China: Under economic globalisation and market socialism, rural health care financing has disappeared and the socialist language of 'equity' has been replaced by the capitalist language of cost. Being predominantly uninsured,

---

[2] These examples are drawn from Lee and Kleinman (2000).

rural people have to pay for medical services out-of-pocket. To do this, however, is frequently to invite financial catastrophe. In the face of competing needs, sick parents may be the first party in the family to sacrifice themselves. This is illustrated by a forty-seven-year-old rural man with a debilitating neurological condition that required medical treatment. In order to save money (that would otherwise be spent on medical care) for his daughter to enter university (an unusual achievement for a rural family), he killed himself by taking insecticide in 1995. His death as a loving father (*ci fu*) was viewed by the community as a filial act of moral courage. It mobilised community members to start a fund to pay for his daughter's education (Phillips et al. 1999). From a family-centred perspective his suicide was seen as a 'successful' strategy of resistance against inequitable access to health care and limited education for rural people as much as a filial act. Increasingly, Chinese media report rural suicides as an example of impulsive actions growing out of relative hopelessness owing to greater rural–urban disparities in health and social conditions.

The high rates of rural suicide in China have drawn the attention of the media, women's associations, and the Chinese government, and have led to the development of new policies and programmes. This is part of a broader recognition of the downside of economic reform which has widened the gap between rural and urban and rich and poor populations and is associated not just with increased material wealth but with worsening health and social inequality and an epidemic of violence, substance abuse, depression, sexually transmitted diseases, HIV-AIDS, and family breakdown (Kleinman and Kleinman 1999; Lee and Kleinman 2000).

Suicide, among young Chinese women and older men and women, has an ancient provenance. While Confucian ethics does not explicitly authorise suicide as a general right, it is unambiguous in its support of suicide under certain circumstances: namely, where the suicide becomes a moral commentary on immoral conditions and where the suicide is the only strategy for dealing with dire social circumstance. Thus, for scholar bureaucrats in traditional Chinese society, their suicide forced the emperor to address their corpse as moral criticism of their times and his reign. (Qu Yuan, whose suicide is commemorated in the rituals of the Dragon Boat Festival each year, is the classic example.) Suicide by women forced into remarriage after being widowed and by women severely abused by husbands and in-laws in oppressive patriarchal relations was authorised as a legitimate means of escaping intolerable conditions.

But cases of suicide usually have multiple and complex sources.[3] There may also be depression, impulsive action, sometimes substance abuse, breakdown

---

[3] For example, Kevin Carter, the white South African photojournalist who received the Pulitzer Prize for his image of the Sudanese child committed suicide three months after being awarded the Prize. Although his suicide note mentioned the burden of responsibility incurred by taking the picture, he also suffered from manic depressive disorder and substance abuse and he had gone through a messy divorce that separated him from his own daughter who was about the age of the starving Sudanese child (see Kleinman and Kleinman 1996).

in social relations and situations of relative hopelessness exacerbated by economic inequality.

During the Cultural Revolution, the greatly devastating era of radical Maoism, it is estimated that the suicide rate may have reached an astronomical 500/100,000 (compared to 30/100,000 today)!

Suicide prevention programmes might be usefully framed by considering health equity and human rights. But to do so means taking into account (1) the empirical, on the ground reality of particular cases of suicide among members of high risk cohorts in particular worlds and the moral processes involved; (2) local indigenous ethical formulations (in the Chinese case Confucian, Buddhist, Taoist, Christian, secular and that of the Chinese Communist Party) and the way they get taken up in historically specific events and local social relations; (3) appropriation of global ethical framings by local participants and the criticism and resistance (or, for that matter, support) offered by them to local moral processes of suicide; (4) the ethnographer's own moral positioning and use of both indigenous and global ethical discourse; (5) the suicide programme's social (read: political, economic, and moral) positioning and use of indigenous and global ethical framings. The upshot is not a simple answer but a process for evaluating particular suicides or types of suicide in terms of the clash or agreement between moral experience and ethical formulations. In this instance that clash or agreement would be stated in terms of how this process concretises questions of health equity and rights.

At the level of national policy, this approach would argue for the inseparability of social and health policies. It would also establish both traditional sources of health inequalities (e.g. patriarchy) and the reasons for their intensification in the era of the so-called market socialism. Indeed, the ethnographic approach would reveal that contrary to the dictates of traditional filial piety, the contemporary situation places elderly Chinese women and men in more ambiguous social positions and at heightened risk for suicide. Finally, ethnography would frame the tension between global ethical perspectives on suicide that would seek to prevent at least certain forms of suicide in China and indigenous authorisation of at least certain of the same kinds of suicide as both morally appropriate and ethically justifiable as an agonistic argument within the same and between distinctive local worlds—an argument that could lead to a negotiated basis for policy and programmes and even for local decision-making, but that could not in advance determine the outcome of that negotiation of policy formulation and programme implementation. In this sense, resolution of issues of equity and rights needs to be seen as emergent in a process of engagement between the moral and the ethical aspects of human conditions.

In the Chinese setting, both local moral experience and indigenous ethical discourse could be critiqued as predicated on patriarchal bias against women. That critique would draw on global ethical discourse, but could also find examples of contestation and criticism offered within Chinese worlds by internal critics who appropriate both indigenous and global arguments (Nie 1999). Indeed, the local anchoring of translocal ethics makes them even more appropriate for Chinese communities. But at the same time, the Chinese emphasis that suicide can be an appropriate moral strategy under immoral conditions needs to be projected into the translocal ethical discourse as a framing that may hold salience for other settings as well. It may be an especially challenging formulation of the relation of values to action in settings in which systematic social and health inequalities have not received the status of moral criticism and indictment that the act of suicide, *inter alia*, may bring. Indeed, the epidemic of suicide among youth in societies undergoing the most rapid economic transformation could be examined as a possible moral commentary on deepening health and social inequality under the latest phase of finance capitalism (see Desjarlais et al. 1995).

I cannot in a short space provide a detailed illustration nor for that matter have I worked through such an example of my own regarding specific instances of suicide in China. Hence I am unable to develop this analysis in the depth it deserves, so that this chapter must remain unfinished. The best I can do is to leave it as an unsettled and unsettling example of why moral and ethical understandings when taken alone are inadequate for addressing social experience that is best apprehended (and responded to) by combining these internal and external perspectives. In other words, issues of health equity are more adequately engaged when moral processes and ethical discourse are understood processually in terms of their interactions. But as noted that does not promise that the tension between these ways of treating values in society can be routinely resolved. Perhaps resolution anyhow is not the outcome to seek to achieve. Rather, as already argued, it is the act of authorising the process of engagement that may be the best ethnography can do. That interaction between the moral and the ethical aspects of health matters also will not in and of itself resolve serious issues of health equity and human rights; at best all it can do is create the conditions in which those issues are more validly grounded in actual human conditions so that the moral and ethical burden of responsibility of policy-makers, programme directors, and professionals and laypersons is made unmistakable, even while the potential outcome of engaging those issues of equity and rights remains as uncertain as is the rest of social experience.

References

Coady, C. A. J. (1992). *Testimony: A Philosophical Study*. Oxford: Clarendon Press.

Cohen, L. (1999). 'Where it Hurts: Indian Material for an Ethics of Organ Transplantation', *Daedalus*, 128(4): 135–66.

Daniels, N., B. Kennedy, and I. Kawachi (1999). 'Why Justice is Good for our Health: the Social Determinants of Health Inequalities', *Daedalus*, 128(4): 215–52.

Desjarlais, R. et al. (eds.) (1995). *World Mental Health*. New York: Oxford University Press.

Farmer, P. (1999). *Infections and Inequalities*. Berkeley: University of California Press.

Kleinman, Arthur (1988). *The Illness Narratives: Suffering, Healing and the Human Condition*. New York: Basic Books.

—— (1995a). 'Anthropology and Bioethics', in W. T. Reich et al. (eds.), *Encyclopedia of Bioethics*, revised edition. New York: Macmillan, Simon and Schuster.

—— (1995b). *Writing at the Margin: Discourse between Anthropology and Medicine*. Berkeley: University of California Press.

—— (1997). 'Everything that Really Matters. Social Suffering, Subjectivity and the Remaking of Human Experience in a Disordering World', *Harvard Theological Review*, 90(30): 315–35.

—— (1999). 'Experience and its Moral Modes', in G. B. Peterson (ed.), *The Tanner Lectures on Human Values*, Vol. 20. Salt Lake City: University of Utah Press, pp. 355–420.

—— and J. Kleinman (1996). 'The Appeal of Experience, the Dismay of Images,' *Daedalus*, 125(1): 1–23.

—— and —— (1999). 'The Transformation of Everyday Social Experience: What a Mental and Social Health Perspective Reveals about Chinese Communism under Global and Local Change', *Culture, Medicine and Psychiatry*, 23(1): 7–24.

——, V. Das, and M. Lock (1997). 'Introduction', in A. Kleinman et al. (eds.), *Social Suffering*. Berkeley: University of California Press.

Lau, D. C. (1970). 'Introduction', in *Mencius*, Vol. 1, (trans.). Hong Kong: The Chinese University Press.

Lee, S. and A. Kleinman (2000). 'Suicide as Resistance in Chinese Society', in E. Perry and M. Selden (eds.), *Chinese Society: Change, Conflict and Resistance*. London and New York: Routledge.

Levi, P. (1989). *The Drowned and the Saved*. New York: Vintage.

Li, J. H. and W. P. Wan (1987). 'An Investigation of Suicide in Puning County, Yunan', *Chinese Mental Health Journal*, 1: 23–5.

Levinas, E. (1988). 'Useless Suffering', in R. Beraconi and D. Wood (eds.), *The Provocation of Levinas*. London and New York: Routledge.

Moody-Adams, M. (1997). *Fieldwork in Familiar Places*. Cambridge: Harvard University Press.

Nie, J. B. (1999). 'Voices Behind the Silence: Chinese Moral Voices and the Experience of Abortion', Philosophy Dissertation Humanities Program. University of Texas Medical Branch, Galveston.

Perkins, J. (1995). *The Suffering Self: Pain and Narrative Representation in the Early Christian Era*. London: Routledge.

Phillips, M., H. Q. Liu, and X. R. Zhang (1999). 'Suicide in China', *Culture, Medicine and Psychiatry*, 23(1): 25–50.

Sen, A. 'External and Internal Views of Health and Illness', paper presented at the Bologna Symposium in Health and Illness: Metaphors for Life and Society, 24–7 October 1998.

Shweder, R. A. (1985). 'Menstrual Pollution, Soul Loss, and the Comparative of Emotion', in A. Kleinman and B. Good (eds.), *Culture and Depression*. Berkeley: University of California Press.

Smith, A. (1983) [1759]. *Theory of Moral Sentiments*. Indianapolis: Liberty Classics.

Taylor, C. (1989). *The Sources of the Self*. Cambridge: Harvard University Press.

Todorov, T. (1993). *On Human Diversity in French Thought*. Cambridge: Harvard University Press.

Tu, W. N. (1979). 'Humanity and Self-Cultivation', in *Essays in Confucian Thought*. Berkeley: Asian Humanities Press.

Wilson, E. O. (1998). 'The Biological Bases of Morality', *The Atlantic Monthly*, 28(4): 53–70.

Wong, S. K. (1969). 'Ching in Chinese Literary Criticism'. Ph.D. thesis (Oxford, unpublished, 1969).

15

Equity of the Ineffable: Cultural and Political Constraints on Ethnomedicine as a Health Problem in Contemporary Tibet

VINCANNE ADAMS

15.1. INTRODUCTION

My goal in this chapter is to show that health can be understood in cultural terms—for everyone, not just for Tibetans, not just for cultural anthropologists. By this I mean not simply that culture is revealed in the subjective experience of suffering that can be understood as narrowly cultural-specific. Health is a product of social, economic, political, and religious social structures that are themselves shaped and constituted culturally and in contested political terrain. Health equity, then, must also be considered in cultural terms.

Recognising the centrality of culture to health can, however, open up a Pandora's box of problems for policy oriented work. Typically, culture is bracketed off and held apart, treated as an independent variable in policy discussions, and then ignored in analysis or recommendations. When culture is directly addressed, it is generally seen as an obstacle to effective health reform. The goal then is usually the elimination of cultural views (seen as superstitious), or behaviours (seen as ignorant), because they impede effective health delivery.

The marginalisation of cultural issues may be a result of the fact that focusing on 'culture' makes visible the ways in which groups of people become incomparable. Culture makes differences of opinion, experience, and even structure significant. It forces tidy universalising policies into the realm of the narrowly

I wish to acknowledge the Wenner Gren Foundation for Anthropological research, the National Science Foundation, and Princeton University for generous support of this research. I also wish to thank Dechen Tsering for her support as a research assistant and Tashi Tsering for his tireless help as liaison. I am indebted to the Mentsikhang, particularly the director and the head of the women's ward and the staff in the women's wards at both inpatient and outpatient wards in Lhasa. I also thank the Harvard Center for Population and Development Studies for inviting me to participate in their Health Equity Workshop. I alone take full responsibility for the presentation and analysis offered here.

contingent and consensually unstable. However, culture does make a difference in health. This chapter offers an example of a non-Western socialist nation that laudably recognised the relationship between culture, basic social structure, and health and then implemented social reforms to attend to health equity but, by limiting cultural freedoms, ultimately became implicated in the production of sickness among its citizens.

Another reason culture is often overlooked in analyses of health equity stems from the materialist biases of western medical science itself. That is, western medical models tend to prioritise the physical and material contours of health and health inequality and to treat cultural phenomena as extraneous. Typically, the cultural dimensions of health and healing are relegated to the realm of psychology or, more commonly, to the realm of 'placebo' or 'belief'. Most often these dimensions are seen as 'ineffable' and external to real medical effects or pathologies.

This chapter argues that using Tibetan ethnomedical perspectives privileges a view of sickness that points to the cultural and social dimensions of health and health equity. For many Tibetans, ill health is associated with the perception of loss tied to secularist reforms. The elimination of suffering is, in turn, tied to issues of religion, specifically to ideas about the losses of the sacred in everyday life. These cultural ideas are, however, as 'ineffable' in the world of modern medical science as they are in the secularist ideologies of the Chinese state. Since Tibetan medicine recognises these cultural phenomena as important to health, it may be better suited to attending to health reforms that will bring about health equity than the western secularist medical models now deployed in the Tibetan Autonomous Region.

The chapter suggests in conclusion that the problem of culture is not just one that presents itself in the case of China, where it is politicised, marginalised, and reformed to achieve health for all. It is also a problem in health policy-making centres of the world wherein taking into account 'culture' demands a level of specificity, particularity, and even an understanding of the power of cultural 'belief'. To overlook culture's role in health, and to overlook the advantage some ethnomedicines may offer in seeing these relationships, is to overlook a cause of health and an extremely important basis upon which to design and theorise interventions to bring about health equity.

The materials I present here are based on research I have done over four visits to Tibet since 1993 at the women's ward of the Traditional Tibetan Medical Hospital in Lhasa. My placement in the women's ward is deliberate in that my research goals have been to understand how Chinese modernisation is worked out through women's bodies and women's health, but in ways that are theorised uniquely by Tibetan medical doctors. In what follows, I first describe Tibetan medicine in the context of a history in which medical practices were first politicised and later, under liberalisation, depoliticised by being deemed 'scientific' in this region of the People's Republic of China (hereafter, China). Today, Tibetan medical theories are being modified by political processes that valorise the secular over the religious. This contrasts somewhat with a Tibetan view of the healthy body that is based on Buddhist cultural foundations. In the latter, cultural concerns about morality and the power of the sacred are tied to bodily well-being. Moreover, Tibetan medicine accounts for the influence of social environment as well as the role of belief and the sacred in producing health. I then ask: if Tibetan suffering is often a result of rapid and repressive secularisation, how well can a secularised medicine provide health or health equity to this population?

Thus, the chapter makes two linked arguments: one that shows how social policies and cultural politics can lead to ill health, as understood by Tibetan medicine, and one that shows how competing medical epistemologies in a world that continuously prioritises biomedical science over all other medical theories might also be discussed as an issue of health equity. Concerns are raised about the links between cultural survival and health, as well as the idea of an equity of epistemology—about the way we theorise health and its causes—in international arenas.

15.2. HEALTH EQUITY AND SECULAR ETHICAL DISCOURSE

Ratification of Alma Ata's commitment to Health for All by the year 2000, occurring as recently as 1992, confirmed WHO's commitment to the ethical proposition that it should be possible to help all people achieve 'a level of health that would permit them to lead a socially and economically productive life' (WHO 1992). The obvious difficulty of uniformly *defining* what this level might be, let alone achieving it, has perhaps only been matched by the difficulty that soon became, and remains, apparent in trying to ensure this outcome by calling for *political will* on the part of participating nations. Placing issues of health equity on the health development map in this particular way has meant raising concerns about the need for political and social reforms as *health* priorities. But doing this has in many cases meant treating health itself as a political instrument and subjecting it to political agendas that actually subvert rather than promote health care (Morgan 1993; Ferguson 1994; Adams 1998).

Despite the overt ethical mandate of Alma Ata, in many ways the missing link in the discussions has been the cultural basis of ethics. What ethical boundaries can be set in relation to universalist ideas about 'complete' or even a minimum level of 'adequate health' given that ethics are not always cross-culturally shared? What are the ethical ambiguities of using productivity (economic or social) as basis for defining health, and how do these ambiguities vary cross-culturally? More specific to my discussion, what ethical measures might be deployed in culturally varied settings to ensure that 'political will' works in the best interests of health rather than vice versa?

Perhaps ethical discussions have been less visible than they might be because of the difficulty in deciding on what cultural basis the discussion of ethics should be grounded: philosophical, religious, scientific? One could argue that human rights discourse has in the field of health become the place-holder for this culturally complicated ethical discussion. Human rights offer a secularist and cross-culturally shared ethical mandate that is seen as transcending particular cultural and political agendas in the same way that health is supposed to. Human rights provide a powerful way to speak about health ethics in a universalist fashion.

The benefits of this particular discussion of ethics, however, is not so much in its ability to speak apolitically or even philosophically but rather in its ability to speak secularly and scientifically. Science offers a secularism that is thought to transcend cultural differences and the complicated terrain of ethical disagreement, especially when such ethical disagreements stem from religious cultural differences.

In medicine too, science and secularism form the basis of truth. Medically scientific languages enable universalist ethical claims that produce consensus and practical action partly at least because their terms of objectivity can be agreed upon (Adams 1998). Thus secularism forms an important part of the liberal humanism behind Alma Ata's efforts to promote universal equality in health. But in this chapter I ask whether secularist ethical discourse is the best way to promote health in all cases. China has prided itself on meeting, better than most other nations, both Alma Ata and secularist mandates for the provision of health for all. It has done this by promoting a socialist ethics that prioritised material needs over spiritual ones, and prioritised meeting the basic needs of all over meeting the exhaustive health needs of a privileged few. In this chapter, however, I want to illustrate how even when basic health care is provided universally and even when a basic level of health for all is attained by deploying a highly secularised public health policy, certain culturally specific ethical foundations of health, and hence health itself, can be compromised. The case of traditional Tibetan medicine points to the importance of bringing cultural concerns back into discussions of health equity.[1] It also argues that Tibetan ethnomedical epistemology might better attend to the health concerns of Tibetans precisely because it sustains ideas of sacred as opposed to secular qualities of health.

---

[1] Murmurings of the question of ethnomedicine were heard throughout the 1980s as health development programmes confronted the matter of 'indigenous healers' and most of the literature with which I am familiar suggests that the question of their involvement was largely shifted from the center to the periphery. Even when researchers did not advocate a complete dismissal of indigenous practices illustrations of their utility were nearly always calculated in terms of a presumed dominance of biomedicine. In sympathetic minds, their utility was tabulated in simple models of harmful versus beneficial health practices that could be seen as ineffective at best, dangerous at worst. In other cases it was thought that the best use of indigenous healers was in retraining them in the methods of scientific medicine, which usually meant undermining their own epistemological bases (Bastien 1992).

15.3. ETHNOMEDICINE IN CHINA'S TIBET: POLITICISATION AND 'SCIENTIZATION'[2]

It seems fitting to return to China in order to pursue the topic of health equity. China's model of the barefoot doctor that came fully into existence during the Cultural Revolution was a source of inspiration for the primary health care movement and Alma Ata's declaration of 1978 (Grant 1992). China tried to provide rudimentary health care 'for all' as part of its larger socialist project to establish an equitable society based on Marxist–Leninist ideals of communism. In fact, achieving this was one of China's primary successes. Moreover, in undertaking to incorporate and attend to the needs of what came to be the five major ethnic minority groups who collectively constituted the new Republic, China adopted aggressive policies that would also attend to cultural diversity in their pursuit of health equity. China paid attention to cultural differences.

In programmes that designated and privileged its nationalities with special state benefits (Gladney 1994), members of the ethnic nationalities (*minzu*) were given access to training in basic biomedical health services. More important, attention was paid to making use of their existing traditional ethnomedical resources in this training. The logic followed in minority regions was that a culturally sensitive medicine would work not only to reach more people, but also effectively demonstrate the benevolence of the state in caring for and accepting all its diverse nationalities.

Given this history, it is not surprising that one can still find state expressions of official forms of tolerance for cultural diversity in a robust medical pluralism in China (Farquhar 1994; Ots 1994). In China's more remote minority regions, like Tibet, the tolerance for ethnomedical traditions must have played a significant role in arousing some loyalty and commitment to the socialist project in the early days. But this glowing picture of a tolerant and equitably oriented state can be differently illuminated in consideration of the state's early and equally strong need to control cultural pluralism through medical institutions, particularly when such culture became a site for opposition to state ideology, or when it fuelled national separatism.

In medicine, as in other areas, a relationship was set in place whereby services were received from a benevolent state so long as unquestioned loyalty to its ideology was continuously shown, even when this meant retraining its practitioners and rewriting its theories (Farquhar 1987). Here, the idea that basic health care should be provided to all of China's citizens became possible only by politicising health care all the way down to its delivery of tinctures of iodine and referrals for tertiary care (New and New 1977). In a very literal sense, the Chinese barefoot doctor programme to promote health equity 'sutured' the public in all its cultural diversity to state political objectives that were presumed by the state to be uniformly desired (Anagnost 1997).

---

[2] See Janes (1995) for my inspiration on this topic.

Unlike in other regions of the developing world, arousing 'political will' was, if anything, not a problem in China. On the contrary, it was enforced. The exemplary model was provided by the Han majority's emphasis on uses of *zhongyi* (traditional Chinese) medical techniques and treatments in the training of the barefoot doctors during the Cultural Revolution. Although traditional Chinese medicine was itself on the wane in the years before the Cultural Revolution, it was revitalised during these years by being remade into a set of practices that served the socialist agenda and were considered ideologically unproblematic, for example, not-elitist, not religious, and materialist in orientation (New and New 1977; Farquhar 1987); primary health care for the masses on an equitable basis. In the case of Tibet, the politicisation of medicine and incorporation of indigenous traditions was enacted most profoundly in and through the denigration of Tibetan medicine's epistemological foundation in Buddhism (Janes 1995).[3] As elsewhere in China, reforms during the Cultural Revolution focused on retaining those aspects of traditional medical systems that were deemed both practical and useful by the state.[4] This meant trying to eliminate the superstitious and religious aspects of Tibetan medicine as part of a widespread persecution of religion during this period.[5] It entailed

[3] In Lhasa, Tibet, efforts to modernise Tibetan medicine actually began before the arrival of the People's Liberation Army. In 1916, the great Khenrab Norbu, physician to the Thirteenth Dalai Lama, sponsored the construction of a secular college for Tibetan medicine and astrology, the Mentsikhang. At the time, there was only one other government college for medicine, the monastery at Chags-po-ri, or 'Iron Mountain,' built in 1694 by the medical visionary Desi Sangye Gyamtso, regent for the Fifth Dalai Lama. The medical college at Chags-po-ri was designed for monastic scholars who would, after learning the esoteric arts of medicine and tantrism, mostly remain in the monastery, serving the public as would other monk scholars and lamas. The Mentsikhang, in contrast, was designed as a college for 'laypersons' who would, after receiving training, return to their rural areas for work as doctors and educators. Although the modernisation envisioned by the lama-physician Khenrab Norbu attended to concerns for the state's interest in the public's health, his project was carried out under the auspices of a theocracy. Thus the modernisation of medicine was at this point not necessarily one that entailed secularisation. Most of the students who were accepted for study at the Mentsikhang received training in religious fields prior to their arrival. In most cases, merely learning to read and write Tibetan script entailed religious study. Moreover, all of the ten fields of scholarship taught at the Mentsikhang, including grammar, logic, technology, medicine, religion, literature, rhetoric, drama, and astrology, were based on religious teachings.

Prior to 1916, the only other way for Tibetans to learn the arts of medicine was by becoming apprentice to, or raised within, a family of practising physicians. The history of family-based lineage practitioners probably dates back to the origins of Tibetan medicine in at least the twelfth century, although even thereafter there was monastic tutoring in medicine (see Meyer 1992 for a nice summary of history). Lineage practitioners learned medicine through oral instruction and memorisation of the four tantras. Although they were not always recognised as religious figures associated with one or another of Tibetan's five Buddhist sects, they were taught the religious components of the tradition. One can surmise that from at least the seventeenth century this entailed receiving initiation and empowerment blessings of the *ningje wong* (*nying rje dbang*) or 'empowerment of compassion'. These teachings were meant to enable practitioners to use their own techniques of meditation as preparation for treating others.

[4] Support for traditional Chinese medicine in other regions of China was on the wane (New and New 1977) due to the large influx of foreign medical services in the 1930s particularly.

[5] For the early years of China's control in Tibet support for traditional medicine was largely uninterrupted, reflecting the government's strategy of 'gradualism' in implementing communist

ideological retraining of professionals to meet the needs of the revolution, including mandatory periods of service in the rural countryside by most of the medical system's only qualified practitioners and teachers. It sometimes included imprisonment. It often entailed traumatic 'thought reform' sessions. Socialist modernisation required all professionals and non-professionals alike to develop an acute sensibility about the legitimacy and illegitimacy of certain forms of traditional cultural knowledge and practice. Knowing what was officially acceptable and what was not, especially in terms of religious practice, became not simply a strategy for successful delivery of health care, but a matter of individual survival. Thus despite China's overt effort to tolerate cultural differences, religious cultural differences became a site for state intolerance early on throughout China and later, in Tibet, a site for state repression.

The persecution of religion during the 1960s and early 1970s marked the beginning of the period of secularist reforms that would be the greatest influence shaping the contemporary practices of Tibetan medicine and affecting Tibetan health. However, the terms of this influence have, since the end of the Cultural Revolution and rise of the period of Liberalisation under Deng Xiaoping and Zhang Zemin, changed somewhat. Two trends are worth noting as post Cultural Revolution reforms in the Tibetan region. The first is the marriage of an existing socialist materialism with an unproblematic importation of Western-based scientific technologies believed to guarantee rapid and uniform modernisation. In the early days, this marriage was carried out as a political mandate within the health system: secularising medicine was a political act, a product of the politicising of the health system. But today, the trend is toward the opposite: instead of making scientific medicine the basis for political indoctrination, the official effort is now to distinguish the *scientific* from the *political* (Rofel 1999). That is, secularism becomes a way of showing that one is not engaged in politics. Secularism stands for state political correctness, while religious adherence stands for potential political splittism.

This trend is cross-cut by a second: official efforts to revitalise specific traditional cultural practices, including selected religious practices no longer believed to threaten the materialist foundations of the nation (Germano 1998). Whereas this trend has led to a genuine flourishing of religious and traditional cultural practices throughout most of China, in Tibet, this trend becomes deeply entangled in persistent state fears of separatism. This trend has meant

reforms in this minority region (Janes 1995; Goldstein 1998). However, with the first signs of political dissent to Communist rule in Lhasa, things changed. In 1959, opposition activities were launched as rumors of threats to the Dalai Lama were circulated. Chags-po-ri medical college was destroyed and the Dalai Lama along with some 100,000 Tibetans fled from Tibet and from communist rule. The monk and lama scholars from Chags-po-ri were sent to the Mentsikhang where agendas for more rapid modernising were already being implemented. For example, it was already clear that efforts to establish separate departments that were modelled after biomedical systems were in place by 1962 (e.g. creation of separate wards). Attempts to restore Tibetan medicine began during the Cultural Revolution (late 1960s, according to Meyer 1992), although the real resurgence seems to have followed the 1978 reforms.

that on the one hand there is a great nostalgia and reverence for the minority cultures on the part of Han majorities, and on the other hand it has led to a fragile sense of security concerning the legitimacy of traditional cultural practices among Tibetans themselves. Increasingly, the minorities are seen as resources for recuperating the lost cultural treasures of the greater Chinese nation (Schein 2000), and even in Tibet medical practitioners are overtly compelled to join the effort to sustain and revitalise their traditional practices. At the same time, the terms of Tibetan involvement in this project are a constant source of anxiety because they are labelled as potential expressions of political dissent that compete with the prevailing effort to modernise through *scientific* progress. Whereas medicine has been 'depoliticised,' by being labelled scientific, religion has been increasingly politicised, making it less possible to be seen as a foundation for medicine. Secularisation, in other words, is the priority for the state, and therefore in its efforts to promote health equity.

In Tibet, this has backfired as an effective political and health policy. It is not surprising that since religion was early on a site for the execution of political reforms within China, religion has remained an important site for political dissent in the years since the Cultural Revolution.[6] In Tibet, religion is frequently tied to official suspicions of Tibetan nationalist and separatist sentiment (Goldstein 1997, 1998). Government fears over national separatism tie religion to perceived desires for political independence and to exile Tibetan activism (particularly to the Dalai Lama) (Human Rights Watch 1996). The state sustains constant paranoia over the meaning of religious expression and so, despite overt official efforts to allow a certain amount of religious freedom in Tibet today, religious activities are still highly scrutinised, regulated, and dangerous for those who do them. As fears of nationalist-separatism rise, the degree to which religion can be sanctioned, even in medicine, is raised as a sensitive issue, leading to severe pressure to secularise traditions, especially medicine.

There are other forces of secularisation in Tibetan medicine. Since the opening of the Tibetan Autonomous Region (TAR) to foreigners in the 1980s, urban Tibetan practitioners have been made aware of the international interest in their work, and in the fairly widespread attention already given to Tibetan medicine in the Tibetan exile community. This interest is matched by the growing state interest in making the virtues of Tibetan medicine known throughout the rest of China. Practitioners, in turn, have become increasingly

[6] By the last years of the 1970s, state efforts in Tibet to rebuild religious institutions, especially monasteries, were quickly compromised (though not abandoned) by unsuccessful negotiations with His Holiness the Fourteenth Dalai Lama, a rise of internal dissent on the part of Tibetan monks toward specific forms of reform, and an ongoing perception on the part of the government that internal dissent was tied to separatist activities of exiled Tibetans. This resulted in creating an intractable suspicion of religion on the part of government officials. The deployment of the exile communities' International Campaign for Tibet does not help assuage their fears. At the same time, exiled Tibetans believe their cause remains justified by what they see as ongoing religious repression and cultural genocide there. The blame for suspicion cannot be placed solely on exile opposition.

interested in assessing their work in the language of medical legitimacy that has since the Cultural Revolution been put forward in the Chinese scientific arena. These are largely based on standards found in the international scientific community associated with biomedicine (and whatever forms these take in this local, regional context).[7]

Both science and Chinese socialism insist on a radical materialism that separates religious 'belief' from objective 'facts' when it comes to health issues. This trend is applauded and supported by the government, not simply as a way of ensuring widespread recognition of the scientific efficacy of Tibetan medicine but also as a way of lessening the importance of its problematic religious aspects. At the same time, the official policies supporting religious freedom work against this trend. The overall effect is one in which practitioners remain sensitive about both what constitutes religious content in their medical practices and how much they should involve themselves with it. Secularisation demands, in other words, work on medical practitioners as well as on the Tibetan public whereupon its effects are, as we will see, sometimes nefarious.

If a secular materialism of Marx and Lenin became the foundation of the socialist state in China, then the materialism of Western science might be seen as offering similar sorts of epistemological interventions in the western world. Both views maintain that scientific knowledge is based on distinguishing fact from belief, objective truth from subjective experience, and the social from the material bases of reality (Shapin and Schaffer 1985). Traditional Tibetan medicine, however, does not do this. Tibetan medicine conflates subjective beliefs with scientific facts (at least what Westerners generally think of as 'scientific'). It recognises that subjective belief plays an important role in producing objective realities of the body. And it places equal emphasis on social and material pathogens. It is precisely this achievement in Tibetan medicine that makes it appear as a failure in Western scientific communities, ensuring it is unlikely to be considered a valid medical epistemology in programmes deployed to achieve health equity. At the same time, it is precisely this 'failure' that enables Tibetan medicine to make visible the role that culture plays in health.

The cultural politics of contemporary Tibet produce a form of suffering that becomes visible through Tibetan medical epistemologies. In what follows, I show how Tibetan medicine renders visible the effects of culture on health. I present the outcomes of a stridently secularist policy on Tibetan health. By showing that Tibetan ethnomedical perspectives make these insights possible, I then pose the question of health equity in terms of culture in two ways that are explored in the remainder of the chapter: how exactly can we take culture into account when discussing health equity and in what ways can a discussion of equity be aided by explorations of non-Western medical epistemologies?

---

[7] I realise that I am leaving the category of 'science' undefined in this chapter. It is the subject of a longer exploration that is still ongoing for me (see Adams 2002).

15.4. WIND DISORDERS AS EFFECTS OF THE DEGRADATION OF SOCIETY

In this section I first explore Tibetan ill health as embodied experiences of social discord tied to secularist modernization. In the second part, I explore how Tibetan medicine approaches the problems of secularisation as a cause of suffering.

Changes in the health of Lhasa Tibetans since the 1960s are directly tied to larger changes occurring within Tibetan society. Traditional practitioners in the women's ward of the Mentsikhang felt that the health of urban women was in many ways worse now than historically. This was because of the rapid changes modernisation had wrought which, they believed, although they had made more basic health resources available, also had created a great deal of pathogenic situations. More varied diet and the consumption of too many imported foods, changes in behaviour, especially among young sexually active women, new demands being placed on them for fertility control, and the presence of new disease agents (especially sexually transmitted agents) were all seen as being on the rise. Women suffered high rates of infertility which doctors associated with frequent abortions, rapid succession pregnancies, lack of sexual and feminine hygiene, too much sex, and resulting reproductive tract infections.

In most cases, women's complaints were seen as having a long history that spanned the period of modernisation ushered in by communism. Current ill health dated back to the years just before the Cultural Revolution when women recounted frequent miscarriages from heavy labour, arduous work conditions in regions unfavourable to patients' constitution, traumatic deaths of family members.[8] In many cases, the diagnoses of these women included imbalances of one of the body's three humours, the wind humour, *rlung*.

Dolma was a fifty-six-year-old woman who had kidney and heart trouble that she felt could be traced to her early reproductive years. At seventeen years of age in the early 1960s, she was working as a labourer in the metal works production unit outside of Lhasa. Workers there had to lift very heavy hammers for this work, and because of this, she said, she miscarried her first pregnancy. She then, with great struggle, delivered a full-term boy who was pronounced dead upon delivery. She explained, 'I am not the only one who

---

[8] The Tibetan medical model of health posits that one is born in a state of non-optimal health. The epistemological grid for Tibetan approaches to healing thus begins from the perspective of chronicity—we are all suffering all the time—therefore the best a doctor can achieve is helping people to live *with* their disorders and attain enough well-being in order to gain merit. This might be seen as distinct from biomedical traditions that treat most disorders as acute and episodic, in the Aristotelian sense, as having beginnings middles and ends, giving rise to much consternation over handling chronic patients (Estroff 1981; Frankenberg, personal communication 1991). Kleinman (1988) suggests interventions in medical care through reading illness histories in patient narratives in a manner that refocuses our attention on the 'life of the patient' as opposed to the 'life of the disease' in approaches to care.

suffered like this. There were many women in my area who worked and had miscarriages because they did very strenuous work that caused bleeding. Many women lost their babies. It was very common.' Later, she was able to conceive again and gave birth to a baby girl who is still alive.

Dolma was later transferred to a road construction labourers unit and there got pregnant again. Here again, because of the hard work requirements for road building, she lost that baby. It began with a lot of bleeding. This time, she had to have surgery. This time, the baby that had died in her womb had to be removed and in the course of this she had to have 'seven people's blood put in her' through transfusions.

In 1975 she was sent to a different county during a time when 'all of the labourers were divided and sent to remote places'. The county she was sent to had no factory work and so she was given a job at the school. Because she told the administrator that she was weak from her enormous blood loss and could not handle manual/physical work, he gave her the job of ringing the school bells. This job, she said, suited her because she had developed a problem with her heart from both the blood loss and the exhaustion from years of heavy manual work.

The symptoms bringing her into the hospital included pain in her kidneys, pains in her uterus, heart weakness. She said that her body had become very weak from all the blood she lost many years ago. Even if she works a little bit, she noted, her face starts to swell and she feels very tired and dizzy. She said that before 'I was a very healthy young girl, but the job was just too hard, physically hard.'

Dolma's doctor explained that she had two problems, a kidney fever with arthritis and a heart-wind disorder (*snying rlung*). Her kidney and joint pains were related to the fact that the region where she was transferred was known as a damp place, and once there, she had to do a lot of washing in cold water (clothes, bathing, etc.). Cold water and cold climate both had an effect on her phlegm humour because phlegm is responsible for cold in the body. Since the kidneys process the cold water, its ingestion will have a cooling effect on them, slowing the phlegm in her body and eventually producing a 'fever' from too much cold at the location of her kidneys. Weakened by all her blood loss, her heart was also disabled. The winds responsible for moving her blood through her body were involved with this. Because of the trauma of her hard work and difficult circumstances surrounding the deaths of her children, Dolma's winds were weak. This added to her excessive blood loss. Here, unfavourable climate and onerous work conditions are linked to humoural imbalances that have a long-term effect on the body. Dolma stayed at the hospital two weeks until her kidney trouble subsided and then became an outpatient for several months while being treated for her *snying rlung*.

Yangki's story showed similar physiological outcomes of harsh social policies. In her mid-fifties now, Yangki was diagnosed with a growth in her uterus and a 'wind' disorder. She explained that when she was young, she had three children. Her husband died when they were all small. The doctor noted that generally a woman's wind will become more easily agitated with age, but Yangki's problems began when she lost her husband. Her periods were generally heavy, meaning she lost a lot of blood. Her winds were weakened by the sadness over losing her husband and stress of raising three children by herself. In particular, her *thursel rlung* (downward expelling wind) was unable to hold back the flow of blood from her body.

Over the years, this wind problem had contributed to the growth of a tumour in her womb, but her condition was exacerbated by her current work situation. Yangki had a job in the government office that was responsible for monitoring religious activities in the Lhasa area. She told us that her job was stressful. She had to go from nunnery to nunnery to ostensibly provide government assistance with their management. Everyone knew, however, that this meant that she was supposed to monitor them for illegal political activities. She was essentially in the position of policing her fellow Tibetans' religious behaviours. This meant sometimes limiting the number of enrolled nuns, literally throwing them out of the nunnery, and undertaking cultural re-education programmes that would ensure politically correct readings of the historical feudal theocracy of Tibet. When asked to talk more about her work, she became quiet and agitated.

During the research with patients, I was told by the doctors that it was important to avoid talking about certain topics with patients who had wind disorders because getting them to think about their difficult life situations could exacerbate their conditions. In her case, like Dolma's above, difficult life conditions manifest themselves as physiological problems—here, excessive bleeding and tumour growth, in Dolma's case high blood pressure and arthritis.

Patients in the women's ward nearly always recounted their suffering in terms that linked physical distress to social conditions over which they had little control. Yangchen was a twenty-five-year-old road construction worker who lived in Lhasa. She was diagnosed with a bile-related infection in her uterus *(mngal-nad mkhris gyur)*. She explained that her problems began when she was twenty-two-years-old and aborted a child. At that time, neither she nor her husband had been living in their government work unit long enough to receive a pass for having a child. So she aborted. Some time later she applied for the pass and, after receiving one, got pregnant again.

Looking back, Yangchen thought that her second pregnancy came too soon after her first. She had a complicated delivery at the People's Biomedical Hospital and had an infection afterward that caused her to be told she could not yet contracept. So, she got pregnant again soon thereafter. By this time, she explained, she could not have the second child because she had already submitted her contract and received a pass to have only one child. Her work unit had provided incentives of money to her to have only one child, and they had also indicated strong disincentives, such as fines and job loss, were she to fail to keep to her contract. So she had to give up that child too by abortion.

She spent two and a half months in the hospital as an inpatient before her health was fully restored.

Yangchen's doctor explained that her infection came about because she failed to take enough rest after her pregnancies and deliveries. Every time a pregnancy is finished the blood needs to be replenished. Again, the blood loss itself will cause the wind humour, *rlung* to be weakened. In Yanchen's case, her blood loss and worries over her infection caused her anxiety. But the doctor also suggested that Yangchen's problems were related to her sexual appetites. Having too much sex can be a problem, she noted. She became pregnant in too rapid succession and never gave herself a chance to rest in between pregnancies. Her sexual appetites were themselves an indication of *rlung* imbalance, but now, the doctor noted, she had become depressed from her 'whole life situation'. Her nervousness and anxiety, in turn, meant that '*rlung* had been recruited and was supporting the bile activity in the infection. This [would] in turn lead to more bleeding'. If it continued, Yangchen might be at risk of developing a more serious wind disorder called *srog rlung* (wind in the life-force channel) that can if untreated lead to madness and even death. The doctor made sure to note that when interviewing her, care must be taken not to get her thinking about the seriousness of her condition. Here, onerous demands for fertility control and her own sexual appetites led to infections of the womb.

The idea that bodies can 'wear' the signs of social discontent is found elsewhere in China (Kleinman 1981, 1987, Ots 1994), but the social conditions of distress were perhaps more oppressive in Lhasa given contemporary governmental political suspicions and the urgency with which they demanded modernisation. Just as medical practitioners have had to develop an acute sensibility about the ideological implications of their actions and utterances, so too have all Tibetans, especially in the urban areas, had to develop this acute sensibility since the late 1950s. This was particularly true of utterances with religious content or content that could be construed as 'religious' superstitious or 'backward' thinking.

The perception on the part of a great many urban Tibetans, though not all, was that matters of life and death were decided for them on the basis of their ability to utter speech and perform actions that were considered conforming to official ideology. Some understood (and some with more ambivalence than others) that the instruments the government had put in place to help ensure a productive and thriving society were also apparatuses of censorship and surveillance over their political speech and degree of loyalty to state agendas. These included, for example, neighbourhood councils and weekly political meetings for confessing irregularities or suspicious behaviours, work units that paid managers to watch over public and private lives of employees, an enormous plainclothes police force that circulated the public zones of the city at all times in order to obtain information about possible separatist opposition. Again, among the most scrutinised zones, they felt, were those involving religious acts of worship (private and public) that could be construed as political. The effects of failing to conform to government policies on appropriate speech and action were severe: arrests and public trials preceding private executions of prisoners whose crimes were expressing open dissent to Chinese rule.

The links between what many Tibetans consider to be repressive historic and contemporary social policies in Tibet, from the Great Leap Forward to the contemporary political repressions, are that in both cases Tibetans are asked to participate in modes of sociality that they find morally problematic. Despite the overt effect of these policies to create a social infrastructure that is more conducive to health equality, their effects have been uneven in China as a whole. One way to describe these effects is by looking at the direct effects of social reforms on the health of women—particularly at reproductive policies that induce high rates of infection and infertility. Another way to describe these effects is through the subtle links between perceptions of social degradation/ desecration and the health of Tibetan women.

For older women who suffered spontaneous abortions, great regret is expressed over the loss of children at the hands of the state. The price paid for rapid modernisation was simply too high for some Tibetans, both in the sense of intellectual regret and in the sense of physical damage to their bodies. Among younger women, attitudes about the demands of modernisation are mixed. Reproductive policies requiring regular abortions lead some to express extraordinary sadness over the taking of a life, noting the karmic effects of killing and the moral burden that will be carried with them into their future lives. For those participating in government jobs that require them to ferret out and punish religiously minded Tibetans, the burdens can be equally severe. While it is certainly true that not all Tibetans feel the same way about the promise and price of modernisation (in fact, some Tibetans applaud the death of religion), there is an equally prevalent sentiment that desecrating religious persons (especially monks and nuns) by refusing to allow them to practice religion constitutes a form of immoral behaviour and infraction that will cause tremendously bad outcomes in one's future lives. The effects of this immorality are physical—degradations and/or agitations of the wind humour in a manner that produces systemic and chronic health outcomes. Wind disorders, in other words, make visible the ways in which sentiments or perceptions of desecration can be a cause of ill health. I will explain this in more detail below.

The medical language of 'winds' was, for political reasons, situated ambiguously between that which was considered 'scientific' and that which was considered 'religious'. Thus, discussion of the humoural bases of disorders was tricky for Tibetan doctors and patients alike. To the extent that criticisms of the effects of government's policies was made visible in diagnoses of wind disorders, Tibetans had to be careful about how the idea of 'winds' was classified. On the one hand, winds could be identified as a medical idea that was by all accounts 'scientific' in a Tibetan sense of the term because it pertained primarily to issues of the body's health. At the same time, winds pointed to the religious foundations of Tibetan medicine, both in the sense that the very idea of a 'wind' humour emerged originally from a Buddhist soteriology (tied to the poison of 'desire') and also in the sense that winds rendered visible the ways in which Tibetan patients suffered from their perceptions of a moral degradation set in motion by government policies of secularisation. Wind disorders, in other words, could be seen as both a kind of religious thinking and as a product of desecrations of religion that were mandated by policies of rigid and inflexible secularisation.

One way to understand the suffering of Tibetan patients like those described above is thus to see them as outcomes of deliberate government policies aimed at producing equality among the masses. The most severe were deployed as repressive mechanisms during the Cultural Revolution. In that era, physical suffering among reproductive women was both expected and taken as a sign of true devotion to the party. Even before and after the Cultural Revolution, however, efforts to modernise rapidly entailed attempts to eliminate all traces of traditional religious culture. This repression is tied to government suspicions of political separatism (tied to religious expressions that can be linked to the former theocratic ruler, the Dalai Lama) (Human Rights Watch 1996) and cause disorders in a different manner that is perhaps best understood through traditional Tibetan medical epistemology.

15.5. WIND DISORDERS AS A TIBETAN MEDICAL THEORY ON THE CULTURAL BASIS OF HEALTH

The paranoia of the state in its perceptions of a potentially volatile Tibetan Autonomous Region trickles down to most Tibetan citizens and re-emerges in a variety of complaints, but, as I have shown, most prominently in wind disorders.[9] Janes identifies this stunningly in a quote from one Tibetan doctor who told him: 'Of course, *rlung* must be more common nowadays because Tibet is no longer free. The Chinese government is the government of *rlung*. The Chinese government makes people unhappy, and so *rlung* must be more common... Tibetans have *rlung* because they are not free' (Janes 1995: 31).

In order to understand the links between secularization, wind disorders, and the cultural basis of health, it is useful to backtrack somewhat into the Tibetan medical theory underlying the wind humour. Tibetan medicine derives from a long history of empirical observation, translations, Tibetan tradition, and Buddhist cosmology.[10] The Buddha's insight on the four noble truths is the

---

[9] This might be considered another 'ineffable' in my analysis—the ill health producing silence imposed by a political regime.

[10] The most compelling evidence of the religious foundations of Tibetan medicine are found in the medical texts themselves, and in the medical thankas depicting the contents of the materia medica commissioned by the regent Desi Sangye Gyatso in the seventeenth century. The first text of Tibetan Medicine was believed to be compiled in the form that comes to us today by Yuthok Yonden Gombo, the younger, in the twelfth century. His text, 'The Tantra of Secret Instructions

generally held to be a basis for understanding the nature of both health and all suffering in Tibetan medicine (Dhonden and Kelsang 1983; Meyer 1992). Evidence for his claim that suffering was inevitable in life is found in his reported understanding that all suffering arises originally from the presence of the three poisons: desire, anger, and ignorance. At the time of conception, the presence of these poisons give rise to the physical body in the form of three humours: wind, bile, and phlegm. Accordingly, the theory argues that the best remedy for suffering is taking refuge in the Buddha and devoting one's life to achieving enlightenment by purifying oneself so as to eliminating the presence of the three poisons.[11]

Beyond this, the basic Tibetan medical theory of anatomy links the material and spiritual worlds in complicated relationship between the five elements (believed to make up all phenomena) and the forces of consciousness that enable the elements to take specific form in, say, a human body. The five elements are wind (responsible for movement), earth (giving substance), water (which holds things together), fire (which transforms or 'cooks' things), and space (providing the place within which things can exist). The elements determine the properties of all substances—hot, cold, heavy, light, stable, unstable, and all the tastes (Clifford 1984; Meyer 1992; Clarke 1995). It is believed that the presence of a variety of winds, operating on a subtle and coarse level, transform these elements into a human body, although not in an obvious way.

The emergence of a human form at the time of rebirth is contingent upon the type of winds circulating in the life-force (e.g. a transmigrating consciousness on its way to rebirth from a human form to another human form) (Meyer 1992; see also Rechung 1973; Dhonden and Kelsang 1983; Dhonden 1986). These can be winds of wisdom or karma. In the being that has karma, the subtle winds give rise to the three channels of the foetal body. They are believed to oscillate as energy fields along the axis of the body: a central channel (*dbu-ma*) a right channel (*roma*) and a left channel (*rkyang ma*). These channels operate in tandem with the presence of ignorance, desire, and anger, respectively (Clifford 1984), which are in the Tibetan system related to moral comportment in relation to others as much as individual emotional states. The places on the body where these energy channels intersect around the central channel (manifesting as ignorance)—that is when desire and anger are present—are known as *chakras* (*kor-lo*). The conceptualisation of this movement is that it takes the form of circulating winds. The winds circulating on a subtle 'energy'

on the Eight Branches, the Essence of the Elixir of Immortality' today known in its short form as the *rGyu bShi*, the four tantras, were based partly on the summarised essence of the Buddha's teachings on medicine, the *gSo wa Rig pa*, or science of health.

[11] It is thus not surprising that the opening chapters of the Tibetan medical texts, called *the rGyu bShi* (Four Tantras) are devoted to worshipping and making and offering and request to Bhaisyagyaguru, the medicine Buddha, Master of Remedies (or King of Medicine), for teachings on how to eliminate these poisons.

level in the body's channels are related to more coarse winds that constitute the body's wind humour, numbering five in all, each one responsible for various types of movement in the body (breathing, muscle, fluids, nerves, senses). These winds are also associated with external winds existing in phenomena outside the body.

Interactions of the elements constituting the internal world with those found in the world outside the body are constant. Therefore, it is believed the body is never in a permanent state, always changing in relation to the climate, the seasons, foods eaten, the emotions in relation to perceptions, and even by the demonic or other harmful forces that exist in the world. What regulates the harmonious relationship between being and environment are the three humours: wind (*rlung*), bile (*mkhris-pa*) and phlegm (*bad-kan*). When the humours are functioning well, the body's waste products emerge in perspiration, faeces, and urine. They also ensure the refinement of ingested products into the seven bodily constituents: chyle, blood, flesh, fat, bones, marrow, and seminal fluid.

When the body sits well in its environment then the potential for material and spiritual well-being is achieved. Ultimate health is achieved by doing things that eliminate bad karma—doing or not doing things in order to transcend samsara—which are the ultimate remedy for states of ill health.[12] Temporary health is achieved by keeping the body's humours in balance through correct diet, behaviour, ingestion of medicines, or other external therapies.

In this view of the three poisons as the basis for the body's three humours, morality is the basis for achieving ultimate health. Controlling desires, aversions, and ignorance pertains to the achievement of health. The average person, however, has little ability to control these winds. Rather, the average person is pushed and pulled by the mind's wandering from one mood to the next, one desire to the next, one aversion to the next. As it moves, so too are the humours activated, creating imbalances that can result in ill health. The external milieu and internal environment are interdependent; the more bilious (bile-tending) one is, the more likely one will perceive of the external world as something over which to have aversion. The reverse is also true: the more anger one feels toward the outside world, the more likely one will crave and eat foods that aggravate the bile because of the ways the winds agitate the digestion processes. These agitations or depletions are put into effect by the body's winds.

Thus, in Tibetan medicine, social conditions that are not conducive to eliminating the poisons are seen as indirectly pathological—as disease producing. Humoural imbalances result in an inability to digest food, think clearly, eat, or even rest properly. This model of health posits that morality is embodied. This

---

[12] In fact, Tibetans often talk about their illnesses and their misfortunes as enabling them to purify bad karma accumulated from past actions (lives). Sickness is not interpreted as outcome of 'sins' but as enabling them to eliminate future suffering caused by their 'sins'.

is not simply in the sense of there being 'sins of the individual', as we might assume from Buddhism's accounting of *kleshas* or disturbing mental states resulting from unvirtuous deeds of the body, speech, mind from past lives. It is in the way that the flesh itself is evidence of past virtues and 'sins' in relation to other beings, while also being a site for the atonement and transcendance of them through actions and intentions toward other beings. People's bodies are literally expressions of their accumulated virtue and non-virtue in relation to other sentient beings in past lives. But the reverse is also true: sicknesses arise from difficult social circumstances and are in some sense an index of the body's internal moral functioning which is, in turn, a reflection of that external milieu. Here, the ethical domain, in so far as it is tied to morality, is not *aggregated* to the physical realm. It is *constitutive* of it. Moral qualities are assigned physiological character because the 'poisons' as humours are assigned elemental properties: bile is associated with fire, phlegm with water and earth, wind with wind. Body constituents are confluent with moral intentions because both are constituted by the same five elements. Understanding this is from a Tibetan medical perspective essential to understanding how to approach the task of making people healthy.

A person whose sickness arises because his or her desires are not fulfilled, because social conditions prevent this, is something of a walking expression of social discord. The harm that results from people behaving unethically toward one another—that is in ways that hurt one another—is here inscribed on patients' bodies in wind disorders. In a world that many Tibetans perceive has become increasingly overrun by concerns for the practical, the political, and the productive as opposed to the sacred and especially the sacred that comes from associating with other beings in virtuous ways, bodies themselves are secularised and traumatised.

For many Tibetans, government policies are largely perceived as having the opposite effect as that which the government ostensibly desires. For most (though certainly not all) Tibetans, modernisation policies are seen as having resulted in a degradation of their society by undermining the religious basis for setting limits and controls on behaviours deemed problematic in a moral or ethical sense. That is, losing children for the sake of building roads, aborting children (killing them) for the sake of meeting government quotas on population growth, and forcing nuns to break their vows and leave their nunneries for the sake of eliminating obstacles to modernisation, or even watching other Tibetans ignore religious precepts, are perceived by many Tibetans as assaults on their religious sensibilities and on their ideal of a humane and equitable society.

Religiously devout Tibetans are being asked to participate in a world that prioritises socialist materialism and secularism. They are aware of their need to refuse or at least self-censor the religious dimensions of their everyday lives, especially in the worlds of work, school, medicine, politics, and even reproduction and sexuality. Such refusals make it less possible for them to contemplate or carry out a morally virtuous life and, consequently, more likely they will suffer from physical diseases as a result of government policies. The particular brand of socialist modernisation they are exposed to is seen by some Tibetans as desecrating the moral basis of society. Problems of political repression arise from treating the world as if it were not morally grounded by removing the imperative to behave toward others in familiar morally virtuous ways.[13]

What Tibetan medical theory makes visible is that secularisation contributes to ill health among Tibetans. Given the scenario in which religious repression is directly tied to physical health, it seemed prudent for some doctors to deploy a medical system that attends directly to the connections between ethical behaviours and physical health. But, given the consequences of overtly discussing the moral basis of medical diagnoses, few Tibetan doctors can do this. China's secularist modernisation of Tibet thus both limits the extent to which Tibetan medical theories can be openly deployed or discussed, at the same time that limitations and restrictions like this are themselves seen as a cause of social suffering and health inequality in the contemporary moment.

This is a tragedy because a medical system that has built its theory around the idea that moral behaviours toward other people are a basis for a healthy body might also effectively engage methods of attending to the ethical health of society. At a minimum this sort of proposition might suggest fruitful discussion of the role of ethnomedical epistemologies in ethical mandates of health for all in that locale.

15.6. CONCLUSION

Medicine was early on in the Chinese socialist project politicised so that it would be configured in a manner that could serve the most people with the most good. Later politicising of religion in Tibet resulted in demands that medicine conform more than ever to the terms of legitimacy set out by the socialist government as scientific. In the medical college and hospital, this has resulted in numerous attempts to make Tibetan medicine speak the language of science, while still attending to the project of seeing health in terms of religious

[13] This is not to suggest that there is not an ethical dimension to secularism. On the contrary, secular social formations have often offered powerful ethical critiques to those based on religions, and many Lhasa Tibetans have wholly adopted this position. But for others, the perception is that modernisation denies the ethical imperatives found in the worlds that were historically sustained by the logic of the sacred under Buddhism. Also, this is not to suggest that ideas of the sacred and the moral imperatives they set in place, historically or ever, penetrated all aspects of everyday Tibetan life, or that all Tibetans ever held uniform and uniformly committed ideas about the sacred. Nor finally am I suggesting that Tibetan Buddhism is not without its ethically problematic areas. Certainly there were instruments of political terror in Tibet's theocracy, and some were rationalised by the Buddhist hierarchy. Certainly there have always been uneven commitments to Buddhism, let alone to a religious life, in Tibet. There is ample evidence of debate over ethical fairness within this religion, although I do not pursue that evidence here.

practices and ideas. Scientising medical theory enables practitioners to participate in the great socialist modernisation in the terms of Western science that have been delivered to them while giving them a basis upon which to claim international recognition for their achievements. But to the extent that 'scientization' promotes secularisation of the social, it can be seen as a source of physical disorders, whether advanced through social policies or through the moral stress they produce.

Tibetan medical theory points to these links between moral sociality and physical disorder, sometimes directly and other times indirectly, but it does so in ways that are often deemed 'ineffable' in the world of science and in the secularist discourse of the Chinese state. Because discussions of wind invariably lead one down the road to open discussions of religiously based morality, such discussions are carefully evaded in Tibet today. I would also suggest that such discussions are difficult in the international community of health and medical scientists. On an epistemological grid that would place bodies opposite minds in the same way that matter is placed opposite spirit, and objective facts opposite subjective beliefs, where do we place the wanderlust wind and its powerful effects on health?

The last half of the twentieth century has ushered in policies that require Tibetans to think of their religion as a distinct domain of life—something one can do on weekends and days off—as opposed to a culturally prescribed way of being that imbues nearly all acts of everyday work and living. How successful this effort has been is unambiguously clear. Secular forms of humanism in many nation-states is seen as that which can protect religious freedom. But in China, a secular humanism offered to ensure modernisation has been effected through policies that have variously deemed religions as problematic and therefore needing to be eradicated. At a minimum, modernisation policies have tried to force a disaggregation of domains of ethnic identity, politics, medical science, and religion in order to forge new political allegiances, only to reunite them as an effect of governmental paranoia over state security. In Tibetan medicine, this disaggregation and aggregation becomes visible in physical disorders of women who have been asked to sacrifice a great deal for the sake of equity and progress within the Chinese nation.

The results of China's restrictions of cultural freedom illustrates the importance of culture to health. With this in mind, it would seem that calls for basic cultural liberties would be fundamental to policy discussions on health equity. But raising the question of cultural freedom in international arenas opens up other debates. For one, what does it mean to ensure cultural freedom and to bring cultural concerns into the policy arena at the same time? How does one guarantee cultural freedom while tying cultural forms to state or even international agendas? Does not culture risk being put in the service of particular political agendas in the same way that health care is often forced into such a position when it is politicised by becoming attached to one political platform over another? Politicisation here does not mean simply mobilising a uniformly accepted idea about how to attend to the social good. Rather, it means privileging one set of political and cultural ideas that are forged through contestation into the position of being (usually temporarily) dominant, whether or not there is consensus. Government policies are in this sense seldom universally consensual, and one could ask whether international agendas can ever be as well. More often, they represent the winning side in political battles that compromise one set of agendas for another. Just as it is difficult to understand how health can avoid politicisation once it is policy-bound, it is also hard to understand how culture can escape this fate once brought into the policy realm (Bastien 1992). Would not one end up doing just what China has done: picking and choosing cultural features for eradication and preservation on the basis of health priorities that are already politically determined?

A second challenge raised by this case is that all medical theories implicitly make ethical and moral claims whether they are secular or religious (Foucault 1973, 1981; Bates 1995), but how do we reconcile those systems of knowledge that are explicitly or even in some way religious with those that are not? In other words, in the international community, how do we fairly determine standards of efficacy that accommodate non-secular, non-Western epistemological claims?

Herein, questions of an equity of epistemology are raised. The Tibetan medical perspective operates as both a theoretical tool and as source of medical intervention. Tibetan medical theory points to the centrality of cultural freedom to health and it offers a mode of intervention that encompasses the social and cultural dimensions of human suffering. But it does so through ideas that are recognised as generally beyond the pale of science, being based on religious cosmology and philosophically specific ideas that appeal to the moral basis of health and healing. They raise fundamental questions about the role of epistemology in an effort to recognise the cultural basis of health. What possibilities are there, then, for recognising that culture and different approaches to healing should not be overlooked in efforts to bring about health equity in the international arena?

References

Adams, Vincanne (1998). *Doctors For Democracy: Health Professionals in the Nepal Revolution*. Cambridge: Cambridge University Press.

—— (2002). 'The Sacred in the Scientific: Ambiguous Practices of Science in Tibetan Medicine', *Cultural Anthropology*, 16(4): 542–75.

Anagnost, Ann (1997). *National Past-Times: Narrative, Representation and Power in Modern China*. Durham: Duke University Press.

Bates, Don (1995). *Knowledge and the Scholarly Medical Traditions*. Cambridge: Cambridge University Press.

Clarke, Barry M. D. (1995). *The Quintessence Tantras of Tibetan Medicine*. Ithaca: Snow Lion Publications.

Clifford, Terry (1984). *Tibetan Buddhist Medicine and Psychiatry: The Diamond Healing*. York Beach, Maine: Samuel Weiser, Inc.

Dhonden, Yeshi (1986). *Health Through Balance: An Introduction to Tibetan Medicine*, (trans. Jeffrey Hopkins). Ithaca: Snow Lion Publications.

—— and Jampel Kelsang (1983). *The Ambrosia Heart Tantra. Journal of Tibetan Medicine*. Dharamsala: Library of Tibetan Works and Archives, p. 6.

Estroff, Sue (1981). *Making it Crazy*. Berkeley: University of California Press.

Farquhar, Judith (1987). 'Problems of Knowledge in Contemporary Chinese Medical Discourse', *Social Science and Medicine*, 24(12): 1013–21.

—— (1994). *Knowing Practice: The Clinical Encounter of Chinese Medicine*. Boulder: Westview Press.

Ferguson, James (1994). *The Anti-Politics Machine: 'Development,' Depoliticization, and Bureaucratic Power in Lesotho*. Minneapolis: University of Minnesota Press.

Foucault, Michel (1973). *The Birth of the Clinic: An Archeology of Medical Perception*. New York: Vintage.

—— (1981). *The History of Sexuality, Volume One, an Introduction*. New York: Vintage.

Germano, David (1998). 'Re-membering the Dismembered Body of Tibet: Contemporary Tibetan Visionary Movements in the People's Republic of China', in Melvyn C. Goldstein and Matthew T. Kapstein (eds.), *Buddhism in Contemporary Tibet*. Berkeley: University of California Press.

Goldstein, Melvyn C. (1997). *The Snow Lion and the Dragon*. Berkeley: University of California Press.

—— (1998). 'Introduction', in Melvyn C. Goldstein and Matthew T. Kapstein (eds.), *Buddhism in Contemporary Tibet*. Berkeley: University of California Press.

Gladney, Dru (1994). 'Representing Nationality in China: Refiguring Majority/Minority Identities', *Journal of Asian Studies*, 53(1): 92–123.

Grant, James P. (1992). 'Introductory Comments', WHO Interregional Seminar on Primary Health Care, Geneva: WHO.

Human Rights Watch (1996). *Cutting off the Serpent's Head: Tightening Control in Tibet, 1994–1995*. New York: Tibet Information Network/ Human Rights Watch Asia.

Janes, Craig (1995). 'The Transformations of Tibetan Medicine', *Medical Anthropology Quarterly*, 9(1): 6–39.

Kleinman, Arthur (1981). *Patients and Healers in the Context of Culture*. Berkeley: University of California Press.

—— (1988). *The Illness Narratives: Suffering, Healing and the Human Condition*. New York: Basic Books.

Meyer, Fernand (1992). 'Introduction: The Medical Paintings of Tibet' in Yuri Parfionovitch, Gyurme Dorje, and Fernand Meyer (eds.), *Tibetan Medical Paintings: Illustrations to the Blue Beryl treatise of Sangye Gyamtso (1653–1705)*. New York: Harry N. Abrams, Inc.

Morgan, Lynn (1993). *Community Participation in Health: The Politics of Primary Care in Costa Rica*. Cambridge: Cambridge University Press.

New, Peter Kong-ming and Mary Louise New (1977). 'The Barefoot Doctors of China: Healers for All Seasons' in David Landy (ed.), *Culture Disease and Healing*. New York: Macmillan.

Ots, Thomas (1994). 'The Silenced Body—the Expressive Lieb: On the Dialectic of Mind and Life in Chinese Cathartic Healing', in T. Csordas (ed.), *Embodiment and Experience*. Cambridge: Cambridge University Press.

Rechung Rinpoche (1973). *Tibetan Medicine*. Berkeley: University of California Press.

Rofel, Lisa (1999). *Other Modernities: Gendered Yearnings in China after Socialism*. Berkeley: University of California Press.

Schein, Louisa (2000). *Minority Rules: The Miao and the Feminine in China's Cultural Politics*. Durham: Duke University Press.

Shapin, Steven and Simon Schaffer (1985). *Leviathan and the Air Pump: Hobbes, Boyle, and the Experimental Life*. Princeton: Princeton University Press.

Sharf, Robert H. (1998). 'Experience', in Mark C. Taylor (ed.), *Critical Terms in Religious Studies*. Chicago: University of Chicago Press.

WHO (World Health Organization) (1992). *A Report on Health for All by the Year 2000*. Geneva: WHO.

Index